高等教育出版社　中国·北京

Higher Education Press, Beijing, China

英漢實用中醫藥大全

趙樸初題

7

TUINA
THERAPEUTICS
推拿治療學

7
推拿治疗学

	中文	英文
主　编	张素芳　王国才	徐象才
副主编	王道全　管　政	
编　者	王永泉　周建国	
	张　太　乔建君	
	李华东	

TUINA THEREPEUTICS

	English	Chinese
Chief Editor	Xu Xiangcai	Zhang Sufang Wang Guocai
Deputy Chief Editors		Wang Daoquan Guan Zheng
Editors		Wang Yongquan Zhou Jianguo
		Zhang Tai Qian Jianjun
		Li Huadong

(京)112 号

The English—Chinese
Encyclopedia of Practical TCM
Chief Editor   Xu Xiangcai

7

TUINA THERAPEUTICS

English Chief Editor   Xu Xiangcai
Chinese Chief Editors   Zhang Sufang
Wang Guocai

英汉实用中医药大全

主编 徐象才

7

推拿治疗学

中文主编 张素芳 王国才

英文主编 徐象才

*

高等教育出版社出版
新华书店总店科技发行所发行
国防工业出版社印刷厂印刷

*

开本 850×1168 1／32 印张 26.75 字数 690 000
1994 年 12 月第 1 版 1994 年 12 月第 1 次印刷
印数 0001— 5 170
ISBN7-04-005074-9／R·32
定价 ▇▇▇ 元

The Leading Commission of Compilation and Translation
编译领导委员会

Honorary Director 名誉主任委员	Hu Ximing 胡熙明		
Honorary Deputy Directors 名誉副主任委员	Zhang Qiwen 张奇文	Wang Lei 王镭	
Director 主任委员	Zou Jilong 邹积隆		
Deputy Director 副主任委员	Wei Jiwu 隗继武		
Members 委员 （以姓氏笔划为序）	Wan Deguang 万德光	Wang Yongyan 王永炎	Wang Maoze 王懋泽
	Wei Guikang 韦贵康	Cong Chunyu 丛春雨	Liu Zhongben 刘中本
	Sun Guojie 孙国杰	Yan Shiyun 严世芸	Qiu Dewen 邱德文
	Shang Chichang 尚炽昌	Xiang Ping 项平	Zhao Yisen 赵以森
	Gao Jinliang 高金亮	Cheng Yichun 程益春	Ge Linyi 葛琳仪
	Cai Jianqian 蔡剑前	Zhai Weimin 翟维敏	
Advisers 顾问	Dong Jianhua 董建华	Huang Xiaokai 黄孝楷	Geng Jianting 耿鉴庭
	Zhou Fengwu 周凤梧	Zhou Ciqing 周次清	Chen Keji 陈可冀

The Commission of Compilation and Translation
编译委员会

Director 主任委员	Xu Xiangcai 徐象才

Preface

I am delighted to learn that THE ENGLISH—CHINESE ENCYCLOPEDIA OF PRACTICAL TRADITIONAL CHINESE MEDICINE will soon come into the world.

TCM has experienced many vicissitudes of times but has remained evergreen. It has made great contributions not only to the power and prosperity of our Chinese nation but to the enrichment and improvement of world medicine. Unfortunately, differences in nations, states and languages have slowed down its spreading and flowing outside China. At present, however, an upsurge in learning, researching and applying Traditional Chinese Medicine (TCM) is unfolding. In order to maximize the effect of this upsurge and to lead TCM, one of the brilliant cultural heritages of the Chinese nation, to the world for it to expand and bring benefit to the people of all nations, Mr. Xu Xiangcai called intellectuals of noble aspirations and high intelligence together from Shandong and many other provinces in China and took charge of the work of both compilation and translation of THE ENGLISH—CHINESE ENCYCLOPEDIA OF PRACTICAL TRADITIONAL CHINESE MEDICINE. With great pleasure, the medical staff both at home and abroad will hail the appearance of this encyclopedia.

I believe that the day when the world's medicine is fully

developed will be the day when TCM has spread throughout the world.

I am pleased to give it my preface.

Prof. Dr. Hu Ximing
> Deputy Ministerof the Ministry of Public Health of the People's Republic of China,
> Director General of the State Administrative Bureau of Traditional Chinese Medicine and Pharmacology,
> President of the World Federation of Acupuncture —Moxibustion Societies,
> Member of China Association of Science & Technology,
> Deputy President of All—China Association of Traditional Chinese Medicine,
> President of China Acupuncture & Moxibustion Society.

December, 1989

Preface

The Chinese nation has been through a long, arduous course of struggling against diseases and has developed its own traditional medicine—Traditional Chinese Medicine and Pharmacology (TCMP). TCMP has a unique, comprehensive, scientific system including both theories and clinical practice. Some thousand years since ito—beginnings, not only has it been well preserved but also continuously developed. It has special advantages, such as remarkable curative effects and few side effects. Hence it is an effective means by which people prevent and treat diseases and keep themselves strong and healthy.

All achievements attained by any nation in the development of medicine are the public wealth of all mankind. They should not be confined within a single country. What is more, the need to set them free to flow throughout the world as quickly and precisely as possible is greater than that of any other kind of science. During my more than thirty years of being engaged in Traditional Chinese Medicine(TCM), I have been looking forward to the day when TCMP will have spread all over the world and made its contributions to the elimination of diseases of all mankind. However it is to be deeply regretted that the pace of TCMP in extending outside China has been unsatisfactory due to the major difficulties in expressing its concepts in foreign languages.

Mr. Xu Xiangcai, a teacher of Shandong College of TCM, has sponsored and taken charge of the work of compilation and translation of The English—Chinese Encyclopedia of Practical Traditional Chinese Medicine—an extensive series. This work is a great project, a large—scale scientific research, a courageous effort and a novel creation. I deeply esteem Mr. Xu Xiangcai and his compilers and translators, who have been working day and night for such a long time, for their hard labor and for their firm and indomitable will displayed in overcoming one difficulty after another, and for their great success achieved in this way. As a leader in the circles of TCM, I am duty—bound to do my best to support them.

I believe this encyclopedia will be certain to find its position both in the history of Chinese medicine and in the history of world science and technology.

Mr. Zhang Qiwen

Member of the Standing Committee of
All—China Association of TCM,
Deputy Head of the Health Department
of Shandong Province.

March, 1990

Publisher's Preface

Traditional Chinese Medicine(TCM) is one of China's great cultural heritages. Since the founding of the People's Republic of China in 1949, guided by the farsighted TCM policy of the Chinese Communist Party and the Chinese government, the treasure house of the theories of TCM has been continuously explored and the plentiful literature researched and compiled. As a result, great success has been achieved. Today there has appeared a world—wide upsurge in the studying and researching of TCM. To promote even more vigorous development of this trend in order that TCM may better serve all mankind, efforts are required to further it throughout the world. To bring this about, the language barriers must be overcome as soon as possible in order that TCM can be accurately expressed in foreign languages.

Thus the compilation and translation of a series of English—Chinese books of basic knowledge of TCM has become of great urgency to serve the needs of medical and educational circles both inside and outside China.

In recent years, at the request of the health departments, satisfactory achievements have been made in researching the expression of TCM in English. Based on the investigation into the history and current state of the research work mentioned above, the English—Chinese Encyclopedia of Practical TCM has been published to meet the needs of extending the knowledge of TCM around the world.

The encyclopedia consists of twenty—one volumes, each dealing with a particular branch of TCM. In the process of compilation, the distinguishing features of TCM have been given close attention and great efforts have been made to ensure that the content is scientific, practical, comprehensive and concise. The chief writers of the Chinese manuscripts include professors or associate professors with at least twenty years of practical clinical and / or teaching experience in TCM. The Chinese manuscript of each volume has been checked and approved by a specialist of the relevant branch of TCM. The team of the translators and revisers of the English versions consists of TCM specialists with a good command of English professional medical translators, and teachers of English from TCM colleges or universities. At a symposium to standardize the English versions, scholars from twenty—two colleges or universities, research institutes of TCM or other health institutes probed the question of how to express TCM in English more comprehensively, systematically and accurately, and discussed and deliberated in detail the English versions of some volumes in order to upgrade the English versions of the whole series. The English version of each volume has been re—examined and then given a final checking.

Obviously this encyclopedia will provide extensive reading material of TCM English for senior students in colleges of TCM in China and will also greatly benefit foreigners studying TCM.

The assiduous efforts of compiling and translating this encyclopedia have been supported by the responsible leaders of the State Education Commission of the People's Republic of China, the State Administrative Bureau of TCM and Pharmacy, and the Education Commission and Health Department of Shandong

Province. Under the direction of the Higher Education Department of the State Education Commission, the leading board of compilation and translation of this encyclopedia was set up. The leaders of many colleges of TCM and pharmaceutical factories of TCM have also given assistance.

We hope that this encyclopedia will bring about a good effect on enhancing the teaching of TCM English at the colleges of TCM in China, on cultivating skills in medical circles in exchanging ideas of TCM with patients in English, and on giving an impetus to the study of TCM outside China.

Higher Education Press

March, 1990

Foreword

The English—Chinese Encyclopedia of Practical Traditional Chinese Medicine is an extensive series of twenty—one volumes. Based on the fundamental theories of traditional Chinese medicine(TCM) and with emphasis on the clinical practice of TCM, it is a semi—advanced English—Chinese academic works which is quite comprehensive, systematic, concise, practical and easy to read. It caters mainly to the following readers: senior students of colleges of TCM, young and middle—aged teachers of colleges of TCM, young and middle—aged physicians of hospitals of TCM, personnel of scientific research institutions of TCM, teachers giving correspondence courses in TCM to foreigners, TCM personnel going abroad in the capacity of lecturers or physicians, those trained in Western medicine but wishing to study TCM, and foreigners coming to China to learn TCM or to take refresher courses in TCM.

Because Traditional Chinese Medicine and Pharmacology is unique to our Chinese nation, putting TCM into English has been the crux of the compilation and translation of this encyclopedia. Owing to the fact that no one can be proficient both in the theories of Traditional Chinese Medicine and Pharmacology and the clinical practice of every branch of TCM, as well as in English, to ensure that the English versions express accurately the inherent meanings of TCM, collective translation measures have been taken. That is, teachers of English familiar with TCM, professional medical translators, teachers or physicians of TCM and even teachers of palaeography with a strong command of English were all invited together to co—translate the Chinese manuscripts and, then, to co—deliberate and discuss the English versions. Finally English—speaking foreigners studying TCM or teaching English in China were asked to polish the English versions. In this way, the skills of the above translators and foreigners were merged to ensure the quality of the English versions. However, even using this method, the uncertainty that the English versions will be wholly accepted still remains. As for the Chinese manuscripts, they do reflect the essence, and give a general picture, of traditional Chinese medicine and pharmacology. It is not asserted, though, that they are perfect, I whole—heartedly look forward to any criticisms or opinions from readers in order to make improvements to future editions.

More than 200 people have taken part in the activities of compiling, translating and revising this encyclopedia. They come from twenty—eight institutions in all parts of China. Among these institutions, there are fifteen colleges of TCM:Shandong, Beijing, Shanghai, Tianjin, Nanjing, Zhejiang, Anhui, Henan, Hubei, Guangxi, Guiyang, Gansu, Chengdu, Shanxi and Changchun, and scientific research centers of TCM such as China Academy of TCM and Shandong Scientific Research Institute of TCM.

The Education Commission of Shandong province has included the compilation and translation of this encyclopedia in its scientific research projects and allocated funds accordingly. The Health Department of Shandong Province has also given financial aid together with a number of pharmaceutical factories of TCM. The subsidization from Jinan Pharmaceutical Factory of

TCM provided the impetus for the work of compilation and translation to get under way.

The success of compiling and translating this encyclopedia is not only the fruit of the collective labor of all the compilers, translators and revisers but also the result of the support of the responsible leaders of the relevant leading institutions. As the encyclopedia is going to be published, I express my heartfelt thanks to all the compilers. translators and revisers for their sincere cooperation, and to the specialists, professors, leaders at all levels and pharmaceutical factories of TCM for their warm support.

It is my most profound wish that the publication of this encyclopedia will take its role in cultivating talented persons of TCM having a very good command of TCM English and in extending, rapidly, comprehensive knowledge of TCM to all corners of the globe.

Chief Editor   Xu Xiangcai

Shandong College of TCM

March, 1990

Contents

Notes

This book is the 7th volume of THE ENGLISH—CHINESE ENCYCLOPEDIA OF PRACTICAL TRADITIONAL CHINESE MEDICINE.

This volume mainly consists of two parts: adult *Tuina* and infant *Tuina*. The former includes the following seven chapters: Brief Introduction to Adult *Tuina*, Commonly Used Manipulations for Adult *Tuina*, Methods and Steps for Training Manipulations, the Fourteen Channels and the Commonly Used Acupoints, Exercises as Basic Training of Manipulations, Treatment of Common Adult Diseases, and Adult *Tuina* for Health—care; while the latter, the following five chapters: Brief Introduction to Infant *Tuina*, Manipulations for Infant *Tuina*, Commonly Used Points in Infant *Tuina*, Treatment of Common Infantile Diseases, and Infant *Tuina* for Health—care; with the stress put on the elaborate introduction to the treatment of 41 adult and 19 infantile common diseases. In addition, 283 figures are added for the convenience of the readers.

The English version of this volume is conciser, preciser and easier to read and understand. Terms of all the manipulations, all the acupoints and all the specific points in infant *Tuina* as well as a few of TCM terms, which have no corresponding words or expressions in English, are expressed in Chinese phonetic words, the first letter of each of which is capitalized. And what is more, except the terms of acupoints and the specific points in infant *Tuina*, the other two kinds are italicized.

Prof. Zheng Fenghu from Shanghai College of TCM once checked the Chinese manuscript. Messrs. Zhang Zhe, Kong Jian, Yan Jingbo, Zhang Dayong and Wang lei, and Misses Guo Jing, Fei Liping, Wang Xin, Ma Jun and Sun Shiping helped do part of translation work. They have been studying both TCM and English in Shandong College of TCM.

All the illustrations were drawn by Mr. Liu Xingchi.

The Chief Editors

Brief Introduction to *Tuina*

Chinese *Tuina* is a subject of medicine guided by the theories of traditional Chinese medicine (TCM), in which manipulations are used to stimulate the points or other parts of the body surface so as to correct the physiological imbalance of the body and achieve curative effects. It is an important component of TCM. In ancient China, therapy was mainly classified into two: external and internal; *Tuina* was included in the former.

Tuina may be applied to treat lots of disorders, among which are not only various injuries of soft tissue but also many other kinds of diseases of medicine, surgery, gynecology, neurology, the five sense organs, pediatrics, etc. It is especially suitable for infantile and old patients. By the present, therefore, Chinese *Tuina* has fallen into several branches such as adult, infant, orthopaedics and traumatology, cosmetology, health–care, rehabilitation, sports medicine, and so on.

Concrete speaking, adult *Tuina* is traditionally used to treat cervical spondylosis, lumbar muscle strain, prolapse of lumbar intervertebral disc, acute lumbar muscle sprain, rheumatoid arthritis, epigastralgia, gastroptosia, constipation, hypertension and sequel of apoplexy. Treatment of diabetes with adult *Tuina* has long since been reported. If allergic colitis and duodenal bulbar ulcer are treated with adult *Tuina*, quicker cure will be attained. In recent years, treatment of chronic coronary insufficiency and angina pectoris with adult *Tuina* has been remarkedly developed, too. Since 1982, the authors have devoted their efforts to researching and treating the above diseases and found that the treated patients' electrocardiogram, cardiac function and subjective symptoms were all greatly improved. As for infant *Tuina*, it comes up with very satisfactory effects when used to treat such infantile disorders of the digestive system as diarrhea, vomiting, abdominal pain and intestinal obstruction, and remarkable effects when applied to treat vitamin D deficiency rickets, dystrophy, anorexia, measles, chin cough, bacillary dysentery, upper respiratory tract infection, bronchial asthma, anemia and fever. In addition, it plays an evident role in increasing infantile immunity. After treated with infant *Tuina*, infants susceptible to common cold due to low immunologic function can be kept from it for a long time.

Tuina has the effect of dual—direction regulation of the body function. For instance, *Tuina* practised on the corresponding points over the abdomen and the back or the upper limbs of the patient with either hyperperistalsis or hypoperistalsis may either decrease or increase the abnormal peristalsis and return it to normal. Abnormal physiological function of the body is usually due to diseases caused by bacteria, viruses, protozoa or physical and chemical factors. Medicines may be used to hold back the growth of the bacteria and viruses or kill them. But it does not follow that the abnormal physiological function will be corrected naturally. That's why cure is late when some diseases are treated only with medicines. In this case, if *Tuina* is added, the cure will come sooner. The theories of TCM believe that *Tuina* acts on the points, channels and collaterals throughout the body, regulating the functioning of the internal organs. That is , *Tuina* may dredge the channels and collaterals, promote blood circulation and regulate *Yin* and *Yang* so as to return the body function to normal.

Modern research has proved that *Tuina* can improve the microcirculation of the blood and lymphatic systems, which brings quicker recovery to various injuries of soft tissue such as sprain and contusion. Furthermore, because the nervous system controlling the microcirculation of the internal organs connects with the skin, *Tuina* practised on certain points over the body surface may also regulate the microcirculation of the internal organs, which adjusts the functioning of the internal organs. Just because *Tuina* can exert effect on the central nervous system, it may be used to bring about anaesthesia, to lower fever of infants by adjusting body temperature and to treat hypertension and neurosism.

Long—time over—intake of chemical medicines may result in drug resis tance, and side effects of some drugs will produce serious sequelae. Yet, *Tuina* has no side effects, not only that, it can increase the immunity of the body, for it works only through adjusting the functions of the body. In addition, it neither gets patients as nervous as acupuncture, nor consumes much materal wealth of the society. So, *Tuina* is a cheap, highly—effective, beneficial and ideal medical means without side effects.

At present, many things remain to be done in the field of *Tuina* . First, the mechanism of *Tuina* needs to be investigated further with modern medical theories. Second, *Tuina* should be used to treat more diseases in clinical practice so as to widen the range of its indications. Third, *Tuina* ought to be introduced to the world to let all the people abroad also enjoy this very ideal medical means. Finally, more instruments used for treatment, experiment, scientific research and teaching of *Tuina* should be developed.

Tuina may be used not only to treat diseases but also to protect health and build up the body so that a disease can be stopped in its beginning. In his book *Jin Kui Yao Lue*, Zhang Zhongjing, a famous physician in the Han Dynasty (206BC–220AD), pointed out: "As soon as the heavy sensation of the limbs is felt, *Daoyin, Tuna, Zhenjiu* and *Gaomo* (massage with ointment as medium), all of which are therapeutic methods, are carried out in order to prevent the nine orifices from being obstructed, thus keeping the disease off in its beginning. " This shows that self–*Tuina* was widely used at that time as a means for preventing diseases and protecting health. Our forefathers kept their *Qi* and blood flowing freely, strengthened their tendons and bones and got rid of their tiredness and restlessness by self–*Tuina* for the purpose of preventing diseases and prolonging life. One of the essences of the science of prevention and cure in TCM is: prevention first and treatment second, which has been fully reflected in the above. The fruits of modern senile medicine and sports medicine suggest that to meet the needs of mental state and disease condition of old people, health–care *Tuina* should be further researched and developed so as to get as soon as possible better methods of health–care *Tuina* more suitable for the aged. For the detail, please read the following.

1 Brief Introduction to the Development of *Tuina* of TCM

Tuina, a medical method with the hands as the tool for treating diseases, is, so to speak, one of the earliest medical forms of mankind. This may be seen in the medical history of every old nation all over the world, because the behavior for our forefathers to rub, press, knead or pound with their hands their own or their fellows/ bodies in order to keep out the cold, warm themselves and get rid of the discomfort due to fatigue, abdominal distension and various injuries is a congenital instinct of self—defense. In the primitive times in which there were neither medical instruments nor treatment of diseases with drugs at all, our ancestors could do nothing but using the spontaneous medical method of self—rubbing, self—kneading or pounding and stepping each other. In fact, this is, even if based on reasoning, the origin of *Tuina* . The Chinese forefathers were human beings with wisdom, they summed up and developed continually their practical experiences accumulated in the long time, which gradually became what is called now a natural therapy—*Tuina* medical subject.

In China, *Tuina* may date back to the remote reign of emperor Huang, during which *Tuina* was called *Anwu*. By the Spring and Autumn and Warring Stages (two thousand years ago), *Tuina,* called as *Anmo* then, had developed into a widely—used and more basically—perfect medical means. For example, Bian Que, an outstanding physician living in that times, once used a comprehensive therapy including *Anmo* to treat a crown prince of the state Guo who was suffering from a disease called corpse—like syncope with miraculous curative effects, drawing him back from the jaws of death.

Up to the Dynasties of Qin and Han and the times of the Three Kingdoms(205 BC—280 AD), the experiences obtained and the methods created both in the past medical practice had been enriched and summed up step by step, which promoted a monograph on *Anmo* entiled *Huang Di Qi Bo An Mó Jing Shi Juan* to come into being. This book is the first one in the history of TCM. It is a great pity that this book has been lost. If it had been handed down from then to now, we could see the whole developed picture of *Anmo* technique at the time. Fortunately, we can still see the general picture in another great work *Huang Di Nei Jing* written in the same ages, which is the earliest medical classics stored now in China. If you read this book through, you will find out that it contains many chapters with plenty of content dealing with nearly all the aspects of *Anmo* therapy then, such as the origin, manipulations, clinical application, indications, therapeutic principles and teaching. In this book, more than ten maneuvers such as *Tui, An, Mo, Qiao* and *Che* are involved, indications including acute and chronic diseases referring to every clinical department such as disorders due to terror, faccidity with cold limbs, cold or heat syndrome, spleen—wind syndrome, conditions due to obstruction of the channels and collaterals and abdominal pain due to cold are mentioned, and, especially, rather penetrating analyses of the therapeutic principles of manupulations are made and some of them are still playing a guiding role in today's clinical and teaching practice. In addition, there appeared, at the time, many non—medical works: *Meng Zi, Lao Zi, Xun Zi* and *Mo Zi,* in which the popularity of *Anmo*—therapy among the folks is recorded. Later, the outstanding physician Zhang Zhong-jing advanced and summarized the method of *Gaomo* first of all in his book *Jin Kui Yao Lue.* By *Gaomo* is meant first smearing an ointment made from herbal medicines on the patient's body surface, on which are the points of choice and beneath which are the corresponding channels, and then carrying out the *Anmo*—therapy over the ointment with manupulations. Owing to the co—working of both the manipulations and medicines, this method not only further ensures the curative effects but also widens the range of indications of *Anmo*—therapy. Hua Tuo, a famous physician in the time of Three Kingdoms, also used this method to treat febrile diseases and get rid of superficial pathogens in the skin. From what has been said above, we can see that by that time, as a commonly—used medical means, *Anmo*—therapy had been widely applied and greatly valued and researched by many famous physicians in that ages, so that its specialized techniques and theory were continually enriched and developed, which was a sign that *Anmo*—therapy at the time had been freed from the spontaneous medical form of the early time with its academic position established in the system of clinical medicine of TCM.

By the time of the West Jin, East Jin and Northern and Southern Dynasties (265—589 AD), *Gaomo* technique had been further developed. For example, in his book *Mai Jing,* Wang Shuhe put forward a way in which pain due to arthralgia—syndrome was treated with an ointment *Fenggao,* and what is more, Ge Hong summed up systematically the prescriptions, drugs, indications and operations of *Gaomo* and the process of ointment used for *Gaomo* for the first time in his book *Zhou Hou Bei Ji Fang,* in which eight prescriptions for *Gaomo* are introduced whose indications cover the common diseases of such clinical departments as medicine, surgery, gynecology and the five sense organs. In addition, in Tao Hongjing's book *Yang Xing Yan Ming Lu,* there is, too, a volume specially dealing with physical and breathing exercises combined with automassage. With many pages and rich content, this volume introduces many sets of massage exercises such as massage how to be done by oneself on the teeth, eyes, ears, hair, face and body, which is the source of automassage aiming at health care and self—treatment of diseases.

The Dynasties of Sui and Tang (581—907 AD) were a flourishing age for *Anmo* to be fully developed when the department of *Anmo* was officially set up in the State Office of Imperial Physicians. The massagists fell into different degrees: doctor (referring to one with doctorate), physician and worker, the doctor being the highest. With the help of physicians and workers, the doctors took charge of the routine medical work and the organized teaching of students' learning massage. By that time, self—massage and *Gaomo*—therapy had been more widely applied and developed. For instance, an introduction to *Anmo* ends every volume of the book *Zhu Bing Yuan Hou Lun* written by Chao Yuanfang in the Sui Dynasty, besides, there are more prescriptions, drugs and indications of *Gaomo* listed in the book *Qian Jin Fang* written by Sun Simiao in the Tang Dynasty. What is specially worth pointing out is that this book systematically discusses the treatment of more than ten infantile diseases with *Gaomo*—therapy, such as convulsive seizure induced by terror manifested as stiffness of the neck and dying, stuffy nose with discharge flowing, morbid night crying, distention and fullness in the abdomen, and poor appetite for milk. As the medical literature in which health care of infants with *Gaomo*—therapy is recorded for the first time, this book also has it to say that *Gaomo*—therapy often practised in the early morning over the fontanel, palms and soles of an infant in good condition may well protect it from being attacked by cold and wind. From the above, it may be seen that *Anmo* for infants was extensively used in the Dynasty of Tang. Sun Simiao also wrote a book *Lao Zi Anmo Fa* dealing with a method of massage. He introduced many other ones of massage and physical and breathing exercises. Only as far as the maneuvers are concerned, dozens of them such as *An, Mó, Ca, Nian, Bao, Tui, Zhan, Da, Lie* and *Na* are involved in those methods. A famous book *Tang Liu Dian* appearing in that period says that *Anmo* may be used to treat diseases due to eight kinds of pathogenic factors: wind, cold, summer—heat, dampness, overhunger, overfill, overstrain and over-rest, which fully proves that by that age, the range of indications of *Anmo* had been greatly broadened. As for the book *Wai Tai Mi Yao*, it makes main contributions not only to the presence of plenty of experience in the treatment of diseases with *Anmo* but also to the record of many prescriptions for *Gaomo*—therapy with their sources indicated one by one. The above historical information provides the evidence that in the Dynasties of Sui and Tang, *Anmo*, as a clinical subject of TCM, was developed to quite a higher level in its system of basic theory, diagnostic technique and treatment. During that time, the exchange of culture between China and other countries was thriving due to the greater development of politics, economy, culture and transportation and it was then that *Anmo* spread to such foreign countries as Korea,

Japan, India, etc.

In the Dynasties of Song, Jin and Yuan, there was no department of *Anmo* in the state medical institution. But there was a department for treating sore in the Bureau of Imperial Physicians of the Northern Song Dynasty, and a specialty of bone–setting and wound in the Institute of Imperial Physicians of the Yuan Dynasty, both of which were also responsible for the affairs of *Anmo* treatment. *Anmo*–therapy then was mainly used to treat disorders of osteotrauma, which layed foundations for the medical system of bone setting *Tuina* afterwards. Physicians in the Song Dynasty also applied, at the time, *Anmo* to expediting child delivery. Up to that time, physicians had not only had a comprehensive knowledge of the effects, methods and applicable range of *Anmo* but also made a breakthrough in researching the basic theories of selection of maneuvers through differentiation of symptoms and of the principles of maneuvers' work. This may be seen in the book *Sheng Ji Zong Lu*. It says that *An* (pressing), a maneuver, or *Mó* (rubbing), another maneuver, may be applied alone, but both of them are usually used together. And that's why the term *Anmo* comes. While *An* is being done, *Mó* is not, and vice versa. *An* is performed only by hand while *Mó*, sometimes with the help of drug effect. Either *An* or *Mó* is employed according to the practical need. ... In general, the effect of *Anmo* has no more than two: smoothing and checking. Smoothing means dispersing obstruction, while checking, restraining hyperfunction. Those remarks contribute a lot to the development of *Anmo* theory.

Anmo saw the second flourishing development in the Ming Dynasty. In the Institute of Imperial Physician, the state medical institution then, there were thirteen departments of TCM, among which was *Anmo* specialty. Thanks to the continual development of *Anmo* as a whole and especially owing to the rich experience accumulated in the treatment of infantile diseases, the first treatise on infant *Tuina*, *Xiao Er An Mo Jing*, came into being in 1601 in China. Not a long time later, the book *Xiao Er Tui Na Fang Mai Huo Ying Mi Zhi Quan Shu* and the book *Xiao Er Tui Na Mi Jue* were published one after the other. This indicates that as an academic branch of *Anmo* with its own specific system of diagnosis, manupulations and points, infant *Tuina* had been formed by that time. Readers may find out that the term *Tuina* has appeared for the first time in the above. Yes, it was just at that time that the subject term *Tuina* officially popular today began to substitute for *Anmo*. This is of profound significance in the developing history of *Tuina*, for the innovation of subject terminology is a sign that this subject has been raised to a high level as a whole.

In the Qing Dynasty, *Tuina* was looked down upon by the government, yet, it was used and spread rather extensively among the people. Especially in infant *Tuina*, remarkable development was obtained in the early and middle period of this dynasty with a great number of infant massagists emerged along with treatises on infant *Tuina* such as the book *Xiao Er Tui Na Guang Yi*, the book *You Ke Tui Na Mi Shu*, the book *Bao Chi Tui Na*, and the book *Li Zheng An Mó Yao Shu*, which taught the later generations more about infant *Tuina*. In addition, great achievements were made in the treatment of disorders of traumatology with *Tuina* in this period. This may be seen in the book *Yi Zong Jin Jian*, in which the maneuvers *Mó* (palpating), *Jie*, *Chuai*, *Ti Tui*,

Na, An and *Mó* (rubbing) were classified as the eight methods for treating fractures and trauma. So to speak, the medical school traumatology *Tuina* was basically formed in that time.

Before the foundation of the People's Republic of China, there was a time during which enough importance was not attached to *Tuina* medicine. But it was still popularly used because of its specific curative effects. Furthermore, many folk massagists did their best to research, inherit and reform *Tuina* in practice so that various *Tuina* academic schools such as *Yi Zhi Chan, Gun Fa, Nei Gong Tui Na, Dian Xue Tui Na* and *Xiao Er Tui Na* were handed down, which serves as a link between past and future.

After the foundation of the People's Republic of China in 1949, the government advocated TCM with great effort and looked at *Tuina* medicine with a new eye. In 1956, the first *Tuina* training class was run in the city of Shanghai. In 1958, Shanghai Clinic of *Tuina* and Shanghai Technical Secondary School of *Tuina* were set up. In addition, folk massagists all over China were assigned to hospitals to work in the clinical departments of *Tuina* which were established one after another. Up to 1960's, a professional contingent of *Tuina* has been basically formed in China. In 1974, the first *Tuina* section appeared at the department of Acupuncture, *Tuina* and Traumatology in Shanghai College of TCM. Later, the same thing happened subsquently in the TCM colleges of Beijing, Nanjing, Fujian and Anhui. This provides conditions for cultivating outstanding *Tuina* physicians. In 1987, All—China Association of *Tuina* was set up. From then on, academic exchanges of *Tuina*, national or international, were conducted vigorously. The number and quality of the monographs and these on *Tuina* written in the last years have reached the summit of the historical records, and scientific researches on the essentials and clinical practice of *Tuina* have been also made successfully. For instance, the curative effects of *Tuina* in treating cervical spondylopathy, prolapse of lumbar intervertebral disc, infantile diarrhea, coronary heart disease and cholecystitis have taken the lead in the world. As for the research on the mechanical information of *Tuina* maneuvers made by the researchers from Shandong province and Shanghai city, from the biomechanical point of view, it has also brought about a lot of valuable fruits.

Today, *Tuina* medicine flourishing in China is playing its active part in various medical fields such as medical service, rehabilitation, prevention and health—care. Its safe, effective and harmless advantages without side effects will be known and accepted day by day by the people all over the world. Looking forward to the future, we believe that old and young Chinese *Tuina* will take on an entirely new look and march from China to the world, serving the people all over the globe better.

2　An Outline of *Tuina* Schools of TCM

Because of the complicated reasons and backgrounds formed in the long history such as different sources, lineages, targets of treatment, politics, economy, societies, culture, geographical areas and human touches, *Tuina* has had such rich and colorful academic schools and systems as *Yi Zhi Chan Tui Na, Gun Fa Tui Na, Nei Gong Tui Na, Zheng Gu Tui Na, Wai Shang An Mó Liao Fa, An Mó Liao Fa, Xiao Er Tui Na, Dian Xue Tui Na, Zang Fu Jing Luo Tui Na, Bao Jian Tui Na, Yang Sheng An Mó, Wei Bing Tui Na, Nie Jin Pai Da Liao Fa, Zhi Ya Tui Na, Zhi Zhen Liao Fa, Zhi Ba Liao Fa, Nie Ji Liao Fa, Zi Wo Tui Na, Gao Mó Liao Fa, Dong Gong An Mó, Yun Dong Tui Na, Mei Rong Tui Na, Tui Na Ma Zui, Zi Wu Liu Zhu Tui Na, Qiao Xue Qi Shu Tui Na, Jing Wai Qi Xue Tui Na,* etc. A general study of them may disclose the fact that they are all the same in the following three points: first, having a longer history, and forming, spreading and thriving within a district; second, guided by a theory, rich in medical practical experience, and having expert indications and unique methods for exercise and specialty training; third, each having a main maneuver, which may be called "school maneuver", usually colored by evident touch of provincialism and local citizens.

Take *Yi Zhi Chan Tui Na* (a manipulation operating with one thumb) forexample. It has been popularized in south China, especially in the provinces of Jiangsu and Zhejiang and the city of Shanghai, ever since the years of Xianfeng (an emperor) in the

Qing Dynasty (1851–1862). Guided by the TCM's theories such as *Yin* and *Yang*, *Wu Xing* (the five elements), *Zang Fu* (viscera), *Jing Luo* (channels and collaterals), *Ying* (nutrition) *Wei* (defense) *Qi* and *Xue* (blood), *Si Zhen* (four diagnostic methods), and *Ba Gang* (the eight sorts of nature of the syndromes), it is operated according to the diagnosis made through differentiating, comprehensively, the all–round condition of both the syndrome and patient with the disease cause stressed. As for the maneuvers, the leading one is *Yi Zhi Chan Tui Fa* (a manipulation operated with one thumb) and the assistant ones are *Na* (grasping), *An* (pressing), *Mó* (rubbing), *Gun* (rolling), *Nian* (twisting), *Chao* (sweeping), *Cuo* (foulage), *Chan* (quick–pushing), *Rou* (kneading), *Yao* (rotating) and *Dou* (shaking). When performed, they should be soft but penetrating, gentle but firm or firm but gentle, both supplementing each other with gentleness more important. *Yi Zhi Chan Tui Na* has a whole set of methods for training professional techniques and attaches special importance to the training of basic skills, because the leading maneuver and some assistant ones are harder to master. The students are required to practise, first of all, external–strong exercise—*Yi Jin Jing*, and then do basic exercises of the maneuvers on a bag filled with rice. This kind of *Tuina* is mainly conducted along the fourteen channels, on the points along them, and on the extrachannel–points and non–fixed points, with great attention paid to "operation performed on the points and along the channels". It can be used to treat more diseases, such as disorders of the channels, collaterals, body or internal organs whether they are due to external or internal cause. Especially, when it is employed to treat miscellaneous diseases of medicine and gynecology such as headache, insomnia, internal injuries due to overstrain, epigastralgia, prolonged diarrhea, constipation, obstruction of *Qi* in the chest, dysmenorrhea and irregular menstruation, better curative effects will be attained.

Take *Dian Xue Liao Fa* (digital—point—pressure therapy) for another example. It is a *Tuina*—therapy which is derived from *Dian Xue* (digital point—pressing), *Da Xue* (point hitting), *Na Xue* (point capturing), *Ti Xue* (point kicking), etc. of traditional Chinese martial art, and thriving in Qingdao city, Laoshan mountainous district and other places of Jiaodong peninsula of north China. Point beating in martial art functions in two ways: attack in striking, and treatment of injuries. In digital—point—pressure therapy, the practical experience of the latter is summarized, the hurtful or mortal overstrong digital hitting in martial art is turned into the safe—strong one which can be beared by the physiology of human body, and is used for treating diseases guided by the theories of TCM such as *Jingluo* (channels and collaterals). As a result, this therapy becomes a *Tuina* school. Its leading maneuver is *Dian Fa* (digital point hitting), its assistant ones are *Pai Da Fa* (patting), *Kou Da Fa* (tapping), *An Ya Fa* (pressing), *Qia Fa* (nipping), *Kou Ya Fa* (smashing—pressing), *Zhua Na Fa* (clutching—grasping), *Chui Da Fa* (pounding) and *Jiao Xing Fa* (orthopedy), with digital pressing, patting, pushing and pounding as the main ones. All the maneuvers are character-istic of swiftness, firmness and powerfulness. A mild digital pres-sure may produce a power of some 10 kg. while a strong one, 60—70kg. In order to perform this kind of *Tuina*, a massagist has to have stronger fingers, arms and enough power to support his whole body. So the beginners need basic training. What they should do first is to practise digital—point exercises. The main ones are as follows: *Dun Qi Gong* (exercise done by squatting and standing up), *Yun Qi Pai Da Gong*(exercise done by directing one's strength to patting), *Dui La Gong* (exercise done by antagonistic pulling), *Yang Wo Gong* (exercise done by lying on the back), *Zhuang Bei Gong* (exercise done by bumping the back), *Wu Gong Tiao* (exercise done by imitating the movement of a centipede), *Ying Zhao Li* (exercise done to make the fingers stronger with them imitating an eagle's claws), *Chui Zhi Gong* (exercise done by beating a collection of hundreds of sheets of paper with the fists), *Tui Shan Gong* (exercise done as if pushing a mountain) and *Zha Yao Gong* (exercise done for strengthening the loins), etc. About the names of the above *Gong* (exercise), they are not hard to express in English according to the literal meaning of their Chinese charaters. But foreigners will be bewildered or misled by such kind of English expressions as " lying—on—the—back" , "hill—pushing", "waist—pricking", etc., because no one can push a hill and *Zha Yao Gong* does not require the exerciser to prick his waist either, That's why we use Chinese spelling words to express the names of *Gong,* which are, of course, exact, following each of which a brief notes is given for the sake of foreigners, which is, of course, incomplete. Only through doing the exercises practically, can one know what the names stand for. By the way, digital—point —pressure therapy is theoretically based on this. The syndromes of flaccidity, numbness and arthralgia and the like result from adverse flow of *Qi* in the channels and collaterals and obstructed movement of *Ying, Wei, Qi* and blood, both of which are caused by imbalance of *Yin* and *Yang* due to the struggle between the resistance of the body and the pathogenic factors, and the treatment is to shake, stimulate and gradually open the blocked point by exerting stronger maneuvers of digital point pressing before it or on its relevant one so that the obstructed *Qi* and blood will pass through it slowly until their flowing returns to normal. Once the channels and collaterals have been dredged, the syndromes will disappear. Therefore, this kind of *Tuina*—therapy is mainly suitable for the treatment of various sorts of paralysis, numbness, arthralgia and obstinate rheumatalgia.

It may be seen from the brief introduction to the two *Tuina* schools in the above that each of *Tuina* schools is characterized by its own historical source, medical theory, treating manipulation, training method, therapeutic feature and indications, all of which contribute to its own system. There are many *Tuina* schools with rich content in TCM, which can not be explained in detail one by one in this book. What we can do is to generalize and outline the academic content of a part of *Tuina* schools such as *Yi Zhi Chan Tui Na, Gun Fa Tui Na, Nei Gong Tui Na, Dian Xue Tui Na, Xiao Er Tui Na* and *Bao Jian Tui Na* in the two parts of this book. But we hope that the readers can " see the whole through knowing the segments", and have their interest aroused in learning TCM *Tuina,* so that it may better serve the health cause of the people all over the globe.

3 The Way to Master *Tuina* of TCM

TCM *Tuina* is a clinical subject of TCM based on more theories and practice. An expert physician of *Tuina* ought to be well versed in the essential knowledge of both Chinese and Western medicines, master the professional theories and skills needed for clinical diagnosis and treatment, and have a strong body constitution and proficient maneuvers of *Tuina* to meet the needs of clinical practice. That's why the students of *Tuina* sections of TCM colleges in China are required to train themselves strictly both in body constitution and basic techniques of manipulation in addition to their study of all the courses dealing with the essentials of both Chinese and Western medicines and the clinical medicine, which are the required ones of undergraduates.

While studying the essential and clinical courses dealing with the TCM content such as *Yin* and *Yang*, *Wu Xing*, *Ying* and *Wei*, *Qi* and blood, *Jing* and *Luo*, *Zang* and *Fu*, pathogenesis, diagnostic methods and "treatment according to overall analysis of both a disease and the patient's condition", and the knowledge of Western medicine such as anatomy, physiology, pathology and physical diagnosis, the students should learn by heart the more practical basic knowledge guiding the clinical practice of *Tuina* such as the routes of the fourteen channels; the relationship between the fourteen channels and the internal organs; the location, selection, nature, function and indications of each of the commonly used points on the fourteen channels or the extrachannel-points; the structure of the human body, and athletic physiology.

In the training of professional techniques, the students have two things to do. The first one is to do what is introduced in the section of "exercise training" of this book, i.e., to do the commonly used exercises according to their training methods and steps conscientiously so as to improve health conditions comprehensively and get better body constitutions needed for *Tuina* specialty. The second is to do what is introduced in the section of "commonly used manipulations" of this book, i.e., to keep in mind the basic movement mechanism and technical essentials of every maneuver, to master the manipulating skills through strictly following the required training methods and procedures, proceeding step by step and practising assiduously and perseveringly, and to fulfil fully and best the training tasks at the three basic stages: practising on a bag filled with rice, on the human body and in the treatment of patients with common diseases.

Generally speaking, one can master *Tuina* surely as long as he studies conscientiously and practises hard according to what has been said above, and it is not difficult for those with sound basic knowledge of medicine to grasp the essentials of *Tuina* within a shorter time. However, to do it as better as a *Tuina* physician and especially to perform more technically difficult manipulations with high proficiency such as those of *Yi Zhi Chan Tui Fa* and *Gun Fa* are impossible unless long-term professional training has been carried out and "special power" has been accumulated.

4 Brief Introduction to the Principle for TCM's *Tuina* to Work

Why *Tuina* has the effect of treating diseases is a very complicated problem to be further researched. It will be some time before such mysteries about the problem are solved as the essence of channels and collaterals, the biomechanical feature of the movement of a manipulation, and bio—physicochemical process during which the stimulus of a manipulation is received, distributed, transformed utilized in the human body, and the effect is then produced, etc. From TCM's point of view, the principle for *Tuina* to work is mainly from the effect produced due to the acting of a manipulation on the channel and point system of the human body. Therefore, why *Tuina* has the effect of treating diseases depends on not more than two sources: manipulations and channels.

Channels and collaterals are everywhere in the whole body, internally in the *Zang* and *Fu* organs, externally in the extremities, connecting all the organs and tissues throughout the body such as *Zang*, *Fu*, orifices, skin, tendons, muscles, skeleton, etc. *Qi* and blood circulating in the channels and collaterals supply nutrients and transmit messages from the interior to the exterior and vice versa. In this way, a whole stereoscopic regulating and controlling system is formed. While performing *Tuina*, the physician concentrates his mind, regulates his breath evenly and gets the "*Qi* and power" of all his body moving to the operating hands. The hands are kept close to the power—bearing point on the operated part and manipulated on the channels and points of the superficies of the body with a certain standardized movement. Thus, the stimulating messages due to the "specific power—pattern" consisting of the quantity, frequency, periodicity, rhythm and direction of the manipulation's force will activate the peculiar function of the channels and their corresponding points. This function is delivered progressively and wavedly to the different layers of the body tissues in the direction of points→ superficial channels and collaterals→internal channels and collaterals→internal organs, so that the whole system of channels and collaterals and the whole system of internal organs enter an activated state in which they function most in self—regulating and self—controlling. That's why *Tuina* may take a therapeutic role in balancing *Yin* and *Yang*, restoring *Qi*, removing excess, regulating *Ying* and *Wei*, smoothing the channels and collaterals, promoting the circulation of *Qi* and blood, coordinating the *Zang* and *Fu* organs, relieving inflammation, stopping pain, lubricating the joints, etc.

In addition, *Tuina* functions in treating local disorders of soft tissues of the human body. For instance, when disorders due to trauma such as dystopia and displacement of muscle and tendon, subluxation of joint, prolapse of nucleus pulposus of lumbar intervertebral disc, narrowed interspace of lumbar vertebrae, disorder of posterior joints of lumbar vertebrae or incarceration of the synovium are treated, different corresponding *Tuina* maneuvers for strengthening the body by regulating the flow of *Qi* and blood or for treating the injured muscles and tendons by activating the channels and collaterals, such as *Yao* (rotating), *Ban* (pulling), *Ba Shen Qian Yin* (traction by pulling and extending), etc., may be used to correct the anatomic abnormalities and restore the function of the injured soft tissues and tendons.

5 Brief Introduction to the Modern Researches in *Tuina* Manipulations

As we have said in the above, "manipulation" is one of the reasons for *Tuina*'s working. And it is necessary to study it. For the purpose of getting the true information of dynamic force of manipulation, exploring the causality between a manipulation and the force it produces, and disclosing the principles and effects of the maneuvers of *Tuina* manipulation, we developed the "TDL−I Analyzer For Determining The Dynamic Force of *Tuina* Manipulation" (See Fig.1)and combined it with a corresponding secondary meter into the "Measuring And Recording System Of The Mechanical Information Of *Tuina* Manipulation" (See Fig. 2) in 1981, and another instrument called as "Computer−process System Of The Mechanical Information Of *Tuina* Manipulation" (See Fig.3) in 1984. Since then on, we have spent several years carrying out systematic sports biomechamical researches, with those instruments, in the manipulations of the modern famous academic authorities of different *Tuina* schools such as *Yi Zhi Chan Tui Na, Gun Fa Tui Na, Nei Gong Tui Na, Dian Xue Tui Na*, etc., recording a lot of tri−dimensional mechanical waviness−curve−diagrams of *Tuina* manipulations (Fig. 4, 5, 6, 7, 8), doing kinematics and dynamics analysing according to a manipulation and its diagram, and making necessary data processing. By so doing, we get the objective quantitive index of

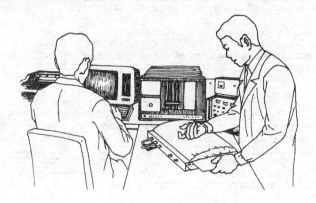

Fig.3

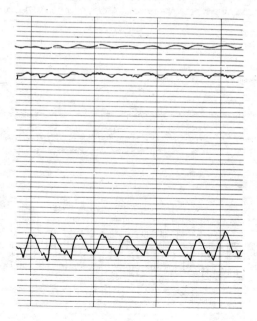

Fig.4

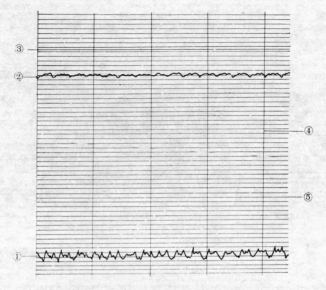

Fig.5

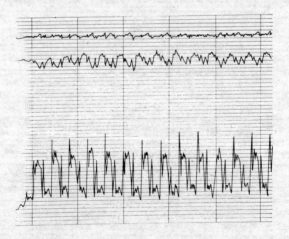

Fig.6

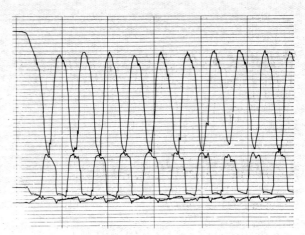

Fig.7

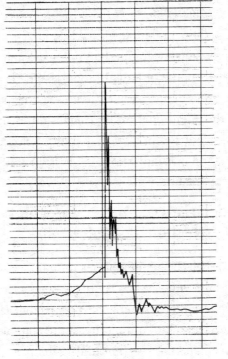

Fig.8

Part One: Adult *Tuina*

1 Brief Introduction to Adult *Tuina*

In ancient times, *Tuina* was not classified as adult and infant ones. Since the Ming Dynasty (1368—1644), however, *Tuina* had developed in treating infantile diseases and a series of *Tuina* therapies mainly suitable for the physiological and pathological characteristics of infants gradually took shape. Then, there appeared infant *Tuina*. Later, adult *Tuina* was advanced to distinguish it from the infant one. Adult *Tuina* is different from infant *Tuina* in manipulation, stimulation quantity, selection of points, therapeutic method and indications. Here is what adult *Tuina* involves in clinical practice.

1.1 Characteristics of Manipulations and Point—selection of Adult *Tuina*

Compared with the manipulations for infant *Tuina,* those for adult *Tuina* of any school, when routinely conducted, are characterized by having larger strength—bearing region, larger motion range and larger stimulation quantity, more suitable for the application on the superficies of an adult's body such as on the points, the routes of the fourteen channels and certain parts of the trunk or extremities. With smaller stimulation quantity, some leading manipulations for infant *Tuina*, such as *Xuan Tui Fa*(revolving—pushing) *Zhi Tui Fa* (finger—pushing) and *Yun Fa* (arc —pushing), are usually limited on certain points of the fingers and palms of an infant and seldom used in adult *Tuina*, while manipulations for adult *Tuina* mainly acting on the points of the body may also be used to treat infantile diseases of surgery and medicine as long as their stimulation quantity is properly regulated and controlled.

Adult *Tuina* plays its treating part mainly through its manipulations performed on the points and along the channels of a patient's body. The points to be selected clinically are mainly the ones on the superficial routes of the fourteen regular channels of the trunk and extremities, extrachannel points and non—fixed points. Before a patient is about to be treated, the physician should choose points and manipulations by differentiating the patient's age, sex, constitution and disease condition as well as the manipulated part, put the selected points and manipulations into order according to certain law so as to make up a *Tuina* prescription, and then carry out the practical treatment. As for the law and method for selecting points to make up a prescription, they are the same as those used in acupuncture therapy: selecting local points, nearby points, distant points along the channel, Shu points and Front—Mu points, or principal points and their assistant ones in the same channel, making up a prescription with mother—child reinforcing—reducing method, according to the principle of "midnight—noon ebb—flow" or by selecting the pain points for local treatment.

1.2　Commonly Used Mediums for Adult *Tuina*

Mediums should be added when many *Tuina* manipulations such as *Ca Fa* (rubbing), *Mó Fa* (palm—rubbing), *Ping Tui Fa*(translation—pushing) and *Zhi Tui Fa*(finger—pushing) are conducted in clinical practice. A medium has two kinds of effect. One is to reinforce the effect of manipulations and raise curative effects through the action of the drugs it contains. The other is to lubricate the manipulated skin of a patient, which may not only benefit the performance of manipulations but also protect the skin from being injured.

Nowadays, commonly used mediums for adult *Tuina* consist of various traditional ones and many other ones made with modern techniques and prescriptions. A brief introduction to them is as follows.

1. Talcum Powder

Functioning in lubricating, it is usually used in summer. When manipulations are conducted on the parts where a lot of sweat tends to appear, local application of talcum powder may protect the skin of both the patient and the doctor (See Fig.9).

2. Sesame Oil

When the manipulation of *Ca Fa* (rubbing) is used, small quantity of sesame oil is often applied on the manipulated part so that the skin can be lubricated and the diathermic effect of the manipulation is increased.

3. Ointment of Chinese Holly Leaf

This ointment is made by mixing *Dongqing* oil (methyl salicylate) with vaseline and often used for *Ca Fa* (rubbing) or *Rou An Fa* (kneading—pressing). It can strengthen the diathermic effect of the manipulations and take its drug role in removing wind–dampness, promoting blood circulation and relieving pain (Fig.9).

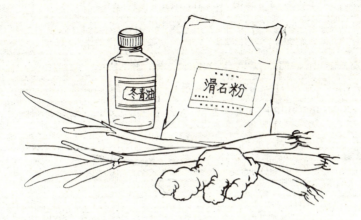

Fig.9

4. Turpentine oil, oil made from *Honghua* (Flos Carthami) and liquid medicine for relieving the rigidity of muscles and activating collaterals may all be applied according to practical condition.

5. Massage Emulsion

Massage Emulsion of Landing Stage Brand is manufactured by Jinan Chemical Plant For Producing Goods of Daily Use. It is a new type of medium for *Tuina* developed with natural perfume oil, extracts of herbal medicines, surface–active agents, etc. Clinical and pharmacological experiments have proved that this massage emulsion applied on the body when the manipulations of *Mó* (palm–rubbing), *Ca* (rubbing) and their like are performed plays its medical and health–protecting part not only in lubricating the skin to prevent it from being injured but also remarkably in promoting blood circulation to stop pain, relieving inflammation to subduing swelling and alleviating fatigue. It was reported that Massage Emulsion had been applied as a medium in *Tuina* to treat 150 cases of acute soft tissue in jury with the curative rate reaching 92%. Compared with the 60 cases in the control group who were treated with mere *Tuina* manipulations, the curative rate was raised by 17% (P < 0.01) with the average treating times 1.9 time fewer (P < 0.01). It is clear that Massage Emulsion is a practical medium (See Fig. 10).

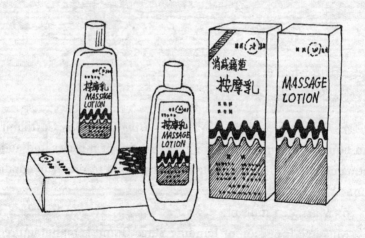

Fig.10

1.3　Points for Clinical Attention in Adult *Tuina*

In *Tuina* clinical practice, to ensure a safe and effective treatment without side effects, to convenience the physician's performance and to provide the patient with better medical service and mental ease are based on the preparation of both the physician and patient before treatment, their coordination during treatment and the essential facilities.

1. Essential Medical Facilities

(1) A commodious and bright consulting room in which there is fresh air, favourable temperature (25°C or so) and convenient water supply.

(2)Clean, tidy, smooth, stable, fixed, not too high and not too low (Reaching the knees of the physician is proper.) beds for *Tuina* medical treatment, around which there are no walls but there is enough space so that the physician can regulate his standing position freely and do his work conveniently.

(3)Get various kinds of commonly used mediums ready and put them where the physician easily reach.

(4)The consulting room should be equipped with different sizes of medical toweling, blanket and soft cushion, which are put beneath or on a patient's body or used for him to lean upon in the course of treatment.

(5)There should be chairs, stools or stools whose height may be adjusted in the consulting room.

(6)One wall of the consulting room should be equipped with several big mirrors whose lower edges are near the floor, in which patients may look themselves when they are doing medical exercise.

2. Points for Physicians' Attention

(1)Before treatment, a physician with warm, affable and sincere attitude should tell the patient in detail what responses are likely to happen while the manipulations are conducted and how he must cooperate. During treatment, the physician should interpret patiently what has happened in order to be trusted by the patient.

(2)A physician should often trim his fingernails, take good care of his hands so as to keep their skin soft and smooth, and remove the ring and the like from the hands before treatment lest the skin of the patient be injured.

(3)While he manipulates, the physician should concentrate his mind, observe attentively the facial expressions and responses of the patient, and experience carefully the feeling of the hands. Once something abnormal is found, timely proper measure should be taken.

(4)According to the disease condition, constitution, age, sex and manipulated part of a patient, the physician should choose an appropriate posture to see that the patient feels comfortable, the performance of manipulations is convenient, and the manipulated part is fully exposed.

(5)While carrying out the manipulations, a physician should always pay attention to coordinating his own movements; bringing his will, breathing and maneuvers into line. Even when sudden exertion of strength is needed, prolonged holding back or controlling breath for managing it is not suggested lest self—injuries occur such as pain in the chest when breathing, chest pain, chest oppressed feeling and overstrain or sprain of the tendons of the joints of the hands.

(6)Be sure to have the manipulated part fully exposed when manipulations such as *Ping Tui* (translation- pushing), *Ca* (rubbing), etc. are carried out directly on the skin of a patient, and to smooth the patient's local dress or the toweling covered on the patient when manipulations such as *Yi Zhi Chan Tui Fa* (one—thumb—operating), *Gun Fa* (rolling), etc. are carried out indirectly on the skin, that is, over the local dress or toweling on the skin. Or else, the maneuvers of the manipulations may not be done freely so that the curative effects will be lowered.

(7)It is better to conduct such therapies as acupuncture, hot compress and infra-red radiation after the *Tuina* one. *Tuina* therapy should be carried out 2 hours after any of the above therapies has been done.

(8)In the course of manipulating, the stimulation quantity and the passive motor scope should be adjusted to the extent that smaller, certain stimulation value needed has been reached; larger, not only the patient can endure but also the human structure, the pathological conditions and the physiological function can stand. Violent manipulating will bring manipulative injuries to patients. For example, over rubbing, pressing, digital-pressing and kneading will break the skin, causing ecchymosis; violent hitting, beating, tapping and pressing will lead to fracture and injury of the internal organs; over pulling, rotating and traction will result in laceration of ligament and subluxation of joint; over manipulating on the spinal column will bring about subluxation of cervical vertebra, intimal laceration of vertebral artery and infarction of cerebellum and brain stem, all of which are severe medical accidents. So, manipulative injuries have to be avoided.

3. Points for Patients' Attention

(1)When treated, trust in the physician, follow his order, get everything ready and cooperate with him closely.

(2)Ask a physician for the treatment not just after strenuous exercise or eating a fill, nor on an empty stomach or in hunger, but one hour later after a meal and after more than ten minutes of rest in the consulting room.

(3)Before treated, go to W.C., take off the coat, remove the belt and tell actively the physician your own health condition such as whether you have exopathy and fever, whether there is rupture, damage or infection on the skin of the manipulated part, and whether you are in menstrul or pregnant period if you are a woman.

(4)During treated, calm the mind, relax the whole body, don' t read or go to sleep, and pay attention to the experience of manipulation stimulation and tell the physician your feeling timely.

1.4 Indications of Adult *Tuina*

1. Disorders due to Trauma

Various sprain and contusion, subluxation of joint, stiffneck, cervical spondylopathy, prolapse of lumbar intervertebral disc, posterior articular disturbance of lumbar vertebrae, retrograde spondylitis, superior clunial neuritis, piriformis syndrome, syndrome of the transverse process of the third lumbar vertebra, scapulohumeral periarthritis, subacromial bursitis, external humeral epicondylitis, tenosynovitis stenosans, meniscus injury, systremma, sternocostal shield injury, disturbance of costovertebral joint and functional disturbance of temporognathic joints.

2. Syndromes of Medicine

Epigastralgia, gastroptosis, gastroduodenal ulcer, headache, insomnia, asthma, pulmonary emphysema, cholecystitis, hypertension, angina pectoris, coronary heart disease, diarrhea, constipation, diabetes, gastrointestinal dysfunction, impotence, uroschesis and neurosism.

3. Diseases of Surgery

Acute mastitis in the early stage, bed sore and postoperative intestinal adhesion.

4. Diseases of Gynecology

Dysmenorrhea, amenia, irregular menstruation, pelvic inflammation and puerperal separation of symphysis pubis.

1.5   Contraindications of Adult *Tuina*

1. Acute and chronic communicable diseases such as hepatitis.

2. Infective diseases such as erysipelas, medullitis and suppurative arthritis.

3. Various hemorrhagic diseases such as gastric ulcer in the bleeding period, hematochezia and hematuria.

4. Various malignant tumors, tuberculosis and pyemia.

5. Scald and localized area of ulcerative dermatitis.

6. Bleeding due to trauma.

7. Lumbosacral and abdominal portions of a woman in menstrul or pregnant period.

2 Commonly Used Manipulations for Adult *Tuina*

The way that a physician manipulates various standardized technical maneuvers on the joints, along the channels and over the specific portion of a patient's body surface with his / her hands or other parts of his / her limbs for medical purpose is called "manipulation", which is the main means of *Tuina* to treat diseases. Good curative effects comes from good clinical choice and performance of manipulations.

The ancient and modern medical specialists have created many effective *Tuina* manipulations, more than 110 of which are recorded in written language. However, no more than 20 or 30 of them are commonly used. Each manipulation is undertaken according to its own pattern of standardized technical movements. This pattern is called "make—up of movement", which mainly includes the following respects: the posture of the whole body, breathing, support and coordination of the will, the preparatory gesture of manipulation movement, stage of movement, essentials of movement, the angle and amplitude and frequency and rhythm and periodicity of each movement link, and the work and interrelation of different acting muscles.

The manipulating technique of traditional *Tuina* medicine is basically characterized by permanence, forcefulness, evenness and softness, all of which get together to producea " deep- going" effect. By permanence we mean that a manipulation should be kept performed for a certain required time, that is, within a certain time, the manipulation should remain the same either in its make-up or in its dynamic pattern; by forcefulness, a manipulation can exert a certain power, whose volume should be changed according to the patient's constitution, disease condition and age, and the manipulated part as well, small, it may ensure the requried stimulation volume and large, the patient can stand it; by evenness, a manipulation should be rhythmic with constant frequency and pressure; by softness, a manipulation should be gentle but not superficial, heavy but not sluggish, powerful but not rough or violent, and smooth with its maneuvers changed naturally; by deep-going, a manipulation should be performed with the direction of its acting force properly adjusted so that the effect of the applied dynamic force may go deep into the body and act on the target tissue where the disorder is located, ensuring the therapeutic effect of *Tuina*. Of course, all the above aspects are not isolated but interrelated closely and organically; They are the technical essentials of every maneuver of every kind of *Tuina* manipulation. Guided by them in practice, a manipulation is trained and whether it has been standard is decided. But manipulations are different in the make-up of maneuver, so, they are also different in technique, each having its own emphasis. For instance, the manipulations of *Yi Zhi Chan Tui Fa* (a manipulation operated with one thumb) and *Gun Fa* (rolling) are firm but gentle, with the latter emphasized; *Ji Dian Fa* (digital hitting) is accurate, resolute, rapid, and gentle but firm, with firmness emphasized; *Mó Fa* is slow, gentle or strong, but moderate, with the last emphasized.

In the course of training themselves in manipulating technique, the students should try to learn about the features unique to any manipulation in addition to having a good master of the movement essentials of every one. Only in this way can they master the manipulations to such a high extent that they perform them not only with their hands but also with their minds, and use them with high proficiency while a patient is being clinically treated.

The following is the introduction to 20 commonly used manipulations and the methods for mastering them through training.

Translator's notes: In this book, the terms of manipulations will be expressed with the Chinese phonetic words, for, usually, there don't exist exactly corresponding words or terms in English which may be used to do so. For example, the manipulation of *Gun Fa* has been translated into "rolling", just because the Chinese word *"Gun"* is equal to the English one *"rolling"* in literal meaning. But *Gun Fa* is done with a hand and the hand cannot be rolled or roll. Besides, the word rolling can not infer what *Gun Fa* really means. Foreign readers should keep the terms expressed in the Chinese phonetic words in mind and learn their exact meanings from the "explanations" of the manipulations to be introduced. By so doing, they will never be misled.

As for the English word or expression in the brackets after each Chinese phonetic term, it is used just for elicitation.

2.1 *Yizhichan Tui* **(operate / operating with one thumb)**

Explanation

Put the whorled or lateral surface of the tip of the thumb on the part to be operated with the shoulder relaxed, the elbow dropped and the wrist raised; flex and stretch the elbow joint cyclically and swing the forearm inward and outward so as to bring about the flexion and extension of the thumb joint (See Fig.11). This is called *Yizhichan Tui*.

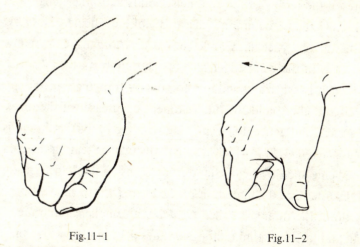

Fig.11—1   Fig.11—2

Essentials

Cup the fist by flexing naturally but not closing tightly the index, middle, ring and little fingers and with the fist hole covered by the thumb. Relax the muscles of the upper limb. Exert acting force naturally and avoid forceful pressure after the thumb is fixed on the operated point. Keep steady the pressure, frequency and amplitude of swing so that the produced force can act on the part being treated rhythmically and continuously. The frequency of this manipulation should be between 120—160 times per minute.

Application

This manipulation is characterized by small force—bearing point, great pressure intensity produced by the acting force, strong deep—going effect, continuous and rhythmic and gentle stimula given to the patient, and stimulation volume possibly regulated according to the needs. It may be performed everywhere on the body, on the channels, points and other parts, and used to treat common diseases of medicine, surgery, traumatology, gynecology and the five sense organs. Concretely, pressing with the whorled surface of the thumb is called *Luowen Tui*, which is especially suitable for the performance on the abdomen and chest, and for the treatment of diseases of the digestive system and gynecology; pressing with the tip of the thumb is called *Zhongfeng Tui*, which is most effective in treating diseases of medicine such as headache, dizziness, insomnia, hypertension and disorder due to stagnation of the liver—*Qi*; pressing with the very tip of the thumb is called *Chanfa* with smaller amplitude of swing and faster rhythm (200—240 times per minute), which may create unique curative effects when used to treat laryngological diseases and surgical carbuncle and furuncle; pressing with the side of the thumb—radius is called *Pianfeng Tui*, which is suitable for the operation on the craniofacial region and often used to treat myopia, rhinorrhea with turbid discharge, stuffy or running nose, headache, distending sensation in the head, tinnitus, facial paralysis, prosopalgia and toothache.

2.2 *Na* (grasp / grasping)

Explanation

The thumb and the two fingers, index and middle or the thumb and the other four fingers exert slow and symmetrical forces to hold and pull, and, meanwhile, twist and knead the treated part, which is then released. This is done again and again (See Fig.12) and called as *Na*.

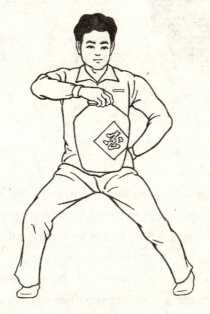

Fig.12-1

Essentials

Stretch each interphalangeal joint of the thumb and the other four fingers and do the work with finger surfaces. Don't flex the fingers lest the treated part be digged and nipped with finger nails. Ensure harmonious and rhythmical movements of the wrist and phalangeal joints. Add force slowly and gently when pulling until it is strong enough and avoid sudden decrease or increase of the force, and sudden and rapid holding and releasing of the part with voilent force.

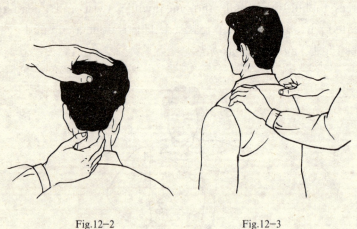

Fig.12—2   Fig.12—3

Application

This manipulation can produce strong stimulation which will make the patient feel remarkedly and strongly sore and distending. It is often applied to the cord—like soft tissues such as muscles and tendons of the neck, shoulder, back, lateral abdomen and limbs. Its effects are as follows: inducing resuscitation and restoring consciousness, relieving superficies syndrome by means of diaphoresis, expelling wind and clearing away cold, relaxing muscles and tendons to promote blood circulation, and relieving spasm and pain. When it is performed in clinical practice, whether one hand or the two hands in involved should be decided on according to the treated part and the disease condition.

2.3 *An* (press / pressing)

Explanation

Press with the finger or palm the operated part vertically, slowly, first gently and superficially and then forcefully and deeply until a certain depth is reached, and take away slowly the finger or palm after the pressing is stopped for a minute or for several times of kneading. Do this repeatedly. Pressing with the thumb is called *Muzhi An;* pressing with the middle finger, *Zhongzhi An;* pressing with the palm, *Zhang An;* pressing with the palm base, *Zhanggen An* (See Fig.13).

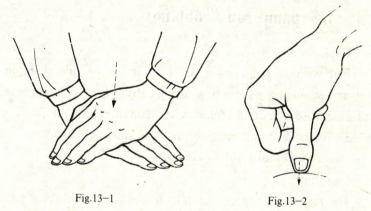

Fig.13—1   Fig.13—2

Essentials

Breathe naturally in the whole course and not hold back breath when emitting force. Exert force steadily, which is small at the beginning, and add it gradually until the patient has got such sensations as soreness, distension, numbness and radiation. Spend 5—10 seconds or so pressing one time. When more powerful and repeated operations are needed, the best way to save strength and achieve better effect is as follows: stretch straight the two arms, put one thumb or one palm on the other and press the operated part one time after another, each time your body inclines a little forward as if you are supporting it on the operated part with your arms so that your body weight can be utilized instead of the force exerted actively by the fingers or arms.

Application

This is a munipulation whose stimulation should be changed from mild degree to moderate one. It should be carried out until the patient has got the above—mentioned sensations. Pressing with the fingers may be conducted on the points of all parts of the body, while pressing with the palm, on the loins, back and abdomen.

2.4 *Mó* (palm—rub / rubbing)

Explanation

Rub with the palm or the palmar sides of the index, middle, ring and small fingers the treated part rhythmically, in a circle, and clockwise or counter—clockwise. Rubbing with the palm is called *Zhang Mó*, while rubbing with the surface of the four fingers (exept the thumb), *Zhi Mó* (Fig.14).

Essentials

The rubbing is carried out in a circle, the acting force is gentle and mild, and the frequency is steady and moderate, usually being 100—200 times or so per minute.

Application

As one of the commonly used manipulations of *Tuina*, this manipulation is mainly applicable to the chest, hypochondrium, epigastrium and abdomen. Because of its following effects:

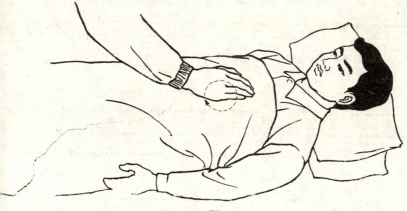

Fig.14-1

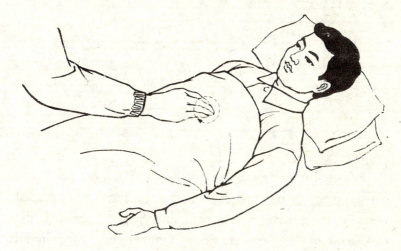

Fig.14-2

relieving the depressed liver and promoting the flow of *Qi*, warming up the middle—*Jiao* to normalize the function of the stomach, removing retained food, and regulating gastrointestinal peristalsis, it is often used to treat epigastric and abdominal pain, distension due to stagnant food, choking sensation in the chest due to stagnation of *Qi,* and impairment of the chest and hypochondrium.

2.5 *Rou* (knead / kneading)

Explanation

Knead the treated part gently, slowly and rotatedly with the fingers, palm base, major thenar and so on. This is called *Rou,* which is subdivided as follows: kneading with the middle finger is called *Zhongzhi Rou;* kneading with the thumb, *Muzhi Rou;* kneading with the palm base, *Zhanggen Rou;* kneading with the major thenar, *Dayuji Rou;* kneading with the elbow, *Zhou Rou* (See Fig.15).

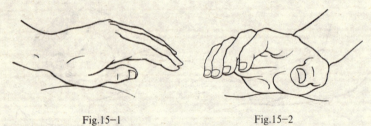

Fig.15—1   Fig.15—2

Essentials

Put the force—exerting part such as a finger, the palm base and so on tightly on the treated part to make its skin kneaded rotatedly in a small circle with the help of coordinating movements of the shoulder, elbow, forearm and wrist joint so that gentle and slow internal friction is caused between the skin and the soft tissue beneath it. It is emphasized that the kneading is gentle, the circle becomes larger gradually, the force grows step by step, and the operating part is fixed on the treated part lest friction and slipping occur between the operating part and the skin of the treated part. It is proper that the kneading frequency is kept within 100—140 times per minute.

Application

Being a commonly used manipulation in clinical pratice, *Rou* may be undertaken all over the body. By and large, *Dayuji Rou* is applicable to the craniofacial area, the thoracica—abdominal region and the local parts of the joints of the limbs, which are swelling and painful due to acute sprain; *Zhanggen Rou*, to the back, loins, buttock and thick muscles of the limbs; *Zhi Rou*, to the channels and points all over the body and the area where digital stimulation is needed; *Zhou Rou*, to the deep layer of tissue. This manipulation has such effects as soothing the oppressed chest, regulating the flow of *Qi*, strengthening the spleen, normalizing the function of the stomach, promoting blood circulation, removing blood stasis, relieving swelling, stopping pain and tranquilizing the mind, and it is often used to treat headache, vertigo, facial paralysis, distending pain in the epigastric and abdominal region, choking sensation in the chest, hypochondriac pain, constipation, diarrhea and swelling and pain of soft tissue due to trauma.

2.6 *Dian* (digital—press / pressing)

Explanation

Pressing more forcefully and vertically the operated part with the very tip of the thumb or the middle finger or with the flexed, protruded and proximal interphalangeal joint of the middle or index finger or the thumb is called *Dian*. Pressing with the tip of the middle finger is called *Zhongzhi Dian;* with the tip of the thumb, *Muzhi Dian;* with interphalangeal joint, *Zhijie Dian*

(Fig.16)

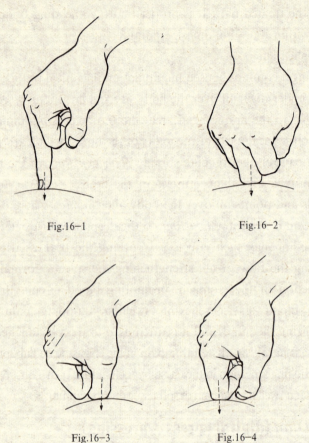

Fig.16—1

Fig.16—2

Fig.16—3

Fig.16—4

Essentials

Breathe naturally and avoid holding back breath when pressing. Add heavy and deep-going force after the light and superficially—going one while exerting force. The force exerted should be strong enough to make the patient have stronger required sensations but it should be within the range that the patient can receive. Over—force is inhibited lest ecchymoma occur or unbearable sufferings be brought to the patient.

Application

Dian is a digital—striking manipulation with strong stimulation, which is commonly used in clinical practice. Its acting points are small and concentrating, its effect is deep—going like what is induced by acupuncture. So, it is often used to strike the mass or pressure pain point which is deep in the muscles or between the bones so as to make the patient strongly feel sore, numb, distending and painful, thus stopping pain by the induced pain. This manipulation is usually applied to the treatment of epigastric and abdominal pain due to spasm, pain of the limbs due to pertinacious stagnation of *Qi* and blood or old injury, and numbness and paralysis.

2.7　*Ca* (rub / rubbing)

Explanation

Rub the treated part to and fro in a straight direction with the palm, minor thenar or major thenar. Rubbing with the palm is called *Zhang Ca;* with the minor thenar, *Xiaoyuji Ca;* with the major thenar, *Dayuji Ca*(Fig.17).

Essentials

Ca requires a large amplitude, a distance as long as possible and a straight direction no matter how it may be done on the surface of the body: straight upward and downward, across from left to right, or obliquely. In addition, the operating hand should be kept closely touching the skin of the operated part, the acting force should be always even along the whole trail of *Ca*. Meanwhile, the force should be moderate, for rubbing with hard pressure tends to injure the skin.

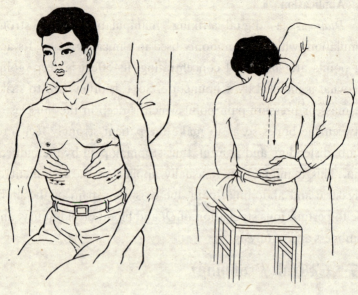

Fig.17-1   Fig.17-2

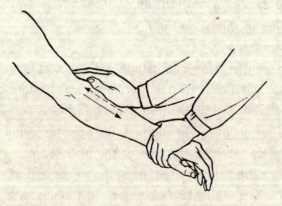

Fig.17-3

Application

Ca and Mó are the same in rubbing but they are different in the following: the former is done in a straight direction, while the latter, in a circle, and the former is more powerful and produces more warming effect than the latter. Clinically, the more powerful and warming effect of Ca contributes to the following curative effects: warming the channels and alleviating pain, expelling wind and dispelling cold, relieving swelling and resolving mass, regulating the flow of Qi and promoting blood circulation. When the practical performance is clinically conducted, attention should be paid to the following: full exposure of the operated part, 1–2 times of gentle and slower rubbing at the beginning followed by more rapid ones which are carried out until local heat occurs. In general, ten times of rubbing are enough for each time of performance and prolonged performance is not advocated lest blisters occur on the skin due to the induced over–heat. In order to protect the skin from being hurt and to help produce heat, medium, such as sesame oil, ointment of Chinese Holly Leaf or massage emulsion, is usually used while this manipulation is being performed.

2.8 *Gun* (roll / rolling)

Explanation

Rotate the forearm outward and inward cyclically to lead to the flexion and extension of the wrist joint, so that the $\frac{1}{3} - \frac{1}{2}$ area of the slightly arched dorsonulnar is made to roll back and forth to the limit on the treated part. This is what *Gun* means (Fig.18).

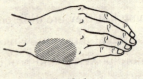

Fig.18-1

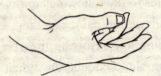

Fig.18-2

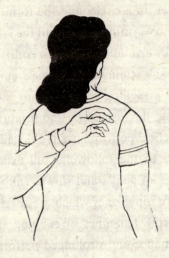

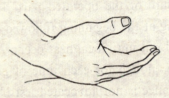

Fig.18-3

Fig.18-4

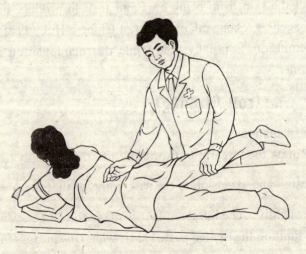

Fig.18-5

Essentials

The hand should be closely attached to the skin of the treated part for fear that rubbing and sliding occur. The pressure should be even, gentle and constant and too powerful push is avoided. The maneuver is done like this: the forearm is kept between prone 45 degrees and supine 45 degrees; the wrist joint, between 45 degrees when flexed and 10 degrees when stretched; the hand, naturally flexed without any active closing and extending; the shoulder relaxed and naturally dropped; the shoulder joint, in the posture of 30 ° —40 ° anteflexion and about 30 ° abduction; the elbow joint, 90 ° —120 ° flexed naturally; the frequency between 140 to 160 times per minute.

Application

This manipulation can involve larger area, produce powerful acting force and result in evident deep—going effect. Except the craniofacial, anterior—cervical and thoracico—abdominal regions, it can be applied on all parts of the body, especially on the loins, the back, the buttock and the areas of the limbs where there are rich and thick muscles. If the area of the second, third, fourth and fifth metacarpophalangeal joints is made to act on the treated part through regulating the posture of the hand, greater stimulation quantity will be produced. *Gun* has the following effects: relaxing muscles and tendons and activating collaterals, expelling wind and dispersing cold, warming channels and removing dampness, promoting blood circulation to dispel blood stasis, relieving spasm and stopping pain, weakening adhesion, and lubricating joints. As one of the most—often used manipulations in clinical practice, it is especially suitable for the treatment of the disorders of the motor and nerve systems.

2.9 *Zhen* (vibrate / vibrating)

Explanation

The tip of the middle finger or the palm is put on the treated part. The extensor and flexor muscles of the forearm are made to contract alternately, rapidly and in a minor range so that gentle and constant vibration is led to. The vibration acts on the body through the tip of the middle finger or the palm on the treated part, and this is called *Zhen*(Fig.19).

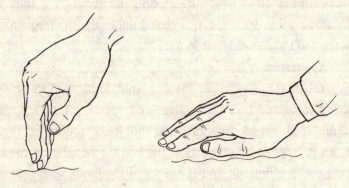

Fig.19−1　　　　　　　　Fig.19−2

Essentials

Active forceful pressing on the treated part is not allowed. The contraction of the muscles of the forearm causes the hand to produce vertical vibration. The frequency of the vibration is between 8−12 times per second. See to it that the vibration is produced by the force, the force is directed by *Qi,* the *Qi* is guided by the mind, and the whole process of the maneuver is natural, consistent, harmonious and integrate. To do so, the physician has to concentrate his mind, lead his *Qi* down to Dantian, regulate his breath even, and, then, get, by way of the mind, the *Qi* going along the inside of the palm to the point of Laogong at the center of the palm or to the tip of the middle finger so that it may direct the force there. Forcing the breath to be held back for the exertion of force is strictly prohibited.

Application

Suitable for the application to all parts of the body, especially to the craniofacial and thoracico—abdominal regions, this manipulation may bring about such effects as tranquilizing the mind, improving eyesight, strengthening intelligence, warming up the middle—*Jiao*, regulating the flow of *Qi*, promoting digestion, and adjusting enterogastric peristalsis. So, better curative effects will be achieved when it is used to treat insomnia, amnesia, gastrointestinal dysfunction, etc.

2.10 *Cuo* (do / doing foulage)

Explanation

Hold and then twist and rub the treated part of the body back and forth rapidly with the two palms, which move upward and downward again and again at the same time. This is called *Cuo* (Fig.20).

Essentials

The physician half—squats with his upper body inclining a little forward. The forces exerted by the two palms are symmetrical. The twisting movements are rapid and their amplitudes are even. The up—down moving of the palms is steady and slightly slow.

Application

As one of the commonly used auxiliary manipulations, *Cuo* is often performed over the upper limb, the hypochondriac region, the loins or the lower limb before a treatment is ended. Its effects are as follows: regulating blood and *Qi*, restoring joints and tendons, and relaxing muscles.

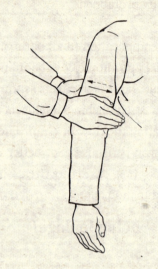

Fig.20—1

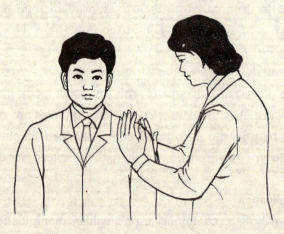

Fig.20—2

2.11 *Mǒ* (wipe / wiping)

Explanation

Rub the treated part in a straight direction, gently, vertically or horizontally, and repeatedly with one or two thumbs, whose surface is closely attacked to the skin of the treated part in the course of rubbing. This is called *Mǒ* (Fig.21).

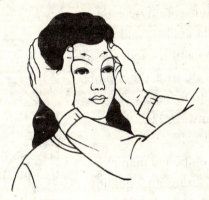

Fig. 21

Essentials

The force exerted should be moderate, for over force will block the movement, but less force will make the movement superficial. The frequency should be even. When rubbing is done along the same vertical straight line, the two thumbs work alternately, while when rubbing is done horizontally, the two thumbs work at the same time. Talcum powder may be used as a medium in summer when sweating tends to occur.

Application

This manipulation is often applied to the craniofacial and cervical regions. It is usually used as the main or an auxiliary manipulation when dizziness, headache, facial paralysis, prosopalgia, and stiffness and pain of the nape are treated. It can play a part in inducing resuscitation, tranquilizing the mind, restoring consciousness, improving eyesight, relaxing muscles and tendons, and promoting blood circulation.

2.12 *Tina* (lift–grasp / grasping)

Explanation

The tendons or muscle bundles of a patient are held and lifted with the thumb and the index and middle fingers or with the thumb and the other four fingers. This is what *Tina* means(Fig.22).

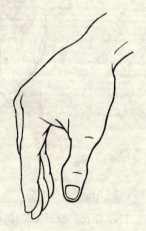

Essentials

This is a compound manipulation in which lifting and holding are combined. Its essentials are the same as *Na'* s in addition to its more powerful lifting.

Application

Fig 22–1

This manipulation will produce stronger stimulation and has the effect of exciting nerves, activating *Yang–Qi,* removing stagnation, expelling wind and dispersing cold. Evident curative effect can be attained when it is used to treat myophagism, nerve paralysis, stubborn arthralgia due to wind–dampness and hemiparalysis.

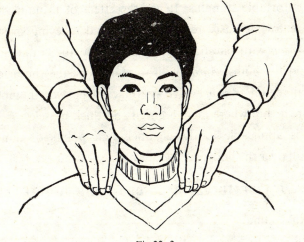

Fig.22—2

2.13 *Anrou*(press—knead / kneading)

Explanation

Kneading is added as pressing is being done, which is called *Anrou*.

Essentials

The manipulations of *An* and *Rou* are combined into this one, whose essentials are those of the above two. The one with three fingers such as the index, middle and ring fingers is called *Sanzhi Anrou*. The one with the two thumbs, one is pressed on the other which has been put on the point and they both exert force together, is called *Shuangzhi Anrou,* which is used when hard pressure is needed on the point. Usually, the thumb, the middle and index fingers are involved when *Sanzhi Anrou* is done.

Application

Having forcefulness and gentleness combined together, this

manipulation can produce a kind of heavy and forceful but gentle and comfortable stimulus. It has the effect of tranquilizing the mind, removing stasis, resolving mass, and relieving spasm and pain. *Anrou* with one finger is applicable to the craniofacial region and the limbs; *Anrou* with three fingers, the thoracico—abdominal region; *Anrou* with two fingers (the two thumbs), the loins or the hip where there are rich and thick muscles. After all, *Anrou* is applicable to the channels and points or non—fixed points all over the body.

2.14 *Boyun* (forearm—knead / kneading)

Explanation

Rubbing or kneading the treated part with the region of the forearm where is located the belly of the upper 1 / 3 ulnar flexor muscle is called *Boyun* (Fig.23).

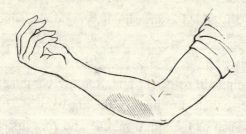

Fig.23—1

Essentials

1. Preparatory Posture: usually sit with the shoulder relaxed (not lifted), extend the upper arm naturally forward with the elbow flexed about 90° —100°, keep the forearm fully in the pronator position with the palm downwards and the fingers free.

2. Performance: Rhythmic extending and flexing movement

within 90 ° −160 ° is done with the elbow joint in order that rubbing and kneading effect may occur on the treated part. While performing, the physician should sit upright with his upper body inclined a little forward, but be sure not to incline the whole upper body too much lest the movement is blocked.

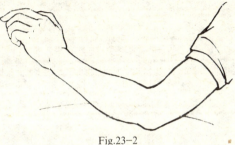

Fig.23−2

Application

The acting surface of this manipulation is larger than that of rubbing with fingers or palm and the pressure of it is larger, too. That's why it is applicable to the loins, back, hip, thigh, other treated parts where large surface needs rubbing or kneading, and the abdominal region as well. Better curative effects will be obtained when it used to treat sprain, contusion, lumbar intervertebral disc and sciatica.

2.15 *Ji* (beat / beating)

Explanation

Beating the treated part rhythmically with the back of a fist, the palmar base, the palm, the minor thenar, the tip of a finger or a mulberry stick is called *Ji* (Fig.24).

Essentials

1. Beating with a fist: Cup the fist, extend the wrist joint straight, and beat the body surface with the back of the fist.

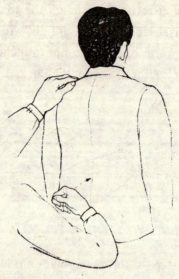

Fig.24—1

2. Beating with a palm: Flex the fingers naturally, extend the wrist joint straight or a little backwards, and tap the treated part with the palm or palmar base.

3. Beating with the minor thenar (also called lateral beating or cutting beating): Extend the hand, palm and wrist joint straight with the thumb naturally abducted and the other four fingers closed, get the forearm and palm upright and beat the treated part rhythmically with the ulnar surface of the minor thenar. The two hands may be used alternately.

4. Beating with the fingers (also called digital beating or tapping): beat the points on the body surface with the tip of the middle finger, the tips of the thumb and the index and middle fingers or the closed tips of the five fingers.

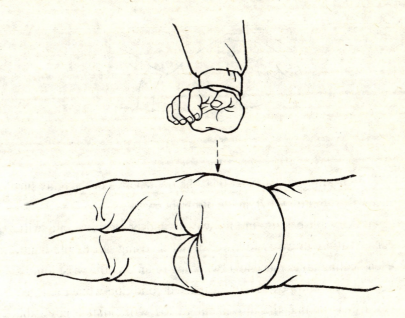

Fig.24-2

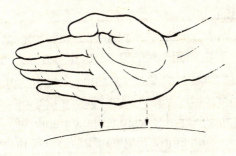

Fig.24-3

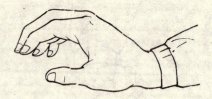

Fig.24—4

5. Beating with a stick: Beat the treated area of the body surface with a treating stick made of mulberry twigs.

All in all, beating in any way should be decisive and swift, each beating—down is followed by each rising—up of the hand, each beating takes place in a twinkling of an eye, the wrist joint is kept in a certain posture and a relaxed condition while the lifted forearm is falling, the movement of the wrist joint follows the beating in order that the force exerted is elastic but not stiff, and to see that beating won't cause any pain.

Application

Beating with the back of a fist is usually applied to the point of Dazhui and the lumbosacral portion; beating with the palm, the anterior fontanelle of the vertex and the point of Baihui; beating with the minor thenar, the lumbodorsal region and the limbs; beating with finger tip, the channels and points of the head, face, chest, abdomen and limbs; beating with a stick, the vertex, shoulder, back, lumbosacral portion and limbs. Due to its following effects: relaxing the tendons and dredging the collaterals, promoting blood circulation to remove blood stasis, and regulating *Qi* and blood, this manipulation can play an evident part in treating arthralgia due to wind and dampness, numbness, muscular spasm, paralysis and myophagism.

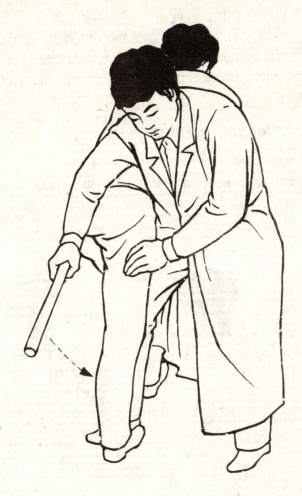

Fig.24–5

Process of Making Mulberry Stick
Strip the peel of each of the twelve pieces of fresh mulberry

twig each of which is about 0.5 cm thick and dry them in the air, roll with mulberry paper and coil with thread each of the dried twigs tightly, put the twelve pieces together and roll them again with mulberry paper round and round into a stick which is coiled with thread and wrapped with a piece of cloth, finally sew the cloth well and the process is over. This stick, 4.5–5 cm in diameter and about 40 cm long, should be moderate in hardness and elasticity.

2.16 *Pai*(pat / patting)

Explanation

Patting the body surface with a hollow palm is called *Pai* (Fig.25)

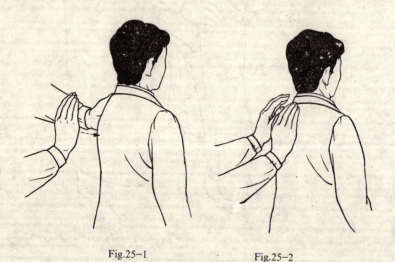

Fig.25–1   Fig.25–2

Essentials

Extend the five naturally-closed fingers with the 2nd, 3rd,

4th and 5th metacarpophalangeal joints a little bent so as to get a concave palm which is called "hollow palm". Pat the treated part with the hollow palm. In doing so, the movement of the wrist joint follows that of the forearm so that the force exerted can be elastic and skillful.

Application

This manipulation is mainly suitable for the performance on the shoulder, back, lumbosacral portion and thigh. Light patting may be conducted on the thoracico—abdominal region. Strong patting lasting a long time may produce the effects of tranquilizing to relieve pain, promoting blood circulation to remove blood stasis, alleviating spasm, and strengthening the body, while light patting lasting a short time, clearing away heat to benefit the mind, exciting the nerves, regulating the intestines and stomach, and soothing the chest oppression and activating the flow of *Qi*. *Pai* is often used to treat various kinds of arthralgia due to wind and dampness, overstrain due to old damage, blood stasis due to new injury, myophagism, hypoesthesia, enteroparalysis, choking and painful sensation in the chest, and involuntary movement due to wrong exercise of *Qigong*.

2.17 *Dou* (shake / shaking)

Explanation

Holding the distal end of an upper limb or a lower limb of a patient with the two hands and shaking it up and down, forcefully, constantly and within a small amplitude is called *Dou* (Fig.26).

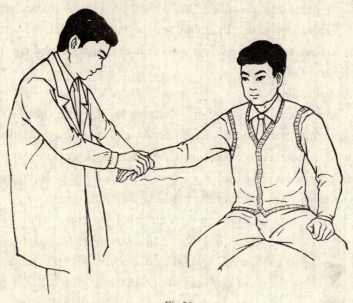

Fig.26

Essentials

Half—squat with the upper body inclined a little forward, stretch the two upper limbs forward naturally with the elbow 130°—160° flexed, hold the wrist or ankle with the two hands and pull the operated limb straight, fix the limb in the abducted position of 45°—60° if it is the upper one, raise the limb until a 30° angle is formed between it and the bed if it is the lower one, exert slow force to shake the operated limb up and down, constantly and narrowly. Be sure neither to close the two hands holding the limb too tightly nor to do over—pulling of the limb so that the limb may be kept in a relaxed condition. The amplitude of shaking should vary from small one to large one and the frequency should be rapid.

Application

Mainly applicable to the limbs and often combined with the manipulation of *Cuo*, this manipulation is usually used before a treatment is ended so as to relax the muscles and regulate the flow of *Qi* and blood. It may also be used to shake the waist like this: raise and pulling—shake the two lower limbs of a patient powerfully to cause the produced vibrating effect to reach straight to the waist. *Dou*, also called *Doula*, is often used to treat prolapse of lumbar intervertebral disc with better curative effects. About ten times of doing is needed to shake the limbs and 3—4 times to pulling shake the lumbar vertebrae in each treatment.

2.18 *Yao* (rotate / rotating)

Explanation

Yao is done like this: Hold the proximal end of the treated joint with one hand and the distal end with the other to cause the joint to do passive movement along its motor axis and within its physiological limit, such as flexing and extending forward and backward, flexing laterally left—ward and right—ward or rotating (Fig.27).

Essentials

Generally speaking, the hand holding the upper proximal end of the rotated joint is the fixing one, whose function is to protect the joint from so in answer to the rotating force as to move beyond its physiological limit and to make it certain that the force is transferred to the treated joint, producing curative effect there. The other hand holding the lower distal end of the rotated joint is the acting or main one, whose function is to cause the joint to do passive movement, which depends on the structure of the motor

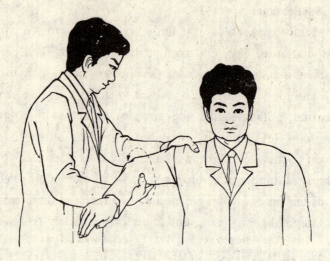

Fig.27-1

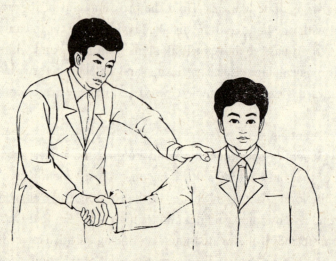

Fig.27-2

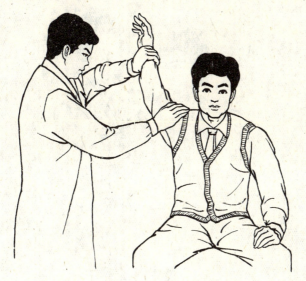

Fig.27—3

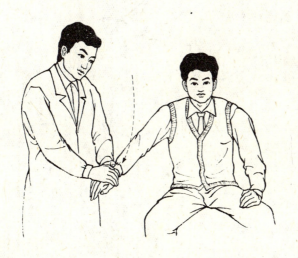

Fig.27—4

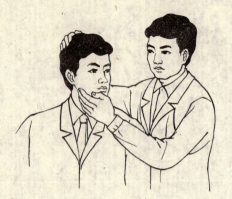

Fig.27—5

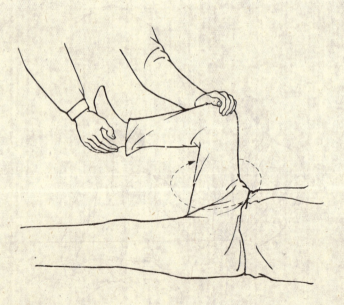

Fig.27—6

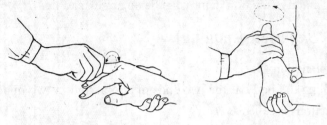

Fig.27-7   Fig.27-8

axis, and is in different direction and amplitude. The above is practised in rotating the joints of shoulder, elbow, wrist, finger, knee and toe and the metacarpophalangeal articulation.

If the rotated joint may be fixed on the bed by the patient's own body weight or by an assistant, the two hands of a physician may be used as the acting ones, which hold the lower distal end of the joint and do rotating. The above is practised in rotating the joints of the wrist, cervical vertebrae and lumbar vertebrae.

In the whole course of rotating, the two hands should work coordinately; the force exerted should be steady and slow, the rotation amplitude should be gradually widened within the physiological limit of the joint. If the rotated joint is in the pathological states such as adhesion, its rotation scope will be remarkedly narrowed. In this case, the rotating of it should begin with the tolerability of the patient. Larger scope of rotating is then followed gradually and haste is stictly forbidden.

Application

Applicable to the joints of the cervical vertebrae, lumbar vertebrae and limbs, this manipulation is the one to cause passive movement of joints. Due to its effect of lubricating joints, releasing adhesion, and improving the function of joint's movement, *Yao* tends to be used to treat ariticular adhesion, stiffness and dysfunction in moving, flexing or extending.

2.19   *Ban* (pull / pulling)

Explanation

Pulling the body at the two ends of a joint and in two opposite directions is called *Ban*.

Essentials

The performance of this manipulation is based on a good command of the features of sports anatomy of the human body such as the structures of various joints and the number, the motion direction, the motion pattern, the motion amplitude and its relevant factors of the motor axises. There is nothing but this command that can lead to correct manipulating position, reasonable maneuver, and effort—saving, safe, painless and effective result. The movement essentials of this manipulation are different due to the difference in the features of sports anatomy of various kinds of joints. The following is the introduction to several ways of *Ban* manipulation.

1. *Ban* Applied to the Neck

(1) Obliquely—pulling of the neck

The patient sits upright with the head about 30 ° inclined forward. The physician props the occiput of the patient with one hand and holds the chin with the other, rotates the head up to the maximum lateral limit (about 45 °) and then does the same in the opposite direction (Fig. 28).

(2) Obliquely—pulling for localizing cervical vertebrae

The patient sits upright with the head 30 ° inclined forward. The physician standing behind the patient does the manipulation like this. His one forearm is used to hold the patient's head, the elbow beneath the patient's chin, the hand on the patient's occiput. The thumb of the other hand is put on the spinous process of the cervical vertebra of the patient which is to be localized, the other four fingers on the patient's shoulder. The elbow exerts strength first to ro tate the head up to the maximum limit (about 45° or so) and then to pull up the cervical vertebra through a rapid rotatedly—pulling action with small amplitude. Meanwhile, the thumb of the other hand exerts strength in the opposite direction to localize the treated vertebra for its reduction (Fig.29).

2. *Ban* Applied to the Chest and Back

(1) Pulling for chest—expansion

This manipulation is the one mainly applied to the sternocostal joints. It is done like this. The patient sits upright with the fingers of the two hands crossed and held on the back of the neck. The physician standing behind the patient holds the two elbows of the patient with his both hands and supports the back of the patient with one of his knees. Then, the patient is asked to throw out his chest and pull his two elbows backwards. The time the patient's active movement has been in the functional position, the physician helps to pull the patient's two elbows backwards with his both hands through a narrow and rapid action, and, meantime, slightly pushes the back of the patient forwards with his knee, thus finishing the pulling for chest—expansion(Fig.30).

(2) Pulling for counterreduction of the thoracic vertebrae

The patient sits upright with his two upper limbs 180° raised. The physician standing behind the patient holds in the front the lower part near the elbow of one of the patient's forearms with Hand A, and presses the affected part of the spine at the back with the thumb of Hand B. Then, the patient is asked to

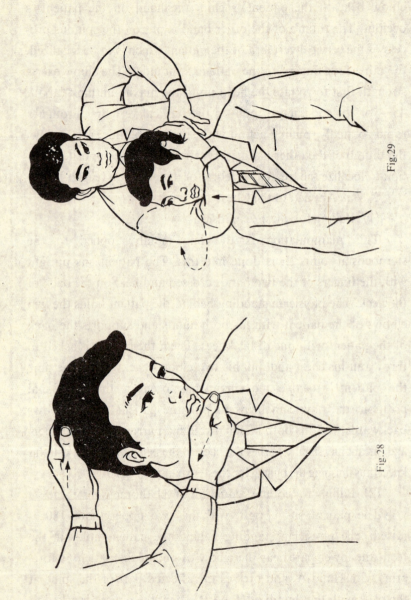

Fig.29

Fig.28

throw out his chest. Following the patient's so doing, the physician pulls the two upper limbs of the patient backwards with Hand A and pushes powerfully the spinous process forwards for its reduction with Hand B (Fig 31).

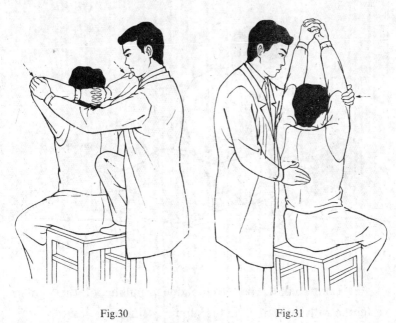

Fig.30   Fig.31

3. *Ban* Applied to the Waist

(1) Obliquely−pulling of the lumbar vertebrae

A. Obliquely−pulling of the lumbar vertebrae with a patient in the lateral recumbent position

The patient lies latericumbently with the leg below extended, the hip and knee of the leg above flexed, the upper arm above put behind the body, and the upper arm below put naturally beside the body. The physician props the scapuloanterior of the patient with Hand A and the hip or the anterior superior spine with

Hand B, and, then, pushes the shoulder with Hand A and pulls the pelvis with Hand B until the lumbar vertebrae are rotated up to the maximum limit, finally, let the two hands exert forces in opposite directions to do a small and rapid pushing—pressing action (Fig.32).

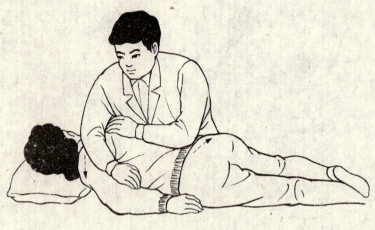

Fig.32

B. Long—handle—pattern obliquely—pulling of the lumbar vertebrae with the patient in the supine position

The patient lies supinely with the right upper limb abducted, the right hip 90 ° flexed, the right knee flexed, the left upper limb put naturally beside the body, and the left leg extended. The physician stands on the left of the patient, presses the scapuloanterior of the patient with his right hand, holds the right knee with his left hand — see Fig.33—1, and, then, does pressing on the scapuloanterior against the bed with his right hand and pulls the right leg leftward with his left hand to rotate the pelvis leftward up to the maximum limit (At this moment, the patient's thigh has been made to be parallel to the bed surface.), finally, push-presses the leg with his left hand which has been on it through a downward, rapid and small action —see Fig.33-2. Pulling right, the physician stands on the right of the patient, all the other being the same as the above except in the opposite direction.

C. Obliquely-pulling of the lumbar vertebrae with a patient in the sitting position

The patient sits upright on a stool with the two legs apart. The physician stands beside one side of the patient, fixes the lower limb of the patient near him with his two legs, props the patient's scapuloposterior near him with one hand, holds the other scapuloanterior of the patient from under the axillary region with the other hand, rotates the upper body of the patient with the force exerted at the same time by his two hands so as to pull up the lumbar vertebrae(Fig.34).

(2) Rotatedly-pulling for reduction of the lumbar vertebrae

The patient sits upright on a stool (Take rotating right for example.). The assistant fixes the patient's left lower limb with his two knees and two hands. The physician stands on the right-back side of the patient, puts the thumb of his left hand near the right of the treated spinous process of the lumbar vertebra of the patient, stretches his right arm from under the right armpit of the patient and holds the left side of the patient's neck with the hand, pulls right with efforts the patient's upper body as soon as the patient is asked to have his waist bent forwards up to the maximum limit in order to rotate his lumbar vertebrae right when they are in the anteflexed position, does a small rapid pulling-rotating action with the right hand following

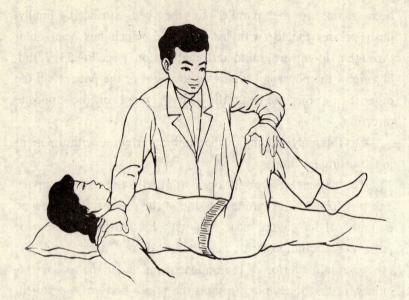

Fig.33—1

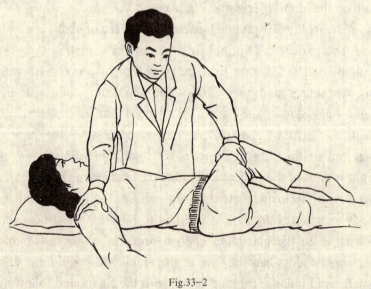

Fig.33—2

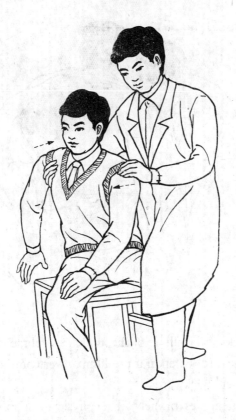

Fig.34

the maximum rotation of the patient's lumbar vertebrae and, meanwhile, push—presses left—upwards the spinous process of the patient's affected lumbar vertebra with the thumb of his left hand, and sets the patient's upper body upright immediately with his right hand as soon as the spinous process feels movable or a crack is heard (Fig.35). The way to rotatedly—pull leftwards is the same as the above except in the opposite direction.

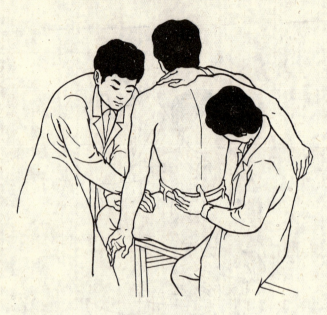

Fig.35—1

(3) Backward—pulling of the lumbar vertebrae

A. Backward—extending the lumbar vertebrae through pulling the two legs backwards

The patient lies pronely. The physician supports the two knees of the patient with Hand A and presses the affected part of the patient's waist with the palm or palm base of Hand B, lifts the knees slowly until the lumbar vertebrae are extended up to the maximum and makes Hand A do a rapid small supporting and lifting action, and, meanwhile, presses forcefully the affected vertebra downwards with Hand B, so that the purpose of pulling up the lumbar vertebrae may be reached (Fig.36).

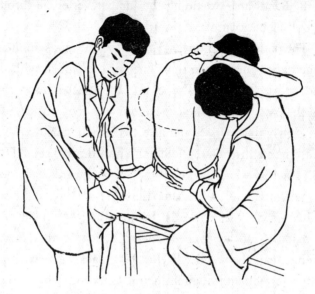

Fig.35-2

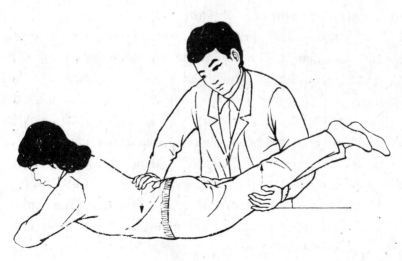

Fig.36

B. Backward—extending the lumbar vertebrae through pulling one leg backwards

The patient lies pronely. The physician stands on the left side of the patient, holds the right knee of the patient with the right hand, presses the spinous process of the affected lumbar vertebra with the palm root of the left hand, raises the right leg of the patient slowly and presses the affected vertebra with efforts afterwards, makes the right hand do an upward rapid small lifting and pulling action when the vertebrae are backwards extended up to the maximum and, at the same time, presses the palm base of the left hand swiftly downwards. In this way, the lumbar vertebrae are made to do an over—extending action so that the affected vertebra can be reduced (Fig.37). Backward—extending the lumbar vertebrae through lifting the left leg may be carried out in the same way.

4. *Ban* Applied to the Shoulder Joint

(1) Pulling the shoulder through abducting

The patient sits upright. The physician squats on the treated side of the patient, with the forearm or elbow of the patient's affected arm on his right shoulder and the above end of the affected shoulder joint pressed with his two hands. The maneuver is done like this. The physician rises slowly so as to abduct the shoulder joint slowly up to the maximum and then stands up abruptly so as to have the shoulder joint 90° abducted. Meanwhile, the shoulder joint is hard pressed downwards and fixed with the two hands. By doing the above, the stress reaches the shoulder joint to remove the articular adhesion and restore the motion function of the shoulder joint (Fig.38).

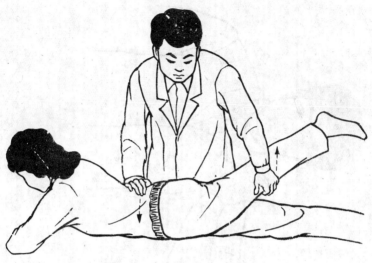

Fig.37

(2) Pulling the shoulder through forward—flexing and back-ward—extending

The patient sitting upright, the physician holds the affected forearm's lower end or the elbow of the patient with Hand A, presses the scapuloposterior with Hand B, and then makes the affected limb slowly flexed forward or extended backward. When the flexion or extension is done to the maximum, he pulls up the affected shoulder joint forward or backward with a sudden force exerted by Hand A, and, meanwhile, fixes the shoulder with Hand B which exerts a force against, and in the opposite direction of, the one exerted by Hand A, in order to strengthen the stress having reached the shoulder joint and ensure the curative effects (Fig. 39, 40).

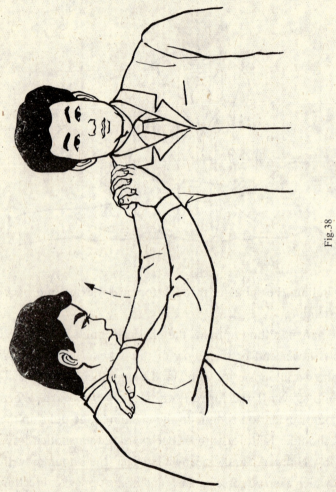

Fig.38

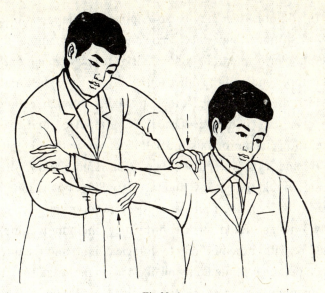

Fig.39—1

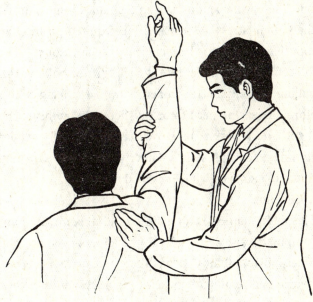

Fig.39—2

In addition, *Ban* may be also applied to the joints of the elbow, wrist, finger, hip, knee, ankle and toe. When any of them is pulled, the principle to be followed is as follows: giving one force to the upper end and the other to the lower one of the joint, both of which are against each other, to make, through pulling, the joint over—extended, over—flexed, over—adducted and over—abducted along its motor axis and within its physiological limit.

By and large, the maneuver of *Ban* manipulation in the beginning should be steady and slow, pulling—up action taking place in the twinkle of an eye must be resolute, rapid and firm, the two hands should work coordinately, the pulling—amplitude should be within the normal physiological limit, and the direction of each pulling is limited only by one chosen motor axis no matter how many motor axises the pulled joint has. When pulling is being done, there will occur a crack in the pulled joint. This is a sign that the pulling stress has reached the required position and the reduction has succeeded. But, clinically, such a sound is not certain to occur to each patient or at each time of pulling. Provided the pulling—amplitude is proper, curative effects will result. Therefore, there is no need to be satisfied only by this sound each time, and it is even more wrong to blindly widen the pulling—range for this sound. Otherwise, unnecessary injury of the joint and ligaments will be resulted in.

Application

This manipulation is applicable to all the moving joints and every amphiarthrosis, especially to the joints of the neck, lumbar vertebrae and four limbs. It has the effect of reducing articular disturbance and semiluxation, releasing adhesion, lubricating the joints, correcting deformity, and restoring the motion function of

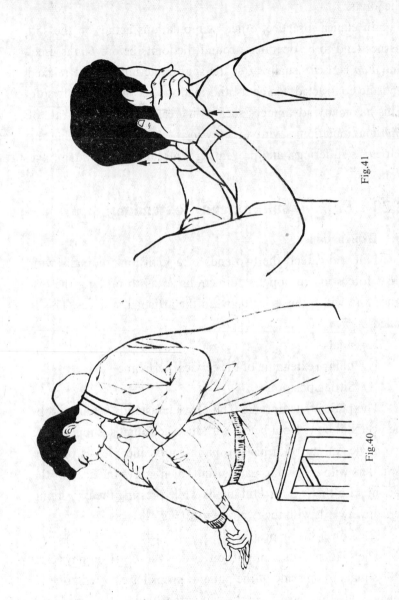

Fig.41

Fig.40

the joints.

In clinical practice, other manipulations acting on the soft tissues tend to be operated around the joints before *Ban* is used, and *Ban* is used usually after the spasmodic muscles are relaxed and the contracted ligaments and tendons become normally soft. This has many advantages such as increasing the success rate of *Ban* manipulation, saving the physician's efforts, decreasing the patient's sufferings, and preventing injury due to *Ban* manipulation.

2.20 *Bashen* (pull—extend / extending)

Explanation

Pull and extend the two ends of a joint longitudinally with great forces in the opposite directions so as to prolong the distance and widen the space between the articular surfaces. This is called *Bashen*.

Essentials

1. Pulling—extending of the cervical vertebrae

(1) Sitting position

The patient sits upright. The physician stands behind, props the occipital bone from below with his two thumbs, supports the two angles of jaw with his two palm roots, and presses the two shoulders with his two forearms, and, then, raises the head of the patient with the two forceful hands while pressing the two shoulders downwards with the two forearms(Fig.41).

(2) Lower sitting position

The patient sits upright on a low stool. The physician half—squats to one side of the patient, props his chin with one elbow, holds his head tightly with the upper arm and the forearm,and supports his occiput with the other hand (Fig.42−1). Then, the physician stretches his upper body straight, holds the patient's head tightly in his arms, orders the patient to relax his whole body, and lifts the patient's upper body away from the stool by changing the half−squatting position into the standing one, thus taking the advantage of the patient's own body weight to fulfil the traction of his cervical vertebrae (Fig.42−2).

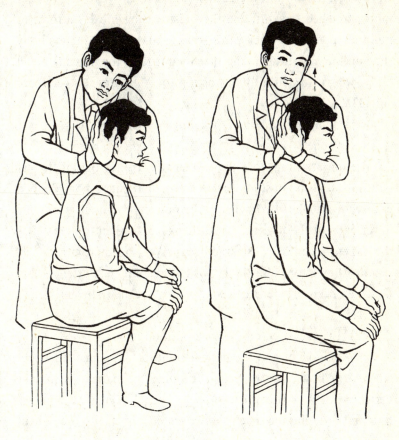

Fig.42−1   Fig.42−2

(3) Supine position

The patient lies supinely without a pillow under the head. The physician sits before the patient's head with the two feet on the floor, the two knees against the two legs of the bed, the upper body inclined a little forward, the spine extended straight, the left hand beneath the occiput of the patient, and the right hand grasping the patient's chin. Then, the physician has the two hands work together to hold the patient's head tightly, the two upper limbs stretched straight, and the waist and back exert a force to pull the upper body backwards so as to make the patient's body slide on the bed, thus taking the advantage of the patient's own body weight to fulfil the traction of the cervical vertebrae (Fig.43).

2. Pulling—extending of the lumbar vertebrae

(1) Prone position

Let an assistant hold the two subaxillary regions of the patient in the prone position (or, order the patient to hold the bed edge with his / her two hands.), the physician himself grasps the lower ends of the patient's two shanks, and, then, pull—extends the patient's lumbar vertebrae by working together with the assistant to give forces in the opposite directions just after the patient has been ordered to have a general relaxation or a cough (Fig.44).

(2) Being-carried-on-the-back position

The physician and the patient stand back against back and elbow in elbow. The physician, proping the patient's lumbar vertebrae or lumbosacral portion to be pull—extended with his hips and ordering the patient to have a cough, carries the patient on his back with the patient's feet off the floor by bending his

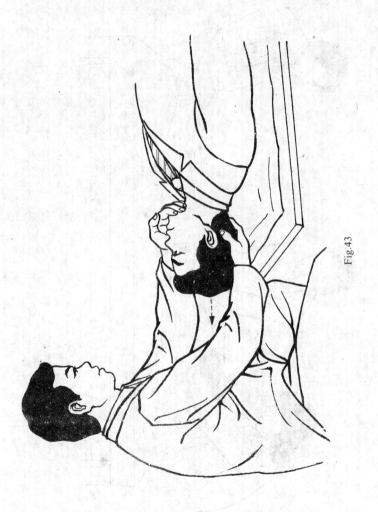

Fig.43

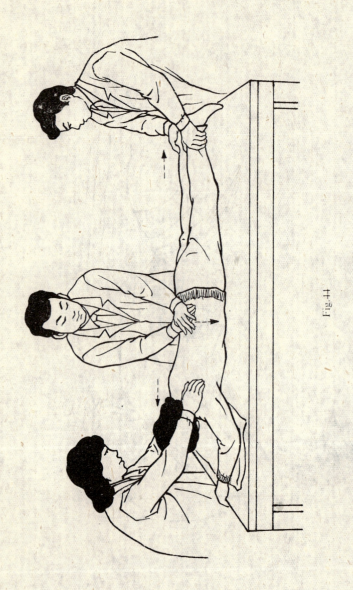

Fig. 44

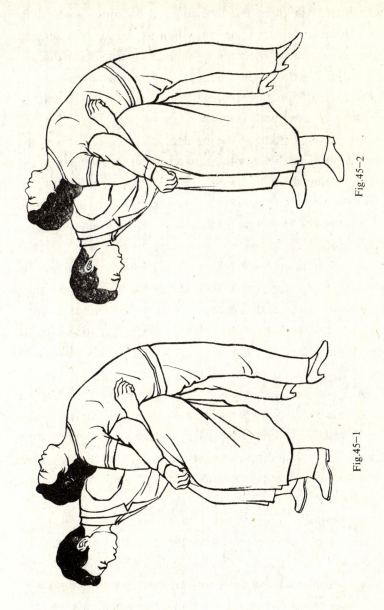

Fig.45-2

Fig.45-1

back, flexing his knees and throwing out his hips just after the cough occurs, and, then, does rhythmical actions of extending knees and throwing out hips to shake or swing the patient's waist, thus having the patient's lumbar vertebrae in backwards—extending position pull—extended by the weight of his / her own lower body (Fig.45).

(3) Pull—extending of the shoulder joint

The physician holds with his two hands the lower part of the forearm of the patient in the sitting position and asks his assistant to fix the patient's body. Then, they both give force in the opposite directions to slowly pull—extend the shoulder joint of the patient (Fig.46).

In addition, pull—extending of such points as the elbow, wrist, finger, hip, knee, ankle and toe may be also done according to the following principle: Holding the proximal end of the joint with one hand and the distal end with the other, the physician pull—extends the joint in the opposite directions so as to widen its space (Fig.47,48).

While *Bashen* manipulation is performed, the force exerted should be even and lasting, the maneuver should be slow and gentle, and voilence is strictly forbidden. As for the direction of the acting force, it should be along the longitudinal axis of the joint. This manipulation must be carefully used if applied to articular deformity and rigidity.

Application

Applicable to the cervical vertebrae, lumbar vertebrae and the joints of the four limbs, this manipulation has the effect of restoring and treating injured soft tissues, reducing dislocated joints, widening joint space, remitting nerve compression, and

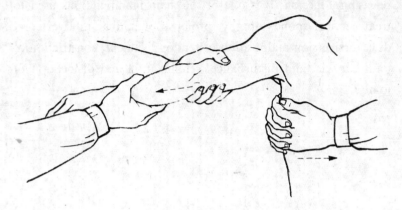

Fig.46

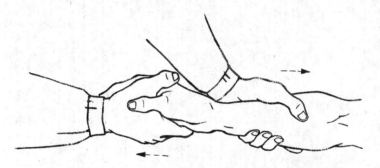

Fig.47

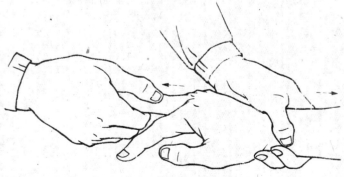

Fig.48

releasing adhesion. It is one of the main manipulations used to treat cervical spondylopathy, prolapse of lumbar intervertebral disc, torsiversion malposition of tendon ligament, constriction of joint capsule, and disturbance, semiluxation and dislocation of joints.

3   Methods and Steps for Training Manipulations

A *Tuina* professional worker should have not only the technical ability to have a good command of the maneuvers of every manipulation but also the ability to carry out everyday arduous task of treatment. These abilities are the specific specialized quality involving both the body and mind that a *Tuina* physician has to possess. This quality can be obtained through doing exercise for *Tuina* training. But more important, it comes from strict practice of manipulations, especially from the practice of those with complex make-up and more difficult skills, such as *Yizhichan Tui, Gun, Mó* and *Zhen,* all of which will be used with high proficiency and made to give curative effects in clinical practice only after the physician has practised them again and again for a long time. That's why the *Tuina* science of TCM has attached great importance to the professional training of manipulations and created and summerized a set of effective training methods in practice. While doing *Tuina* exercise, the beginners have to practise hard, day after day and step by step strictly according to the basic training methods and steps. Only by doing so, can they have the superb techniques of manipulations and all-round specialized quality.

There are three periods in which the basic training of manipulations is conducted. They are practice on a bag filled with rice, practice on the human body and practice through routine performance in treating common diseases. Here is the brief introduction to the training methods and requirements of each period.

3.1 Practice on a Bag Filled with Rice

Except those causing passive movement of joints, all the manipulations need to be practised on a rice bag. Such a bag is made like this: stitch a bag 25 cm long and 16 cm wide, 4 / 5 of which is filled with polished round—grained rice of good quality, which may be replaced with sand washed clean, sew up the bag, coat it with a cloth case whose one end is closed not by sewing up but by tying up with the threads on it so that it may be replaced when dirty. In the beginning, the bag may be tied tight, later on, it may be loosened gradually (Fig.49).

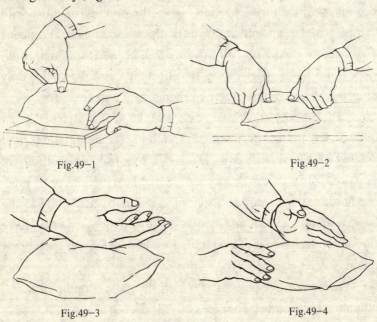

Fig.49—1   Fig.49—2

Fig.49—3   Fig.49—4

The rice bag is put on the table. The student should be in the sitting position if he is going to practise the manipulations of *Yizhichan Tui, Mó, Rou* and *Zhen,* but in the standing position if he is going to practise the manipulation of *Gun.* Then, he does standard and strict training in which great attention is paid to every point from the preparatory posture to movement essentials, including the position of the force—giving point, the angle of every moving joint, the swing amplitude, the frequency, the posture of the whole body, the breathing, and the state of mind as well. The teacher should point out and correct on time the student's wrong maneuver. In the beginning, what is more important is whether the maneuver is correct or not. Before correct maneuvers are mastered, exerting greater force is avoided, for great force from wrong maneuvers will not only keep off the correct ones but also injure the student himself. Only standard maneuvers can lead to "the best mechanical state" of manipulations, and, under this state, the force needed will be produced automatically. Another attention that should be paid to is the alternate practice of the left and right hands.

In addition, in the first period of practice on a rice bag, what is usually practised is the technique of setting operation of every manipulation, that is, the technique of operating in the fixed position. Afterwards, the technique of movable operation is practised. By movable operation is meant that the operating part of the student is moving slowly and straight as the operation is being done to and fro again and again along the longitudinal axis of the rice bag. Practice of these two kinds of techniques may lay a foundation for the future performance on the points and channels of the human body.

Generally speaking, having mastered the standard maneuvers of the main manipulations and highly skilled techniques of operation through practice on the rice bag, the student may start the second period of practice, practice on the human body.

3.2   Practice on the Human Body

The second period of practice on the human body is needed in order to further obtain the technical ability and experience of performing manipulations on the human body and to lay a good foundation for future clinical application. There are two methods for practising manipulations on the human body. One is to practise various manipulations one by one on the selected channels and collaterals and points of the proper parts of the human body. The other is to conduct comprehensive practice of manipulations by grouping many kinds of manipulations applicable to all parts of the body into a routine series of manipulating skills and tricks according to the morphosis of every part of the body, the distribution of the channels, collaterals and points, and certain trails and order.

3.3   Practice through Routine Performance in Treating Common Diseases

What is to be practised in this period is mainly the routine operation of each of the manipulations used in the clinical treatment of various common diseases with *Tuina*. The study of this period can make the student not only have a better command of the manipulations used to treat each common disease, among which there are specific ones for treating specific diseases, but also learn about and have a preliminary master of the rules for selecting points and working out a prescription through differentiation when *Tuina* is used in clinical practice. Therefore, this is a very necessary training period for the student before he really goes to work clinically.

4 The Fourteen Channels and the Commonly Used Acupoints

The Fourteen Channels refers to the twelve regular channels pertaining to the twelve *Zang—Fu,* and the *Ren* Channel and the *Du* Channel of the Eight Extra—channels. The academic content concerning the fourteen channels and the commonly used points is the principal component of all the theories dealing with the channels, collaterals and points. It is the most practical and important basic theory in *Tuina* clinical practice. All the *Tuina* clinical work such as differentiation and diagnosis of diseases, selection of points, composition of prescriptions, choice of manipulations and operation of maneuvers of a manipulation are guided by the theory of channels and collaterals. So, the first thing for a student to do is nothing but knowing the basic content of the fourteen channels and the commonly used points. Otherwise, he will make mistakes now and then.

4.1 An Outline of the Fourteen Channels

1. The Twelve Channels

The twelve channels are the main component of the system of the channels and collaterals. For this reason, they are also called " regular channels ". They respectively belong to the twelve *Zang—Fu.* Each of them connects a *Zang* or *Fu* and is named after the *Zang* or *Fu.* For example, the one connecting the heart is called " the Heart Channel" ; the one connecting the large intestine, " the Large Intestine Channel" . In addition, all the channels belonging to *Zang* are called " *Yin* channel", while those belonging to *Fu*, " *Yang* channel" . Finally, there are also Three *Yin* Channels of Hand, Three *Yin* Channels of Foot, Three *Yang* Channels of Hand and Three *Yang* Channels of Foot; these terms are given according to the distribution of *Yin* and *Yang* channels in the upper and lower limbs.

The regularity for the twelve channels to be distributed on the body surface is as follows. *Yang* channels are mainly distributed on the lateral surface of the upper limb, the lateral surface of the lower limb and the back; *Yin* channels, on the medial surface of the upper limb, the medial surface of the lower limb and the abdominal portion (except that the Stomach Channel of Foot—Yangming crosses the trunk through the ventral surface). The Three *Yin* Channels of Hand start from the chest and run to the hand; the Three *Yang* Channels, from the hand to the head; the Three *Yang* Channels of Foot, from the head down to the foot; the Three *Yin* Channels of Foot, from the foot up to the abdomen.

The twelve channels are connected with each other by their branches (collaterals) so that there appear six pairs of connection relationship among *Zang* and *Fu* and, correspondingly, six pairs of exterior—interior relationship are formed among *Yin* and *Yang* channels. *Yin* channels pertaining to *Zang* but connected with *Fu* and *Yang* channels pertaining to *Fu* but connected with *Zang* are linked together through the Channels of Hand and Foot with the same terms to form the circular system of the twelve channels. This system starts from the Lung Channel, ends at the

Liver Channel and starts again from the Lung Channel, just like a ring in which the *Qi* and blood of the human body circulate endlessly. Here is the diagram showing all the above.

The Lung Channel	The Large Intestine
of Hand – Taiyin (1)	Channel of Hand – Yangming(2)
The Spleen Channel	The Stomach Channel
of Foot – Taiyin(4)	of Foot – Yangming(3)
The Heart Channel	The Small Intestine
of Hand – Shaoyin(5)	Channel of Hand – Taiyang(6)
The Kidney Channel	The Urinary Bladder
of Foot – Shaoyin(8)	Channel of Foot – Taiyang(7)
The Pericardium	The SanJiao
Channel of	Channel of
Hand – Jueyin(9)	Hand – Shaoyang (10)
The Liver Channel	The Gall Bladder Channel
of Foot – Jueyin(12)	of Foot – Shaoyang(11)

Note : " → " shows the connecting order,

" ←-→ " shows the exterior – interior relationship.

Physiologically, the twelve channels mainly function in three aspects; connecting all parts of the body, transporting *Qi* and blood, and regulating the function of the body.

The channels and collaterals, pertaining to *Zang–Fu* internally and going to the extremities externally, closely connect all the tissues and organs of the body, such as the five *Zang*, six *Fu*, limbs, bones, skin, muscles, tendons, and the five sense organs as well, into an organic whole. Implying "route" in Chinese, channels are the main straight passages in the system of the channels and collaterals, while collaterals, having the Chinese meaning of "network", are branches of every kind connecting the channels. They, channels and collaterals, spread crisscross throughout the body, forming a system. In this system, the *Qi* and blood of the body circulate, bringing endlessly various kinds of nutrients to the tissues and organs of all parts of the body so as to maintain the normal physiological function of the human body. Furthermore, owing to the crisscross connection and overall regulation of the channels and collaterals, all parts of the body can work cooperatively and coordinately so that the invasion of pathogenic factors may be resisted and the normal functioning of the organism may be safeguarded.

While the organism is in the state of pathology, the channels and collaterals make the reaction system of symptoms and signs and the transmission route of diseases. Diseases attacking the internal organs may be manifested on the body surface through the channels and collaterals. For example, tenderness, allergic reaction or other pathological manifestations may occur on a specific part of the body surface after some visceral diseases have been brought about. Lumbago due to nephropathy and backache due to gastopathy are such examples. Injuries and disorders of the body surface may also affect step by step the internal tissues and organs at any level through the system of the channels and collaterals. Disease of this organ may lead to disease of that organ, this is still due to the channels and collaterals.

2. The Ren Channel and the Du Channel

The channels of Ren, Du, Chong, Dai, Yangqiao, Yinqiao, Yangwei and Yinwei are called together as the Eight Extra Channels. They are different from the twelve regular channels in that they neither pertain to *Zang—Fu* directly nor have exterior—interior relationship with any other channel. Their main physiological function is to regulate the *Qi* and blood in the twelve regular channels.

The Ren Channel runs along the midline of the abdomen and chest, and upwards to the mandible. On the way, it meets the *Yin* channels of the whole body. That is why it is called "the sea of *Yin* channels". It functions in regulating the *Qi* in all the *Yin* channels.

The Du Channel runs along the midline of the waist, back and nape, and upwards to the cranioface. On the way, it meets the *Yang* channels of the whole body. That is why it is called "the sea of *Yang* channels". It functions in regulating the *Qi* in all the *Yang* channels.

Of the Eight Extra Channels, only the Ren and Du Channels have their own points. All the other six take the points of the regular channels as their own. Because of their features mentioned above, the Ren and Du Channels, together with the twelve regular channels, become one of the bases of Tuina—therapy.

4.2 An Outline of the Acupoints

Locations where *Qi* and blood of the channels and collaterals and of the viscera come in, go out and pool by way of transfusion are called points. They fall into the following three: "channel points" usually called points for short, each of which has a specific name and a specific location on the route of any of the fourteen channels; "extra—ordinary points", each of which has a specific name anda specific location not on the route of any of the fourteen channels; "Ashi points" or "Tianying points", none of which has a specific name or a specific location and each of which is located according to where there is tenderness or other reactions.

All the points, no matter what kind they are included in, are closely related to the channels and collaterals, and by means of the channels and collaterals, they closely connect with the *Zang* and *Fu* organs and the tissues of the whole body. They can not only reflect the physiological and pathological changes of the organs and tissues so as to provide a basis for clinical differentiation, diagnosis, selection of *Tuina* points and composition of *Tuina* prescription, but also serve as the stimulated spots of *Tuina* manipulations. Stimulating the points with manipulations may bring into play the adjusting function of the corresponding channels and collaterals so that the function of *Qi* and blood of the *Zang−Fu* organs can be in turn regulated, the inherent ability of the body to resist diseases can be activated, and the purpose of preventing and treating diseases can be reached.

Whether the positions of the points are identified right or not affects directly the curative effects in clinical practice. To ensure right locations of the points, right methods are needed. Here are several commonly used ones.

1. Proportional Measurements

The width or length of various portions of the human body is divided respectively into definite numbers of equal units each of which is termed as one *Cun*. The method to locate points with this measurement is called "proportional measurements". This method is applicable to patients of different ages and body sizes. See Fig. 50 and the following table to find how many *Cun* each portion of the body is divided into.

Body Part	Distance	Proportional Measurement	Method	Explanation
Head	From the anterior hairline to the posterior hairline	12 *Cun*	Longitudinal measurement	The distance from the glabella to the anterior hairline is taken as 3 *Cun*; from the Dazhui (DU 14) to the posterior hairline, 3 *Cun*. If the anterior and posterior hairlines are indistinguishable, the distance from the glabella to Dazhui (DU 14) is then taken as 18 *Cun*.
	Between the two nipples	8 *Cun*	Transverse measurement	The distance between the bilateral Quepen (ST 12) can be used as the substitute of the transverse measurement of the two nipples.
Chest and Abdomen	From the end of xiphoid process to the centre of the umbilicus	8 *Cun*	Longitudinal measurement	
	Between the centre of the umbilicus and the upper margin of pubic bone	5 *Cun*	Longitudinal measurement	
Back	Between the medial borders of the two scapulae	6 *Cun*	Transverse measurement	Transverse measurement used to locate points on the loins and back

Region	Location	Distance	Measurement		Application
Upper Extremities	Between the end of the axillary fold and the transverse cubital crease	9 Cun	Longitudinal measurement		Applicable to the measurement of both the medial and lateral aspects of the upper limb
	Between the transverse cubital crease and the transverse wrist crease	12 Cun	Longitudinal measurement		
	From the prominence of the great trochanter to the middle of patella	19 Cun	Longitudinal measurement	For measurement of the thigh	For measurement of the anterior, lateral and posterior aspects of the lower limbs
	Between the centre of patella and the tip of lateral malleolus	16 Cun	Longitudinal measurement	For measurement of the shank	
Lower Extremities	From the level of the upper margin of pubic bone to the upper border of the medial epicondylic ridge	18 Cun	Longitudinal measurement	For measurement of the thigh	For measurement of the medial aspects of the lower limbs
	From the lower border of the medial condyle of tibia to the tip of medial malleolus	13 Cun	Longitudinal measurement	For measurement of the shank	

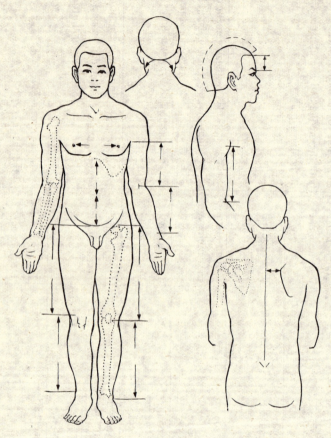

Fig.50

2. Finger Measurement

This is a method used to locate points with the length or width of the patient's finger(s). The physician's finger(s) may be used instead if his body size is similar to that of the patient. Generally speaking, when the patient's middle finger is flexed, the distance between the two medial ends of the creases of the interphalangeal joints is taken as one *Cun*, or the width of the interphalangeal joint of the patient's thumb is taken as one *Cun*. In addition, the width of the proximal interphalangeal joints of the closed four fingers (index, middle, ring and small) is taken as three *Cun* (Fig.51).

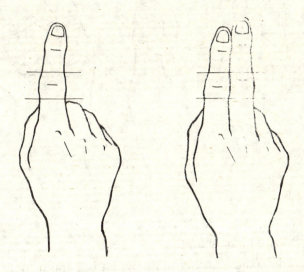

Fig.51−1

3. Measurement Depending on Anatomical Landmarks

Locating points according to various anatomical landmarks on the body surface is the basic method for point location. Those landmarks fall into two categories.

(1) Fixed Landmarks

Fixed landmarks are those whose positions will not change with body movement. The five sense organs, nipples, umbilicus, and the prominences and depressions of various bones are such ones.

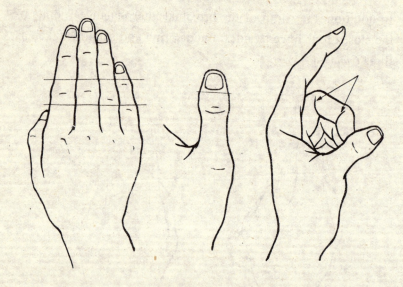

Fig.51—2

(2) Moving Landmarks

Moving landmarks refer to those that will appear only when a body part keeps in a specific position. The depression and prominence of the muscles, the appearance of the thendons, and the creases of the skin seen when a movement is being done are such examples.

4.3 Introduction to the Fourteen Channels and Commonly Used Points and *Tuina* Manipulations

1. The Lung Channel of Hand—Taiyin

This channel originates from the middle—*Jiao*, runs downward to connect with the large intestine, winds back and goes upward into the lung—the organ it pertains to, comes out transversely from the lung system to reach Zhongfu (LU 1), descends along the radial border of the medial aspect of the upper limb, and ends at Shaoshang (LU 11) at the radial side of the thumb. Its branch emerging from Lieque (LU 7) runs to the radial side of the tip of the index finger, where it meets the Large Intestine Channel of Hand—Yangming, to which the Lung Channel of Hand—Taiyin is exteriorly—interiorly related. Located along either of the left and right routes of the Lung Channel of Hand—Taiyin are 11 points, of which the following ones are commonly used (Fig. 52).

Zhongfu (LU 1)

Location: 6 *Cun* lateral to the midline of the chest, at the level of the interspace between the 1st and 2nd ribs.

Indications: cough, choking sensation in the chest, chest pain, and pain in the shoulder and back.

Manipulation: *Yizhichan Tui, An, Rou* and *Mó*.

Chize (LU 5)

Location: in the middle of the cubital crease and on the radial side of the tendon of the biceps muscle of the arm.

Indications: spasmodic pain of the elbow and arm, cough, fullness in the chest and the hypochondriac region, and infantile convulsions.

Manipulation: *An, Rou, Na* and *Yizhichan Tui*.

Lieque (LU 7)

Location: superior to the styloid process of the radius, 1.5 *Cun* above the transverse crease of the wrist. When the index fingers and thumbs of the two hands are crossed with the index finger of one hand placed on the styloid process of the radius of the other, the point is in the depression right under the tip of the index finger.

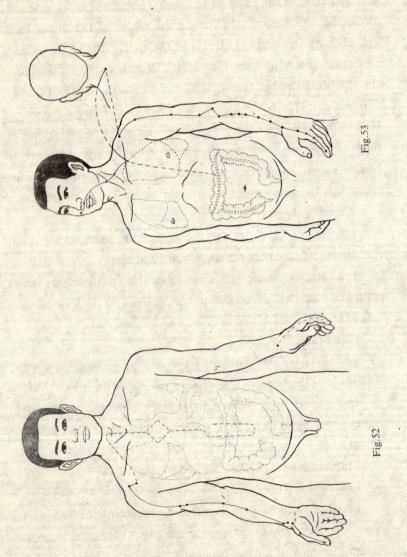

Fig.53

Fig.52

Indications: headache, facial paralysis and hemiplegia.

Manipulation: *An* and *Qia* (nipping).

Yuji (LU 10)

Location: at the midpoint of the first metacarpal bone and on the junction of the red and white skin.

Indications: pain in the chest and back, headache, vertigo, sore throat, fever with chills.

Manipulation: *An, Rou* and *Qia* (nipping).

Shaoshang (LU 11)

Location: on the radial side of the thumb and about 0.1 *Cun* posterior to the corner of the nail.

Indications: swollen and sore throat, cough with dyspnea, apoplexy, coma and infantile convulsions.

Manipulation: *Qia* (nipping) and *Qiarou* (nipping-kneading).

2. The Large Intestine Channel of Hand—Yangming

This channel originates from Shangyang (LI 1) on the radial side of the index finger, runs upward along the radial border of the lateral side of the hand and arm up to the anterior border of the acromion, winds backward and reaches Dazhui (DU 14), turns back and arrives at the supraclavicular fossa, descends to pass through the lung, and at last enters the large intestine—the organ it belongs to. Its branch starts from the supraclavicular fossa, goes upward to the neck, passes through the cheek and the gum of the lower teeth, winds backward to the upper lip, meets Renzhong (DU 26), goes forward again, and ends at Yingxiang (LI 20), beside which it connects with the Stomach Channel of Foot—Yangming. The Large Intestine Channel of Hand—Yangming is exteriorly—interiorly related to the Lung Channel. Along the left route of it there are 20 points; along the right one, there are the same other 20. The commonly used ones are as follows (Fig. 53).

Hegu (LI 4)

Location: on the dorsum of the hand and at the midpoint between the 1st and 2nd metacarpal bones.

Indications: headache, toothache, fever, swollen and sore throat, pain in the shoulder and arm, finger spasm and facial paralysis.

Manipulation: *Na, An* and *Rouqia* (kneading—nipping).

Yangxi (LI 5)

Location: on the radial transverse crease of the dorsum of the wrist and between the vagina tendinum musculorum abductoris longi et extensoris brevis policis and tendinous sheath of long extensor muscle of thumb.

Indications: headache, tinnitus, toothache, swollen and sore throat, conjunctival congestion and wrist pain.

Manipulation: *An, Rou, Qia* (nipping) and *Na*.

Shousanli (LI 10)

Location: 2 *Cun* below Quchi (LI 11) and on the line between Yangxi (LI 5) and Quchi (LI 11).

Indications: spasmodic elbow with difficulty in flexion and extension, and numbness and soreness of the arm.

Manipulation: *Na, An, Rou* and *Yizhichan Tui*.

Quchi(LI 11)

Location: When the elbow is flexed, the point is in the depression at the lateral end of the cubital transverse crease.

Indications: fever, hypertension, swollen and painful elbow and arm with difficulty in flexion and extension, and paralysis.

Manipulation: *Na, An, Rou* and *Qia* (nipping).

Jianyu (LI 15)

Location: in the depression anterior and inferior to the acromion when the arm is abducted.

Indications: pain in the shoulder, motor impairment of the shoulder joint, and hemiparalysis.

Manipulation: *Yizhichan Tui, An, Rou* and *Gun*.

Yingxiang (LI 20)

Location: in the nasolabial groove and at the point 0.5 *Cun* lateral to the ala nasi.

Indications: rhinitis, stuffy nose and facial paralysis.

Manipulation: *Qia* (nipping), *An, Rou* and *Yizhichan Tui*.

3. The Stomach Channel of Foot−Yangming

This channel originates from the lateral side of the ala nasi, runs upward to meet the Bladder Channel of Foot−Taiyang at the radix nasi and to arrive at Chengqi (ST 1) at the infraorbital margin, descends then through the upper gum, round the lips and along the mandible and Jiache (ST 6), and finally winds upward again to reach Touwei (ST 8) at the preauricular frontal angle. The facial branch starts from the mandible, descends into the supraclavicular fossa along the neck, descends again and passes through the diaphragm, enters the stomach—the organ it pertains to, and connects with the spleen. The branch travelling along the exterior route starts from the supraclavicular fossa, descends through the nipple and abdomen, meets the branch arising from the lower orifice of the stomach at Qichong (ST 30) in the inguen, runs downward again along the anterior side of the thigh and the anterolateral aspect of the tibia, and ends at Lidui (ST 45) on the second toe. Located along this channel and on its both routes are

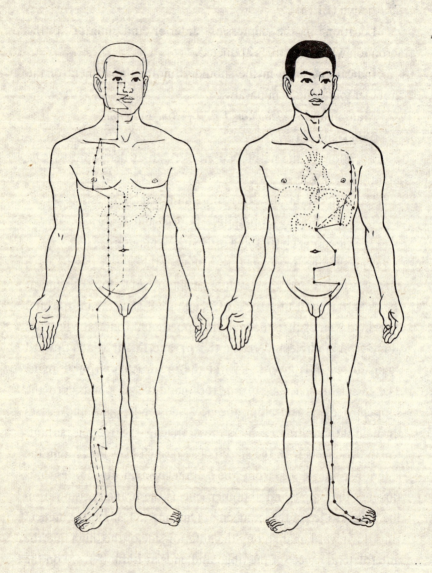

Fig.54

Fig.55

90 points. The following are commonly used. (This channel is exteriorly—interiorly related to the Spleen Channel.). See Fig.54.

Sibai (ST 2)

Location: in the depression of the infraorbital foramen and directly below the pupil while one is looking straight forward.

Indication: facial paralysis, spasm of the facial muscles, and reddened, painful and itching eye.

Manipulation: *An, Rou* and *Yizhichan Tui.*

Dicang (ST 4)

Location: 0.4 *Cun* lateral to the corner of the mouth, directly below Juliao (ST 3).

Indications: facial paralysis and salivation.

Manipulation: *Yizhichan Tui, An* and *Rou.*

Jiache (ST 6)

Location: in the depression one finger—breadth anterior and superior to the lower angle of the mandible.

Indications: toothache, swelling of the cheek and facial paralysis.

Manipulation: *Yizhichan Tui, An* and *Rou.*

Xiaguan (ST 7)

Location: in the depression on the lower border of the zygomatic arch.

Indications: facial paralysis, toothache and temporomandibular joint inflammation.

Manipulation: *Yizhichan Tui, An* and *Rou.*

Touwei (ST 8)

Location: 0.5 *Cun* directly above the anterior hairline at the corner of the forehead.

Indications: headache, vertigo and ophthalmalgia.

Manipulation: *Mǒ, An, Rou* and *Saosan* (kneading–sweeping).

Renying (ST 9)

Location: 1.5 *Cun* lateral to the laryngeal protuberance.

Indications: swollen and sore throat, asthma, choking sensation in the chest, emesis and hiccup.

Manipulation: *Na, Rou* and *Chan* (twining).

Shuitu (ST 10)

Location: 1 *Cun* inferior to Renying (ST 9) and on the anterior border of m. sternocleidomastoideus.

Indications: fullness sensation in the chest, cough, asthma, swollen and sore throat and shortness of breath.

Manipulation: *Na, Mǒ* and *Chan* (twining).

Quepen (ST 12)

Location: in the depression of the midpoint of the supraclavicular fossa and directly above the nipple.

Indications: fullness sensation in the chest, cough, asthma, sore throat, and pain and numbness of the upper limb.

Manipulation: *An, Tanbo* (flicking–poking) and *Rou*.

Tianshu (ST 25)

Location: 2 *Cun* lateral to the umbilicus.

Indications: constipation, diarrhea, irregular menstruation and abdominal pain.

Manipulation: *Rou, Mó* and *Yizhichan Tui*

Biguan (ST 31)

Location: on the line jointing the anterior superior iliac spine and the lateral border of the patella and at the level of the gluteal groove.

Indications: soreness of the loins and legs, numbness and

weakness of the lower limbs with spasmodic tendons which lead to difficulty in flexion and extension, and myoatrophy of the quadriceps muscle of thigh.

Manipulation: *An, Na, Rou, Dian, Gun* and *Tanbo* (flicking—poking).

Futu (ST 32)

Location: 6 *Cun* above the laterosuperior border of the patella.

Indications: pain, coldness and numbness of the knee, and paralysis of the lower limbs.

Manipulation: *Gun, An* and *Rou.*

Liangqiu (ST 34)

Location: 2 *Cun* above the laterosuperior border of the patella.

Indications: pain, coldness and numbness of the knee, stomachache and mastitis.

Manipulation: *Gun, An, Dian* and *Na.*

Dubi (ST 35)

Location: in the depression lateral to the patellar ligament and on the lower border of the patella.

Indications: pain and weakness and motor impairment of the knee joint.

Manipulation: *Dian, An* and *Rou.*

Zusanli (ST 36)

Location: 3 *Cun* below Dubi (ST 35), one finger—breadth apart from the anterior crest of the tibia.

Indications: abdominal pain and distension, diarrhea, constipation, coldness and numbness of the lower limbs and hypertension.

Manipulation: *An, Dian, Rou* and *Yizhichan Tui.*

Shangjuxu (ST 37)

Location: 3 *Cun* directly below Zusanli (ST 36).

Indications: pain around the navel, diarrhea, appendicitis, soreness and numbness of the lower limbs, and paralysis.

Manipulation: *An, Na, Gun* and *Rou.*

Jiexi (ST 41)

Location: on the dorsum of the foot, at the midpoint of the transverse crease of the ankle joint, in the depression between the tendons of m. extensor digitorum longus and hallucis longus.

Indications: sprain of the ankle joint, numbness of the foot and toes, and headache.

Manipulation: *An, Na, Qia* (nipping) and *Dian.*

4. The Spleen Channel of Foot—Taiyin

This channel originates from Yinbai (SP 1) at the tip of the big toe, runs along the medial aspect of the foot, goes upward from the medial aspect of the ankle, ascends along the anterior border of the medial aspects of the tibia and the thigh up to Chongmen (SP 12) in the groin. The line going along an exterior route runs upward into the abdomen, ascends along a line 2 *Cun* lateral to the midline of the abdomen to the chest, and then descends to Dabao (SP 21) at the hyponchondrium. The line going along an interior route runs inside, enters the spleen, the organ it pertains to, connects with the stomach, then ascends alongside the esophagus, and finally reaches the root of the tongue and spreads over the lower surface of the tongue. The branch arising from the stomach goes upward, passes through the diaphragm, enters the heart and connects with the Heart Channel of Hand—Shaoyin. This channel is exteriorly—interiorly related to the Stomach Channel. Located along either of the left and right routes are 21 points, of which the following are commonly used (Fig.55).

Gongsun (SP 4)

Location: on the medial aspect of the tarsal bones of the foot, in the depression of the anterior and inferior border of the base of the first metatarsal bone.

Indications: diarrhea, abdominal pain, vomiting, and swelling and pain on the medial aspect of the foot.

Manipulation: *An, Rou, Dian* and *Yizhichan Tui*.

Sanyinjiao (SP 6)

Location: 3 *Cun* directly above the tip of the medial malleolus, on the posterior border of the medial aspect of the tibia.

Indications: insomnia, enuresis, weakness of the spleen and stomach, uroschesis, nocturnal emission, impotence, irregular menstruation, and hypertension.

Manipulation: *Rou, An* and *Yizhichan Tui*.

Yinlingquan (SP 9)

Location: in the depression of the hypocondylar border on the medial aspect of the tibia.

Indications: soreness of the knee joint and difficulty in urinating.

Manipulation: *Rou, An, Dian, Na* and *Yizhichan Tui*.

Xuehai (SP 10)

Location: 2 *Cun* above the mediosuperior border of the patella.

Indications: irregular menstruation and soreness of the knee.

Manipulation: *Na*, *An* and *Dian*.

Daheng (SP 15)

Location: 4 *Cun* lateral to the centre of the umbilicus.

Indications: diarrhea due to cold of insufficiency type, constipation and pain in the lower abdomen.

Manipulation: *Yizhichan Tui, Mó, Rou* and *Na*.

5. The Heart Channel of Hand—Shaoyin

This channel originates from the heart, spreads over the "heart system"—the tissues connecting the heart with the other *Zang—Fu* organs after coming out of the heart, and descends to connect with the small intestine. The portion of this channel ascending from the "heart system" runs alongside the esophagus to connect the eye and the tissues that connect the eye with the brain. The other portion of this channel coming out of the "heart system" runs upward to the lung, goes transversely to the left and right, emerges from Jiquan (HT 1) at the axilla, travels downward along the upper arm, the elbow joint and the palmar ulnar border of the forearm into the palm, ends at Shaochong (HT 9) at the tip of the medial aspect of the small finger and links with the Small Intestine Channel of Hand—Taiyang. This channel is exteriorly—interiorly related to the Small Intestine Channel. Along it, there are 18 points, 9 on the left route, the same other 9 on the right route. The following are its commonly used points (Fig.56).

Jiquan (HT 1)

Location: in the centre of the axilla.

Indications: choking sensation in the chest, pain in the hypochondriac region, and soreness, coldness and numbness of the arm and elbow.

Manipulation: *Na* and *Tanbo* (flicking–poking).

Shaohai (HT 3)

Location: When the elbow is flexed, the point is located in the depression of the ulnar end of the transverse cubital crease.

Indications: spasmodic pain in the elbow joint and tremor of the hand.

Manipulation: *Na* and *Tanbo* (flicking–poking).

Shenmen (HT 7)

Location: at the ulnar end of the transverse crease of the wrist, in the depression on the radial side of the tendon of m. flexor carpi ulnaris.

Indications: palpitation due to fright severe palpitation, insomnia, amnesia and arrhythmia.

Manipulation: *Na, An* and *Rou.*

6. The Small Intestine Channel of Hand–Taiyang

This channel originates from Shaoze (SI 1) on the ulnar side of the tip of the small finger, runs upward along the ulnar border of the dorsum of the hand and forearm to the shoulder joint, circles around the scapular region and goes further to meet Dazhui (DU 14), then, turns downward to Quepen (ST 12) in the supraclavicular fossa. From there, its branch going inside descends to connect with the heart and further to enter the small intestine—the organ it belongs to. The branch going superficially from the supraclavicular fossa ascends to the neck and further to the cheek, enters the ear, and ends at Tinggong (SI 19) at last. The branch from the neck runs upward to the infraorbital region and further to the lateral side of the nose, reaches the inner canthus and links with the Bladder Channel of Foot–Taiyang. The Small Intestine Channel of Hand–Taiyang is exteriorly—interiorly related to the Heart Channel. Located along it are 38 points, 19 on the left route, the same other 19 on the right route. The commonly used ones are as follows (Fig.57).

Shaoze (SI 1)

Location: on the ulnar side of the small finger, about 0.1 *Cun* posterior to the corner of the nail.

Indications: fever, coma due to apoplexy, hypogalactia and sore throat.

Manipulation: *Qia* (nipping).

Xiaohai (SI 8)

Location: When the elbow is flexed, the point is located in the depression between the olecranon of the ulna and the medial epicondyle of the humerus.

Indications: toothache, pain in the neck and soreness of the upper limbs.

Manipulation: *Na* and *Rou*.

Bingfeng (SI 12)

Location: in the centre of the suprascapular fossa, directly above Tianzong (SI 11).

Indications: pain in the scapular region, and soreness and numbness of the upper limbs with difficulty in raising.

Manipulation: *Yizhichan Tui, Gun, An* and *Rou*.

Jianwaishu (SI 14)

Location: 3 *Cun* lateral to the lower border of the spinous process of the first thoracic vertebra.

Indications: cold pain in the shoulder and back, rigidity of the neck, and soreness and numbness of the upper limbs.

Manipulation: *Yizhichan Tui, Gun, An* and *Rou*.

Jianzhongshu (SI 15)

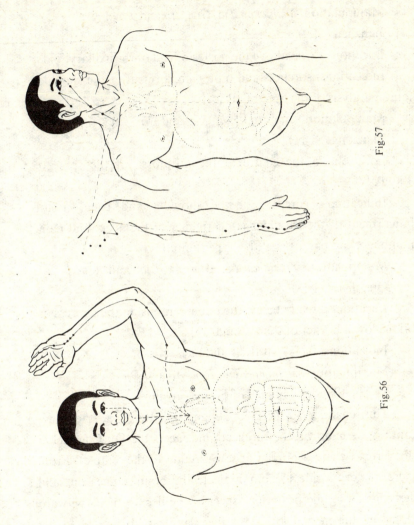

Fig.57

Fig.56

Location: 2 *Cun* lateral to Dazhui (DU 14).

Indications: cough, asthma, pain in the shoulder and back, and blurred vision.

Manipulation: *Yizhichan Tui, Gun, An* and *Rou*.

Jianzhen (SI 9)

Location: 1 *Cun* above the posterior end of the axillary fold.

Indications: soreness and motor impairment of the shoulder joint, paralysis of the upper limb.

Manipulation: *Gun, An, Dian, Rou* and *Na*.

Tianzong (SI 11)

Location: in the centre of the infrafossa of the spine of scapula.

Indications: soreness of the shoulder and back, motor impairment of the shoulder joint, rigidity of the neck, and pain, numbness and paralysis of the upper limb.

Manipulation: *Yizhichan Tui, Gun, An, Dian* and *Rou*.

Quanliao (SI 18)

Location: directly below the outer canthus, in the depression on the lower border of the zygoma.

Indications: facial paralysis and facial spasm.

Manipulation: *Yizhichan Tui, Rou, An* and *Dian*.

7. The Bladder Channel of Foot—Taiyang

This channel starts from Jingming (BL 1) at the inner canthus, ascends via the forehead and meets the Du Channel at the vertex (where a branch arises, running to the temple). From there, it goes inside to communicate the brain, comes out and descends along the posterior aspect of the neck, runs downward alongside the medial aspect of the scapula and parallel to the vertebral column to the lumbar region (where another branch arises, descending). From there, it goes inside the body cavity, connects with the kidney and enters the urinary bladder, the organ it pertains to.

The branch from the lumbar region descends via the buttock into the popliteal fossa.

There is still another branch arising from the posterior aspect of the neck. It runs straight downward along the medial border of the scapula, passes the buttock and the lateral aspect of the thigh, meets the branch from the lumbar region in the popliteal fossa. From there, it makes its way downward again via the shank, emerges from the posterior aspect of the lateral malleolus, runs along the tuberosity of the fifth metatarsal bone, and ends at Zhiyin (BL 67) at the lateral side of the tip of the small toe, where it connects with the Kidney Channel of Foot—Shaoyin.

The Bladder Channel of Foot—Taiyang is exteriorly—interiorly related to the Kidney Channel. Along it, there are 134 points located all over the body, every two of which have the same name. The commonly used ones are as follows (Fig. 58).

Jingming (BL 1)

Location: 0.1 *Cun* lateral to the inner canthus.

Indications: eye disorders.

Manipulation: *Yizhichan Tui, An* and *Zhen.*

Cuanzhu (BL 2)

Location: in the depression on the medial extremity of the eyebrow.

Indications: headache, insomnia, pain in the supraorbital region, and redness and pain of the eye.

Manipulation: *Yizhichan Tui, An, Rou* and *Mo.*

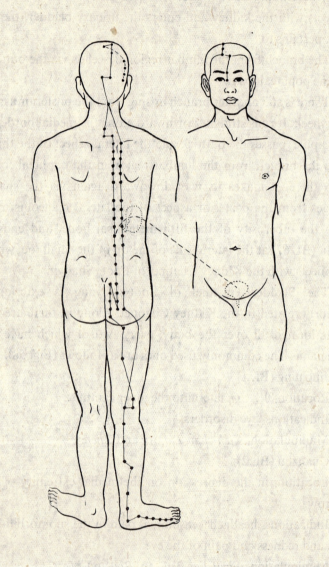

Fig.58

Tianzhu (BL 10)

Location: 1.3 *Cun* lateral to Yamen (DU 15), in the depression on the lateral border of m. trapezius.

Indications: headache, rigidity of the neck, stuffy nose and pain in the shoulder and back.

Manipulation: *Yizhichan Tui, An, Rou* and *Na.*

Dazhu (BL 11)

Location: 1.5 *Cun* lateral to the lower border of the spinous process of the first thoracic vertebra.

Indications: fever, cough, rigidity of the neck and pain in the shoulder and back.

Manipulation: *Yizhichan Tui, Gun, An* and *Rou.*

Fengmen (BL 12)

Location: 1.5 *Cun* lateral to the lower border of the spinous process of the second thoracic vertebra.

Indication: cold, cough, rigidity of the neck and pain in the shoulder and back.

Manipulation: *Yizhichan Tui, Gun, An* and *Rou.*

Feishu (BL 13)

Location: 1.5 *Cun* lateral to the lower border of the spinous process of the third thoracic vertebra.

Indications: cough, asthma, stuffiness and pain in the chest and strain of the muscles of back.

Manipulation: *Yizhichan Tui, Gun, An, Rou* and *Tanbo* (flicking—poking).

Xinshu (BL 15)

Location: 1.5 *Cun* lateral to the lower border of the spinous process of the fifth thoracic vertebra.

Indications: insomnia, amnesia, hemiparalysis, palpitation

and irritability.

Manipulation: *Yizhichan Tui, Gun, An, Rou* and *Tanbo* (flicking—poking).

Ganshu (BL 18)

Location: 1.5 *Cun* lateral to the lower border of the spinous process of the ninth thoracic vertebra.

Indications: distending—pain in the hypochondriac region, hepatitis and eye disorders.

Manipulation: *Yizhichan Tui Gun, An, Rou* and *Tanbo* (flicking—poking).

Danshu (BL 19)

Location: 1.5 *Cun* lateral to the lower border of the spinous process of the tenth thoracic vertebra.

Indications: distending and full sensation in the hypochondriac region, bitter taste of the mouth, jaundice and disorders of the biliary tract.

Manipulation: *Yizhichan Tui, An, Rou* and *Tanbo* (flicking—poking).

Pishu (BL 20)

Location: 1.5 *Cun* lateral to the lower border of the spinous process of the eleventh thoracic vertebra.

Indications: distending—pain in the epigastric region, indigestion, and chronic infantile convulsion.

Manipulation: *Yizhichan Tui, Dian, An* and *Rou.*

Weishu (BL 21)

Location: 1.5 *Cun* lateral to the lower border of the spinous process of the twelfth thoracic vertebra.

Indications: gastropathy, vomiting of milk in infants and indigestion.

Manipulation: *Yizhichan Tui, Dian, An, Rou,* and *Gun.*

Sanjiaoshu (BL 22)

Location: 1.5 *Cun* lateral to the lower border of the spinous process of the 1st lumbar vertebra.

Indications: borborygmus, abdominal distension, vomiting, and rigidity and pain in the waist and back.

Manipulation: *Yizhichan Tui, An, Rou, Dian* and *Gun.*

Shenshu (BL 23)

Location: 1.5 *Cun* lateral to the lower border of the spinous process of the 2nd lumbar vertebra.

Indications: deficiency of the kidney, lumbago, nocturnal emission and irregular menstruation.

Manipulation: *Yizhichan Tui, Gun, An, Rou* and *Dian.*

Qihaishu (BL 24)

Location: 1.5 *Cun* lateral to the lower border of the spinous process of the 3rd lumbar vertebra.

Indications: lumbago and hemorrhoid.

Manipulation: *Yizhichan Tui, An, Rou* and *Gun.*

Dachangshu (BL 25)

Location: 1.5 *Cun* lateral to the lower border of the spinous process of the 4th lumbar vertebra.

Indications: pain in the loins and legs, lumbar muscle strain and enteritis.

Manipulation: *Yizhichan Tui, An, Rou* and *Gun.*

Guanyuanshu (BL 26)

Location: 1.5 *Cun* lateral to the lower border of the spinous process of the 5th lumbar vertebra.

Indications: lumbago and diarrhea.

Manipulation: *Yizhichan Tui, An, Gun, Rou* and *Dian.*

Baliao

Location: Baliao is a collective term of Shangliao, Ciliao, Zhongliao and Xialiao which are located respectively in the 1st, 2nd, 3rd and 4th posterior sacral foramen.

Indications: pain in the loins and legs, and diseases of the urogenital system.

Zhibian (BL 54)

Location: 3 *Cun* lateral to the lower border of the spinous process of the 4th sacral vertebra.

Indications: pain in the lumbosacral region, flaccidity of the lower extremities, difficulty in micturition, and constipation.

Manipulation: *Gun, Na, An, Rou, Dian* and *Tanbo* (flicking—poking).

Yinmen (BL 37)

Location: 6 *Cun* below the centre of the gluteal groove.

Indications: sciatica, paralysis of the lower extremities, and pain in the loins and legs.

Manipulation: *Gun, Dian, Ya* and *Na*.

Weizhong (BL 40)

Location: at the midpoint of the transverse crease of the popliteal fossa.

Indications: lumbago, difficulty in flexing and extending the knee joint, and hemiparalysis.

Manipulation: *Gun, Na, An, Rou* and *Yizhichan Tui*.

Gaohuang (BL 43)

Location: 3 *Cun* lateral to the lower border of the spinous process of the 4th thoracic vertebra, in the depression on the spinal border of the scapula.

Indications: cough, asthma, tidal fever, mania, amnesia and

nocturnal emission.

Manipulation: *Gun, An, Rou* and *Yizhichan Tui*.

Zhishi (BL 52)

Location: 1.5 *Cun* lateral to Shenshu (BL 23).

Indications: nocturnal emission, impotence, irregular menstruation, enuresis and chronic lumbago.

Manipulation: *Gun, Rou, An* and *Yizhichan Tui*.

Chengshan (BL 57)

Location: at the top of the depression between the two bellies of m. gastrocnemius.

Indications: pain in the loins and legs, systremma and diarrhea.

Manipulation: *Gun, An, Rou, Na* and *Ca*.

Kunlun (BL 60)

Location: in the depression between the lateral malleolus and the Achilles tendon.

Indications: headache, rigidity of the neck, lumbago and sprain of the ankle joint.

Manipulation: *An, Na* and *Dian*.

8. The Kidney Channel of Foot—Shaoyin

This channel starts from the inferior aspect of the small toe, goes obliquely towards Yongquan (KI 1) in the centre of the sole, emerges from the lower aspect of the tuberosity of the navicular bone, travels behind the medial malleolus and reaches the heel, ascends along the medio—posterior aspect of the shank, the popliteal fossa and the thigh and enters the vertebral column, ascends further in the column, arrives at the kidney—the organ it belongs to, connects with the urinary bladder, and, then, re—emerges from the pubic bone, runs upward through the abdomen, and ends at Shufu (KI 27) below the clavicle of the thorax at last.

The branch from the kidney runs straight up through the liver and the diaphragm, enters the lung, ascends along the throat, and terminates at the two sides of the root of the tongue.

The branch from the lung joins the heart and runs into the chest to link with the Pericardium Channel of Hand—Hueyin.

The Kidney Channel of Foot—Shaoyin is exteriorly—interiorly related to the Bladder Channel. Along the two routes of it, there are 54 points, of which the following are commonly used (Fig. 59).

Yongquan (KI 1)

Location: on the sole, in the depression when the foot is in plantar flexion.

Indications: migraine, hypertension, infantile fever, vomiting, diarrhea and insomnia.

Manipulation: *Ca, An, Rou* and *Na*.

Zhaohai (KI 6)

Location: in the depression on the lower border of the medial malleolus.

Indications: irregular menstruation, pain in the lower abdomen, dry throat, aphasia and retention of urine.

Manipulation: *An* and *Rou*.

9. The Pericardium Channel of Hand—Jueyin

This channel originates in the chest, enters the pericardium, the organ it belongs to, after emerging, descends through the diaphragm, and passes the abdomen to connect successively with the upper, middle and lower *Jiao*.

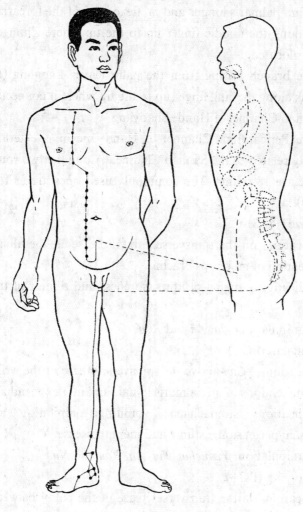

Fig.59

The branch arising from the chest runs inside the chest, comes out from Tianchi (PC 1) in the costal region, travels transversely to the axillary fold, descends into the palm along the middle line of the medial side of the upper arm and between the tendons of m. palmaris longus and m. flexocarpi of the forearm, and passes along the middle finger up to the tip where Zhongchong (PC 9) is located.

The branch arising from the palm leaves Laogong (PC 8) and runs along the ring finger up to the tip where it connects with the Sanjiao Channel of Hand—Shaoyang.

The Pericardium Channel of Hand—Jueyin is exteriorly — interiorly related to the Sanjiao Channel. Along the two routes of it, there are 18 points. The commonly used ones are as follows (Fig. 60)

Quze (PC 3)

Location: on the transverse cubital crease, at the ulnar side of the tendon of m. biceps brachii.

Indications: angina pectoris, soreness and tremor of the upper limb.

Manipulation: *Na, An* and *Rou*.

Neiguan (PC 6)

Location: 2 *Cun* above the transverse crease of the wrist, between the tendons of m. palmaris longus and m. flexor radialis.

Indications: stomachache, vomiting, palpitation, angina pectoris, hypertension, asthma and mental disease.

Manipulation: *Yizhichan Tui, An, Rou* and *Na*.

Laogong (PC 8)

Location: on the transverse crease of the palm, between the 2nd and 3rd metacarpal bones.

Indications: psychosis, palpitation, heatstroke and vomiting.

Manipulation: *An, Qia* (nipping) and *Na*.

Zhongchong (PC 9)

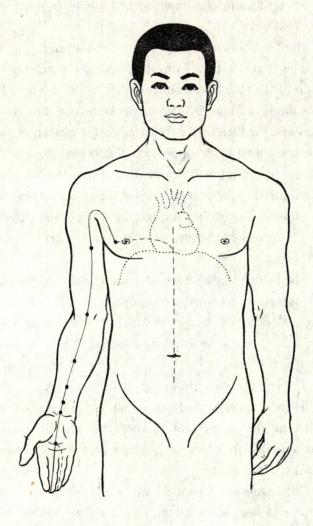

Fig.60

Location: at the tip of the middle finger.

Indications: coma, fever, heatstroke, and difficulty in speaking due to stiff tongue.

Manipulation: *Qia* (nipping) and *Qiarou* (nipping – kneading).

10. The Sanjiao Channel of Hand–Shaoyang

This channel starts from the point of Guanchong (SJ 1) at the tip of the ring finger, runs upward to the shoulder from between the 4th and the 5th metacarpal bones and then between the radius and the ulna of the forearm, via the olecranon and along the lateral aspect of the upper arm, finally goes forward from the shoulder to the supraclavicular fossa. From the fossa, it comes down into the chest and spreads there, connecting with the pericardium. Descending and passing through the diaphragm, it enters in succession the three *Jiao* in the abdomen — the organ it pertains to.

The branch arising from the chest ascends, comes out of the same supraclavicular fossa, ascends to the neck, runs along the posterior border of the ear, winds to the anterior border of the ear, descends along the temple to the cheek, and terminates in the infraorbital region.

The branch arising from the retroauricular region enters the ear. Then, it emerges in front of the ear, crosses the previous branch at the cheek and reaches the outer canthus where Sizhukong (SJ 23) is located, linking with the Gallbladder Channel of Foot–Shaoyang.

The Sanjiao Channel of Hand–Shaoyang has the exterior–interior relationship with the Pericardium Channel. Along the two routes of it, there are 46 points altogether. The following are the commonly used ones (Fig. 61).

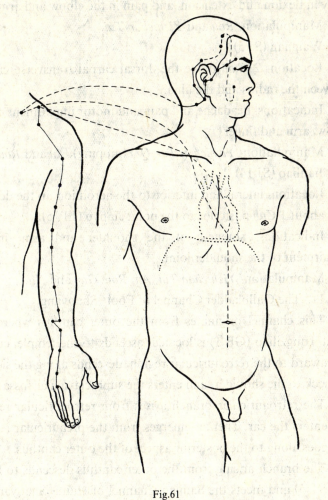

Fig.61

Zhongzhu (SJ 3)

Location: When the fist is naturally clenched, the point is on the dorsum of the hand, in the depression between the posterior borders of the small ends of the 4th and 5th metacarpal bones.

Indication: migraine, pain in the palm and finger with difficulty in flexion and extension, and pain in the elbow and arm.

Manipulation: *Rou* and *Yizhichan Tui*.

Waiguan (SJ 5)

Location: 2 *Cun* above the dorsal carpal transverse crease, between the radius and the ulna.

Indications: headache and pain and motor impairment of the elbow, arm and finger.

Manipulation: *Yizhichan Tui, Qia* (nipping), *An* and *Rou*.

Jianliao (SJ 14)

Location: lateral and inferior to the acromion, in the depression about 1 *Cun* posterior to the point Jianyu (LI 15).

Indications: soreness of the shoulder and arm, motor impairment of the shoulder joint.

Manipulation: *Yizhichan Tui, An, Rou, Gun* and *Na*.

11. The Gallbladder Channel of Foot—Shaoyang

This channel originates from the outer canthus where the point Tongziliao (GB 1) is located, ascends to the temple, curves downward to the retroauricular region, descends along the side of the neck to the shoulder, and enters the supraclavicular fossa.

The retroauricular branch arises from retroauricular region and enters the ear. Then, it emerges from the preauricular region and goes along to the posterior aspect of the outer canthus.

The branch arising from the outer canthus descends to Daying (ST 5) and meets the Sanjiao Channel of Hand—Shaoyang in the infraorbital region, goes downward to pass through Jiache (ST 6) and to arrive at the shoulder, enters the supraclavicular fossa where it meets the main channel, falls into the chest, travels through the diaphragm, connects with the liver, and enters the gallbladder—the organ it pertains to. Then, it runs downwards along the inner side of the hypochondrium, comes out of the groin, passes through the vulva, and goes transversely into the hip joint region.

The branch going straight down from the supraclavicular fossa passes in front of the axilla along the lateral aspect of the chest and hypochondrium to the hip region where it meets the previous branch. Then, it descends along the lateral aspect of the thigh and knee, the anterior aspect of the fibula and the anterior aspect of the lateral malleolus and reaches the lateral side of the tip of the 4th toe where the point Zuqiaoyin (GB 44) is located.

The branch starting from the dorsum of the foot connects with the Liver Channel of Foot—Jueyin.

The Gallbladder Channel of Foot—Shaoyang is exteriorly—interiorly related to the Liver Channel. Along the two routes of it, there are 88 points altogether. The following ones are commonly used (Fig. 62).

Tongziliao (GB 1)

Location: lateral to the outer canthus, on the lateral border of the orbital bone.

Indications: migraine, conjunctivitis, myopia and optic atrophy.

Manipulation: *Rou, An* and *Yizhichan Tui*.

Yangbai (GB 14)

Location: When looking is directed straight ahead, the point is 1 *Cun* directly above the midpoint of the eyebrow.

Indications: facial paralysis, headache and prosopalgia.

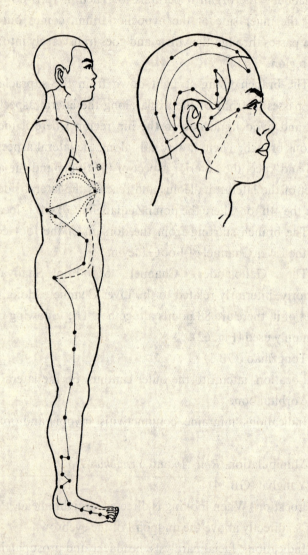

Fig.62

Manipulation: *An, Mo, Pianfengtui* and *Rou.*

Fengchi (GB 20)

Location: between the sternocleidomastoid muscle and the trapezial muscle, at the same level of Fengfu (DU 16).

Indications: migraine, headache, common cold, neurosism, mental disease, rigidity of the neck, myopia and hypertension.

Manipulation: *Yizhichan Tui, An, Rou, Dian* and *Na.*

Jianjing (GB 21)

Location: on the midway between Dazhui (DU 14) and the acromion and at the highest point of the shoulder.

Indications: rigidity of the neck, soreness of the shoulder and back, mastitis and motor impairment of the arm.

Manipulation: *Na, Rou, Yizhichan Tui* and *Gun.*

Juliao (GB 29)

Location: on the midway between the anterosuperior iliac spine and the great trochanter of femur.

Indications: pain in the loins and legs, soreness of the hip joint, sacro—iliilis, and inflammation of the superior clunial nerves.

Manipulation: *Gun, An, Dian* and *Ya* (heavy pressing).

Huantiao (GB 30)

Location: at the junction of the lateral 1 / 3 and medial 2 / 3 of the distance between the great trochanter of femur and the hiatus of sacrum.

Indications: pain in the loins and legs and paralysis of the lower extremities.

Manipulation: *Gun, Dian, An* and *Ya* (heavy pressing).

Fengshi (GB 31)

Location: on the midline of the lateral aspect of the thigh, 7

Cun above the transverse popliteal crease.

Indications: paralysis of the lower extremities, soreness of the knee joint, and inflammation of the lateral cutaneous nerve of the thigh.

Manipulation: *Gun, Dian, An* and *Ca.*

Yanglingquan (GB 34)

Location: in the depression anterior and inferior to the small end of the fibula.

Indications: painful knee, hypochondriac pain, paralysis of the lower limbs, and cholecystitis.

Manipulation: *Na, Dian, An* and *Rou.*

Xuanzhong (GB 39)

Location: 3 *Cun* above the tip of the lateral malleolus, on the anterior border of the fibula.

Indications: headache, rigidity of the neck, soreness of the lower limbs, paralysis and disorders of the ankle joint.

Manipulation: *Na, Dian, An* and *Rou.*

Qiuxu (GB 40)

Location: Anterior and inferior to the lateral malleolus, in the depression on the lateral side of the tendon of m. extensordigitorum longus.

Indications: pain of the ankle joint, paralysis of the lower limbs, and pain in the chest and hypochondriac region.

Manipulation: *An, Dian, Na* and *Rou.*

12. The Liver Channel of Foot—Jueyin

This channel originates from the point Dadun (LR 1) at the tip of the big toe, runs upward along the dorsum of the foot, the anterior border of the medial malleolus and the medial aspects of the shank, the knee and the thigh to the pubic hair region, curves around the external genitalia, and goes upward to the lower abdomen. From there, it divides into two. One goes obliquely to the point Qimen (LR 14) between the two ribs inferior to the nipple. The other runs upward and curves around the stomach to enter the liver, the organ it belongs to, and connects with the gallbladder. Then, it continues to ascend, passing through the diaphragm and branching out in the chest and hypochondriac region. Further upward, it reaches the nasopharynx region along the posterior aspect of the throat, connecting with the "eye system". Finally, it ascends along the forehead to meet the Du Channel at the vertex.

The branch arising from the "eye system" runs downward into the cheek and curves around the inner surface of the lips.

The branch arising from the liver goes upward to pass the diaphragm, enters the lung and links with the Lung Channel of Hand—Taiyin.

The Liver Channel of Foot—Jueyin is exteriorly—interiorly related to the Gallbladder Channel. Along it, there are 28 points altogether, 14 on the left route, the same other 14 on the right route. The commonly used ones are as follows (Fig.63).

Taichong (LR 3)

Location: on the dorsum of the foot, in the depression distal to the juction of the 1st and 2nd metatarsals.

Indications: headache, vertigo, hypertension, pain in the hypochondriac region, infantile convulsion, mental disease and swelling and pain in the dorsum of the foot.

Manipulation: *An, Dian Rou* and *Yizhichan Tui.*

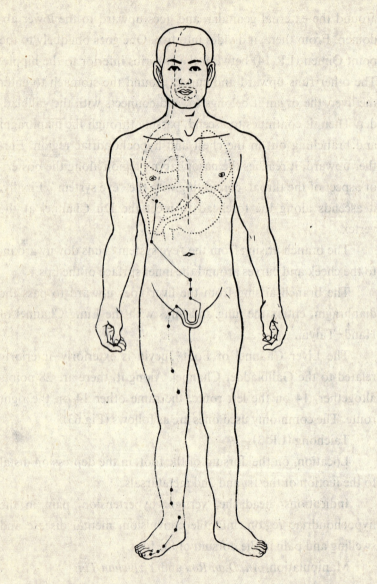

Fig.63

Zhangmen (LR 13)

Location: at the free end of the 11th rib.

Indications: distending pain in the chest and hypochondriac region, choking sensation in the chest and cholecystitis.

Manipulation: *An, Rou* and *Mó*.

Qimen (LR 14)

Location: directly below the nipple, in the 6th intercostal space.

Indications: distending pain in the chest and hypochondriac region, mastitis and disorders of the biliary tract.

Manipulation: *An, Mó* and *Rou*.

13. The Ren Channel

This channel originates in the lower abdomen and emerges from the perineum, It goes straight upward to the throat along the midline of the abdomen and chest. From there, it ascends to the point Chengjiang (RN 24). Ascending further, it curves around the lips, passes the cheek and enters the infraorbital region. (Fig. 64). Along it, there are 24 points altogether. The commonly used ones are as follows.

Qugu (RN 2)

Location: on the midline of the abdomen and on the upper border of the symphysis pubis.

Indications: nocturnal emission, impotence and retention of urine.

Manipulation: *An, Dian* and *Rou*.

Zhongji (RN 3)

Location: on the midline of the abdomen, 4 Cun below the umbilicus.

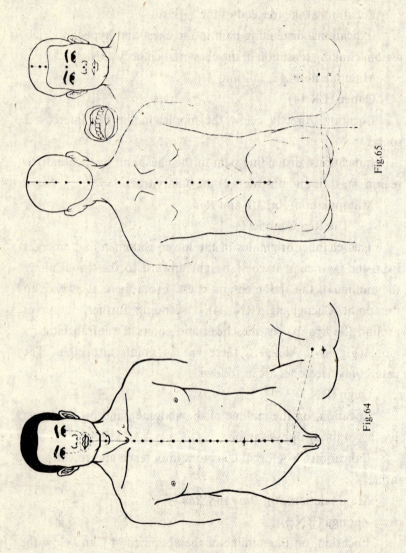

Fig.65

Fig.64

Indications: pain in the lower abdomen, enuresis, retention of urine, irregular menstruation and pelvic inflammation.

Manipulation: *Yizhichan Tui, Mó, Rou, Dian* and *An.*

Guanyuan (RN 4)

Location: 3 *Cun* below the umbilicus.

Indications: irregular menstruation, dysmenorrhea, nocturnal emission, impotence, enuresis and chronic diarrhea.

Manipulation: *Mó, Rou, An, Dian* and *Yizhichan Tui.*

Qihai (RN 6)

Location: 1.5 *Cun* below the umbilicus.

Indications: nocturnal emission, impotence, dysmenorrhea, diarrhea, enuresis, irregular menstruation.

Manipulation: *Mó, Rou, An, Zhen* and *Yizhichan Tui.*

Shenque (RN 8)

Location: in the centre of the umbilicus.

Indications: abdominal pain and diarrhea.

Manipulation: *Mó, An, Rou* and *Zhen.*

Zhongwan (RN 12)

Location: 4 *Cun* above the umbilicus.

Indications: stomachache, abdominal distension, vomiting and indigestion.

Manipulation: *Mó, An, Rou* and *Zhen.*

Danzhong (RN 17)

Location: on the midline of the abdomen, at the level of the 4th intercostal space.

Indications: cough and asthma, stuffiness and pain in the chest, hiccup, mastitis and angina pectoris.

Manipulation: *Yizhichan Tui, Mó, An* and *Rou.*

Tiantu (RN 22)

Location: at the centre of the suprasternal fossa.

Indications: cough with dyspnea, difficulty in coughing up sputum, aphasia and hiccup.

Manipulation: *Rou, An, Qia* (nipping) and *Dian.*

Lianquan (RN 23)

Location: above the Adam's apple, in the depression of the upper border of the hyoid bone.

Indications: aphasia, stiff tongue, difficulty in swallowing and laryngopharyngitis.

Manipulation: *An, Rou, Dian* and *Tanbo* (flicking–poking).

Chengjiang (RN 24)

Location: right in the centre of the mentolabial sulcus.

Indications: facial paralysis, prosopalgia and toothache.

Manipulation: *An, Rou* and *Qia* (nipping).

14. The Du Channel

This channel starts from in the lower abdomen and emerges from the perineum, and then goes backwards to the point Changqiang (DU 1). From there, it runs upward along the interior of the spinal column all the way, passing Fengfu (DU 16), entering the brain and reaching the vertex. Going furter, it winds along the forehead to the columnella of the nose, passes the point Renzhong (DU 26) or the groove of the upper lip, and ends at the point Yinjiao (DU 28) at the upper labial frenum (Fig. 65). Along this channel, there are 28 points, of which the following are commonly used.

Changqiang (DU 1)

Location: 0.5 *Cun* interior to the tip of the coccyx.

Indications: diarrhea, constipation, prolapse of the rectum, and pain in the waist and spine.

Manipulation: *Rou* and *An*.

Yaoyangguan (DU 3)

Location: below the spinous process of the 4th lumbar vertebra.

Indications: pain in the loins and spine, and paralysis of the lower limbs.

Manipulation: *Gun, Yizhichan Tui, An, Rou* and *Ca*.

Mingmen(DU 4)

Location: below the spinous process of the 2nd lumbar vertebra.

Indications: pain in the waist and spine, nocturnal emission, impotence, chronic diarrhea, irregular menstruation and dysmenorrhea.

Manipulation: *Gun, Yizhichan Tui, An, Rou* and *Ca*.

Shenzhu (DU 12)

Location: below the spinous process of the 3rd thoracic vertebra.

Indications: cough and backache.

Manipulation: *Gun, An, Rou* and *Yizhichan Tui*.

Dazhui (DU 14)

Location: below the spinous process of the 7th cervical vertebra.

Indications: common cold, fever, stiff neck, cough, asthma, and pain in the neck and back.

Manipulation: *Gun, An, Rou* and *Yizhichan Tui*.

Fengfu (DU 16)

Location: 1*Cun* directly above the midpoint of the posterior hairline.

Indications: neck rigidity, mental disorders and sequel of apoplexy.

Manipulation: *Yizhichan Tui, An, Rou* and *Dian.*

Baihui (DU 20)

Location: 7 *Cun* directly above the posterior hairline, on the midpoint of the line connecting the apexes of the two auricles.

Indications: headache, dizziness, coma, hypertension, prolapse of the rectum, and mental disorders.

Manipulation: *An, Rou, Yizhichan Tui* and *Zhen.*

Shuigou (DU 26) (This point is also called as Renzhong.)

Location: at the junction of the upper 1 / 3 and the lower 2 / 3 of the midline of the nasolabial groove.

Indications: infantile convulsion, facial paralysis, mental disorders, and acute sprain of the waist.

Manipulation: *Qia* (nipping) and *Rou.*

4.4 Commonly Used Extraordinary Points and the *Tuina* Manipulations Performed on Them

Yintang (EX−HN 3)

Location: at the midpoint between the medial ends of the two eyebrows.

Indications: headache, rhinitis and insomnia.

Manipulation: *Yizhichan Tui, Mŏ, An* and *Rou.*

Taiyang (EX−HE 5)

Location: in the depression about 1 *Cun* posterior to the midpoint between the lateral end of the eyebrow and the outer canthus.

Indications: headache, common cold and eye disease.

Manipulation: *An, Rou, Mó* and *Yizhichan Tui.*

Yuyao (EX—HN 4)

Location: at the midpoint of the eyebrow.

Indications: pain in the supraorbital region, redness, swelling and pain of the eyes, and twitching of the eyelids.

Manipulation: *Mó, Yizhichan Tui* and *An.*

Yaoyan (EX—B 7)

Location: in the depression 3 Cun lateral to the inferior border of the spinous process of the 3rd lumbar vertebra.

Indications: lumbar sprain and aching of the loins.

Manipulation: *Gun, An, Na* and *Ca.*

Jiaji (EX—B 2)

Location: on the line 0.5 *Cun* lateral to the inferior border of each spinous process from the 1st thoracic vertebra to the 5th lumbar vertebra.

Indications: pain and stiffness in the spinal column and diseases of the internal organs.

Manipulation: *Gun, Ca, Ya* (heavy pressing), *Tui* and *Yizhichan Tui.*

Shiqizhui (EX—B 8)

Location: below the spinous process of the 5th lumbar vertebra.

Indications: pain in the loins and legs and dysmenorrhea.

Manipulation: *Dian, Gun* and *An.*

Shixuan (EX—UE 11)

Location: at the tip of each of the ten fingers, 0.1 *Cun* away from the nail.

Indications: coma.

Manipulation: *Qia* (nipping).

Heding (EX−LE 2)

Location: in the depression at the centre of the upper border of the patella.

Indications: swelling and pain in the knee joint.

Manipulation: *An, Rou* and *Dian*.

Lanwei (EX−LE 7)

Location: about 2 *Cun* below the point Zusanli (ST 36).

Indications: appendicitis and abdominal pain.

Manipulation: *An, Rou* and *Dian*.

Jianneiling

Location: at the midpoint of the line connecting the tip of the anterior axillary fold and the point Jianyu (LI 15).

Indications: pain and motor impairment of the shoulder joint.

Manipulation: *Yizhichan Tui, Gun, Na, An* and *Rou*.

See Fig. 67, 68 and 69 for the location of the above points.

Qiaogong a special points

Location: along the line between the inferior and anterior of the temporal process and the point Quepen (ST 12) at the supraclavicular fossa.

Indications: headache, dizziness and hypertension.

Manipulation: pushing downwards with the thumb.

5 Exercises as the Basic Training of Manipulations

Traditional Tuina medicine attaches great importance to basic training through exercises, thinking that "the more the training, the better the curative effects". So, a *Tuina* learner has to do it for the following.

1. To improve the level of his health, especially to develop directionally his constitution, involving strength, durability, sensibility and flexibility which are what a *Tuina* physician has to have.

2. To obtain the breathing, the mind, the supplement of nutrients and energy, and the coordinating working between the nervous system, the endocrine system, the internal organs and the muscles, joints, ligaments of the manipulating organs, which are needed when he is performing any manipulation.

3. To reform and improve the local structure and function of the manipulating organs so as to ensure the effect and quality of manipulations.

4. Any exercise, if a patient does it in the clinic, will enhance the manipulations to raise the curative effects, which is called "treatment in the exterior integrated with exercise in the interior".

In troduced in the following are part of the skills of the main exercises as basic training— *Yijinjing* and *Shaolinneigong*.

5.1 *Yijinjing*

Yijinjing has twelve forms altogether, five of which are in the following.

1. Posture of *Weituoxianchu* (Fig. 69)

Description in the Original

Be in the standing posture with the body as upright as possible,

Curve the arms with the hands cupped each other before the chest,

Set the breathing even with the mind calmed,

Purify the spirits with the look naturalized.

Movements

Preparatory posture: standing upright.

(1) Step a pace leftward with the left foot to set the feet apart at the shoulders' width, with one foot parallel to the other, the soles and toes fixed on the ground, the legs erect, the popliteal portion slightly relaxed, the head as if supporting an object, the eyes looking straight ahead, the chest harbored, the abdomen restrained, the tongue against the palate, and the mouth slightly open. Following that, raise the arms laterally to the shoulder level to form a straight line, with the palms facing the ground and the five fingers of each hand closed.

(2) Move the two arms forward slowly to make the two palms meet together, with the fingertips pointing to the front.

(3) Make, slowly, the elbow joints 90° flexed, with the wrists, elbows and shoulders at the same level and the fingertips pointing upward.

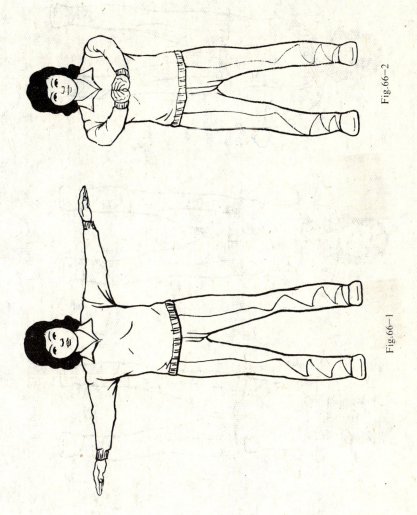

Fig.66—2

Fig.66—1

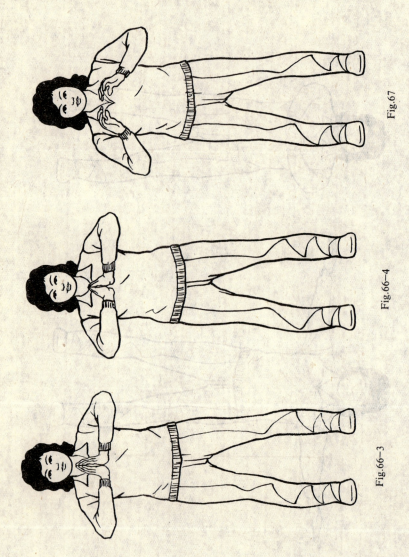

Fig.66-3   Fig.66-4   Fig.67

(4) Turn the arms and hands slowly inward to get the fingertips toward the chest and at the level of the point Tiantu (RN 22).

Essentials

Do the exercise with rapt attention, relax the muscles of all parts of the body, breathe by way of the abdomen with the inhaling quickly through the nose and the exhaling slowly through the mouth, concentrate the mind on Dantian and gather *Qi* in the lower abdomen. In the beginning, do it for 3 munites each time. 1—2 weeks later, the time may be increased by 1—2 munites each week up to 20 munites each time.

Note

Doing this exercise persistently may help develop the strength and durability of the shoulder girdle and the circumflex muscles of the forearm and improve the flexibility of the wrist joint so that the ability of the shoulders to suspend can be strengthened along with the durability and flexibility of the forearms to swing.

In addition, this exercise may be done by a patient like this.

(1) Do the same as (1) in the above.

(2) Move the hands forward until they are as if holding a ball before the chest, with either of the shoulders 45 ° abducted, the five fingers of either of the hands naturally apart and slightly flexed, the palms sunken and the five fingertips and the point Laogong of one hand pointing to those of the other one (Fig. 67).

2. Posture of *Zhaixinghuandou* (Fig.68)

Description in the Original

Put one palm over the head as if supporting the sky, Stare at the palm as if setting the eyes in its centre, Regulate the breath

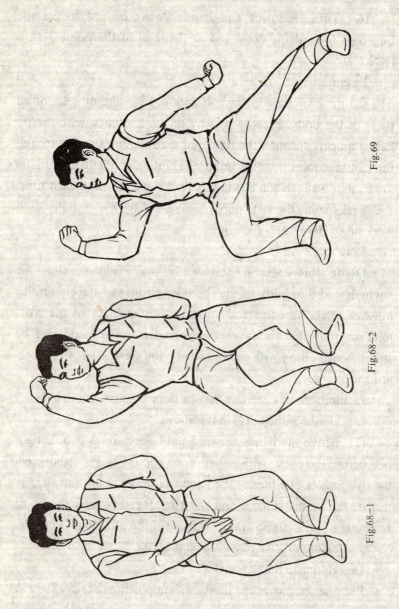

Fig.69

Fig.68—2

Fig.68—1

frequently by nasal inhaling, And shift the eyesight with effort to the other, Which has been put over the head instead.

Movements

Preparatory posture: standing upright.

(1) Step out a little forward-laterally with the right foot to form a T-shaped stance, the heel of the right foot pointing to the midpoint of the interior border of the left one with a space of one fist in between. The left hand is cupped and made to rest against the lumbosacral portion through flexing the elbow backward, at the same time, the right hand hangs anterior to the medial aspect of the right thigh.

(2) Bend the left leg to squat down slowly with the knee about 120°-160° flexed, and, meanwhile, lift the heel of the right foot with the tiptoe on the ground. The upper body is kept erect, its leaning forward or backward is not allowed.

(3) Raise the right hand, whose palm faces the ground and whose fingertips get together to look like a hook, slowly from between the two legs and along the midline of the abdomen and chest. When it reaches the level of the head, adduct the upper arm, rotate the forearm outward, hook the hand and flex the wrist until the shoulder is 90° protruded, the elbow 90° flexed and the wrist 90°-100° bent. Then, keep the right upper limb in this posture at the right side of the body.

(4) Turn the hooked fingertips slightly outward as far as possible, and, meanwhile, lift the head slightly right-upward to stare at the centre of the palm.

The above is consulted when this exercise is done with the left hand.

Essentials

Don't make the knees exceed the toes vertically when squatting. Support the weight of the whole body mainly with the back leg, leaving about 30% of the weight for the front leg to bear. Don't raise the hand too high and keep it only one-fist high above the head. Pinch the five fingers evenly and manage to make the forearm and the laterally-rotated fingertips abducted and the wrist flexed as far as possible for about 10 seconds to sense the soreness and distension produced in this way.

Then, repeat the above every 10 seconds or so until the time required for practice is up. While doing this exercise, be attentive, breathe in the same way as in "Posture of *Weituoxianchu*", ensure natural breathing, and do not hold breath when rotating the arm and generating strength. In the beginning, do this exercise for 1–2 munites each time. One week later, add 1 munite to each time per week until the time amounts to 7 munites. Then, add 1 munite to each time every two weeks until the time of practice for each time comes to 10–15 munites.

Note

This exercise may play a part in strengthening the supporting ability of the lower limbs, especially in developing the strength and endurance of the greater pectoral muscle, the deltoid muscle, the biceps muscle of the arm, the circum-lateral muscle of the forearm, and the flexor groups of the wrist, and in prolonging the posterior ligament of the wrist and the circum-medial muscle of the forearm to improve their flexibility and anti-pulling ability. As a result, doing this exercise may enhance the supporting ability of the shoulder to perform manipulations, the amplitude and durability of the suspended wrist to conduct *Yizhichan Tui*, the swinging strength and speed of the forearm to carry out *Gun*, and the ability of long—time standing to fulfil the long—time standing work. This exercise must be done perseveringly and mastered fully, for it takes an important place in the specialized training of *Tuina*. However, it should be done step by step and acting with undue haste is forbidden.

3. Posture of *Daozhuaijiuniuwei* (Fig.69)

Prescription in the Original

One leg is anteflexed and the other posteroextended,

In the lower abdomen relaxed *Qi* is cherished,

It is the shoulders that exert strength,

And the eyesight is set into the fist.

Movements

Preparatory posture: standing upright.

(1) Turn the upper body right—ward.

(2) Step out a big pace forward with the right leg, whose knee is then 90 ° flexed to form a forward lunge. The upper body is kept upright and a little sunken.

(3) The two hands are clenched into fists with their centres facing upward. The two arms are stretched, one forward and the other backward, with the two wrists slightly flexed and the two elbows 140 ° —150 ° flexed. The front fist is not higher than the level of the brows, the back fist is as high as the level of the lumbosacral region.

(4) Stare at the centre of the front fist. Vertically, the front elbow is kept not to exceed the front knee, and the front knee not to exceed the front foot. Turn with efforts the forearm outwards, the backarm inwards as if either of them was twisted like a string. (The strength exerted to do so is called spiral strength.) Harbor the chest a little straighten the back and gather *Qi* in the lower

abdomen.

Turn round with the left leg in the front and do the same as above.

Essentials

The muscles of the shoulder girdle are kept relaxed without lifting the shoulder. Strength is exerted by the arm intermittently, i.e., twisting an arm up to the time when soreness, distension and pain are sensed and keeping this situation for about 10 seconds, then starting another twisting 10 seconds later. Breathing is in the same way as that in the above posture. In the first week, do this exercise for 3 minutes each time. Later on, add 1 minute to each time every one week till 8—10 minutes for each session.

Note

This exercise plays its part mainly in developing the strength, endurance and antitension ability of the intorter and extortor of the forearm. It is of great help to the grasp of the manipulations *Gun, Tui, Ca*, etc.

4. Posture of *Sanpanluodi* (Fig.70)

Prescription in the Original

The tongue is rested tightly on the palate,

The eyes are open and the teeth are minded,

The feet are apart and the hips are lowered,

The lowering hands seem to get things held,

The rising palms seem supporting added weight,

The eyes are opened wide with the mouth closed,

The body is kept straight with the feet firmly—set.

Movements

Preparatory posture: standing upright.

(1) Step out a pace laterally with the left foot to set the feet

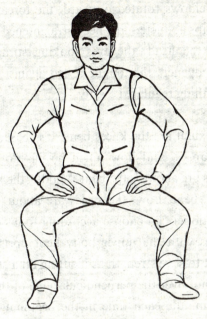

Fig.70

apart at the shoulders' width or a little more, with the toes slightly inward.

(2) Flex the kness and lower the hips. At the same time, turn the palms upward and raise them slowly to the level of the shoulders from the sides of the body and along the chest.

(3) Turn the palms upside down and lower them slowly with the fingers naturally relaxed as if pressing something. Put the palms above the knees with the part between the thumb and the index finger towards the body as if holding something. Incline the upper body a little forward.

(4) Turn the upper body upright with the chest slightly

sticked out, the back bow—like, the muscles of the shoulder girdle relaxed, the shoulders not raised, the shoulder joints about 50 ° abducted, the elbows rotated outward, the forearms rotated inward, the thumbs abducted, the neck straightened as if there were something on the head, the eyes looking straight ahead, the mouth slightly opened, the tongue rested aganist the palate, and the nasal—breathing regulated evenly.

Essentials

To what extent are the knees bent? It is based on how much a practioner can do and how much he has done the exercise. High, the knees are about 160 ° bent. Middle, the knees are about 150 ° — 140 ° bent. Low, the knees are about 100 ° — 120 ° bent. The practioner can choose according to his own condition. Bend the knees with the upper body kept upright without inclining forward to save strength as if sitting on a stool. The knees are protruded not over the perpendicular line of the toes. Do this exercise for 1 minute each time in the beginning. Later, add 1 minute to each time every one week until the time for each time comes to 5 minutes.

Note

Doing this exercise can enhance the strength, endurance and anti—tension ability of the muscles of the axillae and arms, develop long—time supporting ability of the lower extremities and strengthen the legs and waist, thus making it easy to exert strength and saving the energy of the arms while manipulations are being performed.

5. Posture of *Wohupushi* (Fig.71)

Prescription in the Original

Set the feet apart and squat with the body inclined forward,

Flex and stretch the legs with the left **bent and the** right straight,

Hold the head high with the chest thrown forward,

And strengthen the back, lower the waist to get the body stable,

Inhale and exhale by the nose with the breathing evenly regulated,

Support the body with the fingertips put on the ground,

Mimic the posture of a prone tiger being ready to pounce,

And master this exercise for the health*'s sake.

Movements

Preparatory posture: standing upright.

(1) Step out a big pace forward with the left foot and bend the knee at an angle of 90 degrees, stretch the right leg with the toes aganist the ground, thus forming a left forward lunge.

(2) Extend the arms forward and place the fingers on the ground for support with the palms not touching the ground, lift the heel of the back foot, raise the head and look straight ahead.

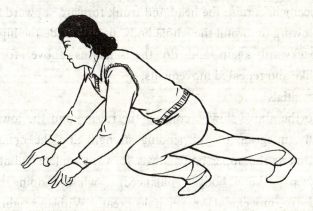

Fig.71-1

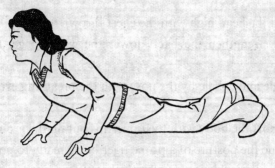

Fig.71-2

(3) Retire the front foot and extend the leg backward, put the dorsum of the retired foot on the heel of the back foot, harbor the chest and abdomen a little, straighten the trunk, and hold the head up.

(4) Pull the body backward with the hip portion protruded backward and the elbows straightened. Then, bend the elbows slowly and lower the head and trunk to the front as if a prone tiger were about to pounce on its prey. When the head is lowered up to about 2 *Cun* from the ground, stretch the elbows slowly, and, meanwhile, raise the head and trunk forward—upward slowly. Following that, pull the whole body and protrude the hip portion backward again and do the same as above, forming wave—like and repeated movements.

Essentials

Do the above slowly, connect the raising and the lowering naturally, integrate the suspending strength and the breathing closely, move the upper body slowly forward while exhaling, try to keep the body balanced, while doing the to—and—fro—movements, never hold breath. With the right foot in the front, the same is done. In the beginning , the fingers and palms may be used together for support, only the fingers are used after the arms and fingers become stronger, and, finally, it is best to use the three fingers: the thumbs, the index fingers and the middle fingers. Make advances step by step in doing this exercise according to your own condition.

Note

Doing this exercise can enhance the strength and endurance of the muscles of the shoulder girdle, the brachial triceps muscle and the biceps muscle of the arm and develop the supporting and anti—tension ability of the fingers. Long—time practice of it can thicken, strengthen and toughen the joints, ligaments and joint capsules of the fingers. All the above will help a *Tuina* physician to exert strong and persistent finger's strength and forearm's pushing—pulling force and to protect himself from being hurt while he is performing the manipulations *Tui, Na, Dian, An, Ca, Gun,* etc.

5.2　Shaolinneigong

Shaolinneigong consists of many forms. Introduced in the following are only four common forms of the exercise and the basic stances. They can be practised independently or alternately.

1. Basic Stances

(1) Posture of standing (Fig.72)

Preparatory Posture　Standing upright.

Movements

Set the feet apart with the distance in between a little longer than that between the shoulders and the toes of either one turned inward. Fix the lower limbs with great effort, with the head upright, the eyes looking straight ahead, the breathing natural, the shoulders dropped, the chest sticked out, the scapulae closer to the spinal column, the loins relaxed, the lower abdomen restrained, the hip portion a little harbored, the arms akimbo, the thumbs at the back and the other fingers in the front, thus being ready for the exercise.

Essentials

"Fix the lower limbs with great effort" refers to getting the ten toes sticking to the ground while directing outward–rotating and tightly–holding strength to the heels and thighs so as to stand firmly.

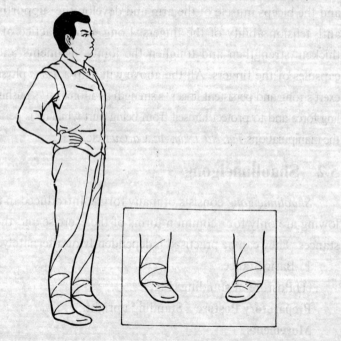

Fig.72

(2) Posture of Horse–riding (Fig.73)

Preparatory Posture Standing upright.

Movements

Set the feet apart with the distance in between a little longer than that between the shoulders and the toes turned inward. Bend the knees which do not exceed the toes vertically and squat down, with the head upright, the eyes looking straight ahead, the chest thrown out, the waist straightened, the hips sunken but not protruded backward, and the arms akimbo (Fig.73), thus being ready for the exercise.

Essentials

The extent of squatting falls into three: high, middle and low. For the details, see 5.1, 4. please. One can choose any of them according to his own condition.

(3) Posture of Forward Lunge (Fig.74)

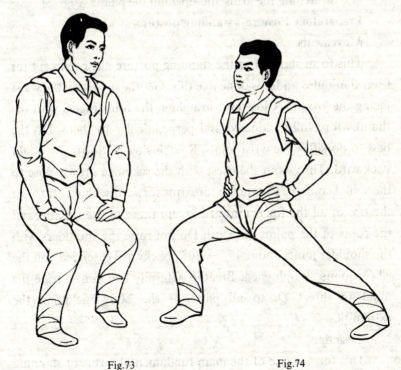

Fig.73   Fig.74

Preparatory Posture   standing upright.

Movements

Set the feet apart with one in the front and the other at the back, the distance between them being about 1 time longer than that between the shoulders. Bend the front knee with the toes turned inward and the shank about vertical. Straighten the back leg with effort, the toes being slightly abducted. Keep the head upright, the eyes looking straight ahead, the chest thrown out, the waist relaxed, the abdomen harbored, the hips restrained, and the arms akimbo, thus being ready for the exercise.

2. Common Forms of *Shaolinneigong*

(1) Stretching the arms and opening the palms (Fig.75)

Preparatory Posture   standing posture.

Movements

This form starts after the standing posture has been kept for several minutes and it is done like this. Get the palms on the waist facing the ground. Close and straighten the four fingers with the thumbs forcefully abducted and perpendicular to them. Do the best to dorsiflex the wrist joints. Stretch slowly the arms straight backward. Throw out the chest with the scapulae drawn close to the spinal column. Rotate the forearms forward with effort to get the tips of all the fingers inward except those of the thumbs and the roots of the palms outward. Do not raise the shoulders with the shoulder joints about 45 ° —30 ° backward extended and the elbow joints straightened. Breathe naturally and concentrate the mind to direct *Qi* to all parts of the body including the extremities.

Essentials

This form is one of the main fundamental forms of standing

posture of *Shaolinneigong*. It requires "three straightness and four levelness", i.e., the straightness of the arms, the trunk, the legs and the levelness of the head, the shoulders, the palms and the feet. It may start following the posture of horse–riding or the posture of forward lunge. The time to do it each time is 1 minute in the beginning and increases gradually up to 10 minutes.

Effect

Long–time of practising this form may have *Qi* directed at will, essence produced by *Qi*, vitality enriched by essence, the mind in full swing, *Zang* and *Fu* functioning well, *Qi* turned to strength, the body and the limbs provided with strength, and the force and endurance of the arms, waist and legs increased.

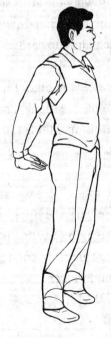
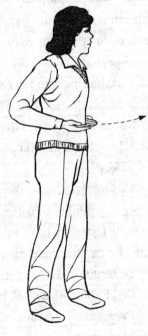

Fig.75   Fig.76

(2) Pushing eight horses forward (Fig.76)

Preparatory Posture standing posture, posture of horse—riding or posture of forward lunge.

The two elbows are 90° flexed with the palms turned upward, the thumbs abducted and strengthened to make them nearly perpendicular to the other four fingers.

Movements

A. Direct strength to the arms and the fingertips and push the arms slowly forward with effort. Meanwhile, rotate the arms inward until they are at the level of the shoulders with the palms facing each other, the thumbs pointing upward and the elbows fully stretched.

B. While flexing the elbows and withdrawing the arms slowly with effort to get the hands returned to the hypochondriac portions, rotate the arms outward and turn the palms upward.

Essentials

Pushing—pulling the two arms or one after the other for 3—5 times is conducted each time. The way of breathing and of leg—force—exerting are the same as what is mentioned in (1) "stretching the arms and opening the palms".

Effect

Ensuring that the lower extremities have stable supporting—ability and they can coordinate with the upper ones while the latter are moving. And that the strength—exerting of the upper limbs and the mainipulations can be smoothly conducted may be resulted in if long—time practice is undertaken.

(3) Pulling nine oxen backward (Fig.77)

Preparatory Posture the same as the above.

Movements

A. While pushing the arms slowly forward, rotate the forearms slowly inward until the elbows are fully stretched, the palms being turned outward with the dorsums of the hands facing each other and thumbs pointing downward.

B. While changing the palms into clenched fists and flexing the elbows to retire the fists, rotate the forearms outward as if pulling a strong ox backward by the tail until the fists reach the costal regions, and, then, extend the fingers with the palms pointing upward (returned to the preparatory posture). Do the above after a pause and repeating 3—5 times is enough.

(4) An overlord who is holding up a tripod (Fig.78)

Preparatory Posture　the same as the above.

Movements

A. Raise with effort the palms facing upward slowly upward as if sustaining a heavy object. As soon as the palms are high above the shoulders, rotate the arms slowly inward until the elbows are fully stretched, with the four fingers of one hand closed and pointing to those of the other, the thumbs abducted and straightened, the palms upward, and the roots of the palms outward.

B. After a pause, rotate the forearms slowly outward and get the palms facing the face with the fingertips upward. Lower the palms with effort from before the chest to the costal regions. After a while, repeat the above 3—5 times.

(5) A lotus leaf which is being swaying by the wind (Fig.79)

Preparatory Posture　the same as the above.

Movements

A. Push the palms facing upward slowly for—up—ward with effort until the elbows are fully stretched. Then, cross the palms

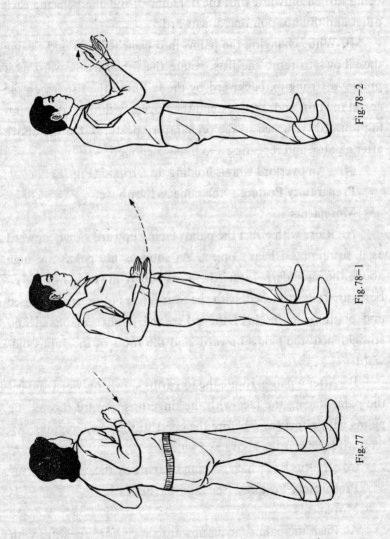

Fig.78-2

Fig.78-1

Fig.77

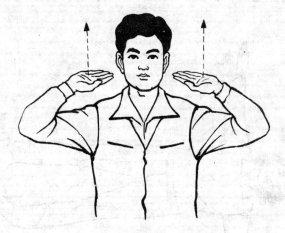

Fig.78-3

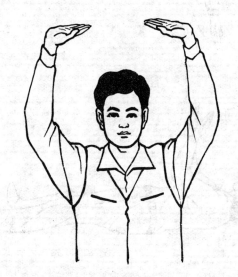

Fig.78-4

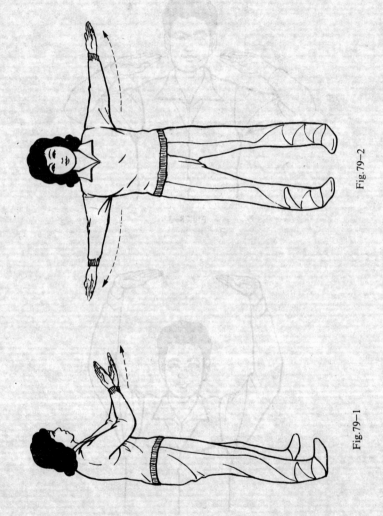

Fig.79-2

Fig.79-1

in front of the chest with the left above the right or vice versa, the distance between them being 1−2 *Cun*.

B. Get the arms apart, one leftward and the other rightward. While doing so, the palms are kept in the pose of holding up an object. After the shoulder joints are 90° abducted, get the arms moving inward until they reach the front. Then, cross the palms again and draw them to the sides of the waist. Keep the ending pose for a while, and do the above again. 3−5 times of re−doing is enough.

(6) The black dragon which is entering a cave (Fig.80)

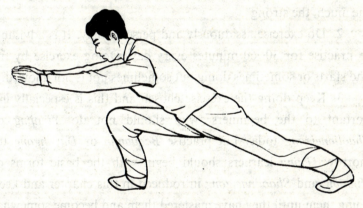

Fig.80

Preparatory Posture   keeping oneself in the pose of wide forward− lunge with the elbows bent and the palms stretched at the sides of the waist.

Movements

A. As pushing the palms facing each other slowly forward, turn them inward gradually until they face the ground, the fingertips pointing forward. The upper body inclines forward fol−lowing the forward−pushing palms. But stand firm with the bent tips of the toes.

B. After the elbows are fully stretched, rotate the arms outward and get the palms gradually facing upward. At the same time, flex with effort the elbows to withdraw the palms to the sides of the costal regions. Keep the ending pose for a while, do the above again, and repeating 3—5 times is enough.

5.3 Points for Attention in Doing Exercises

1. Do exercise in an orderly way and step by step. Arrange reasonably the duration and amount of exercise—doing. Follow the principle "from the simple, the less, the mild to the complex, the much, the strong".

2. Do exercise assiduously and perseveringly. It is advisable to practise for 30—60 minutes every day. Doing exercise by fits and starts or sometimes doing but sometimes not is not allowed.

3. Keep doing the exercise chosen and this is especially important to the beginners, who should not do *Yijinjing* or *Shaolinneigong* today but practise *Baduanjin* or *Dayangong* tomorrow. *Tuina* learners should begin with the basic forms of *Yijinjing* and *Shaolinneigong* introduced in this chapter and keep doing them until they have mastered them and become somewhat skilled. Then, try some others.

4. In the course of doing exercise, concentrate your mind and avoid making joke, holding breath, pressing yourself to do or doing unreasoningly. No matter whatever abnormality may occur such as dizziness, chest stuffiness or pain and irritability, ask the teacher for help in order to prevent deviation or injury.

5. The room in which exercise is done should be quiet, well—lit, air—conditioned and well—ventilated. The exerciser

should be protected from being exposed to cold wind.

6. Loose clothes and cloth shoes with soft soles, gym shoes or special exercise shoes are suitable for doing exercise but much or tight clothes and leather shoes or high−heel shoes are not.

7. Morning is the best time for doing exercise. Do not do exercise when the following just occur: over−intake, empty stomach, stenuous exercise or tiredness. When finishing or stopping to have a rest, wipe the sweat with a dry towel and put on the taken−off clothes, but do not be fanned or take a cold bath immediately, and do not take cold food or drink either. After the practice is ended, the body may be limbered so as to regulate *Qi* and blood, warm tea or nutritious drinks may be taken so as to supplement body fluid and nutrients.

8. Female should not do exercise in periods and pregnancy.

6 Treatment of Common Adult Diseases

6.1 Common Cold

As an exopathic disease common in the four seasons, especially in winter and spring, common cold is manifested mainly as headache, nasal obstruction, running nose, aversion to wind, and fever. Its course is usually 3—7 days.

Etiology and Pathology

It is mainly due to weakness of vital—Qi, sudden change of weather and affection of wind—cold or wind—heat. In winter, it is usually due to wind—cold, while in spring, usually due to wind—heat.

1. Type of Wind—cold: attack of the superficies of the body by pathogenic cold, obstruction of sweat pores, shut of striae of skin, and dysfunction of the lung—Qi.

2. Type of Wind—heat: heat produced due to retention of wind—cold, the heat staying in the superficies of the pulmonary system, and dysfunction of the lung—Qi.

Clinical Manifestations

1. Type of Wind—cold: chills, fever, absence of sweat, headache, soreness of the limbs, nasal obstruction, running nose, cough, watery sputum, thin and whitish tongue coating, and floating and tense pulse.

2. Type of Wind—heat:fever, slight aversion to wind, disturbed sweating, pain and distension in the head, cough with yellowish and thick sputum, sore throat, dry mouth with desire for drink, thin and yellowish tongue coating, and floating and rapid pulse.

Treatment

1. Therapeutic Method: facilitating the flow of the lung—*Qi* to relieve exterior syndrome, and expelling wind—cold or wind—heat.

2. Manipulation: *Yizhichan Tui, Mó, Na, An* and *Rou.*

3. Point Selection: Fengchi (GB 20), Fengfu (DU 16), Tianzhu (BL 10), Fengmen(BL 12), Feishu (BL 13), Yintang (EX—HN 3), Taiyang (EX—HE 5), Touwei (ST 8) and Hegu (LI 4).

4. Operation:

(1) *Tui* or *An* and *Rou* each of the points Fengchi, Fengfu, Tianzhu Dazhu (BL 11) and Fengmen 5—7 times with the parts around the points manipulated for longer time.

(2) *Tui* or *An* and *Rou* is done along the line where the points Yintang, shenting (DU 24), Touwei and Taiyang are located and along the line where the points Yintang, Yuyao (EX—HN 4) and Taiyang are distributed.

(3) *Mó* is done from Yintang to Shenting, from Yintang to Taiyang and along the line where the points Touwei, Shuaigu (GB 8), Naokong (GB 19) and Fengchi are distributed.

(4) *Na* Fengchi, the posterior major tendons of the neck and Jianjing (GB 21).

(5) *An* and *Rou* Fengmen, Jianjing, Feishu, and finally *Na* Jianjing and Hegu.

5. Supplement:

(1) For type of wind-cold, *Gun* is done on Jianjing, Fengmen and Feishu, and *Tui* is done with the palm over the interscapular region until heat is produced.

(2) For type of wind-heat, *Tui* or *An* and *Rou* Fengfu and Dazhui (DU 14) and *Qia* (nipping) and *Rou* Hegu.

(3) For obstruction of the nose, *An* and *Rou* Yingxiang (LI 20).

(4) For sore and swollen throat, *Qia* (nipping) Shaoshang(LU 11) and Shangyang (LI 1).

(5) For difficulty in coughing up sputum, *Rou* Tiantu (RN 22) and Danzhong (RN 17).

6. Treatment Course: Treatment is given once daily. 3 times make 1 course of treatment.

6.2 Headache

Headache is a subjective symptom. It is common in many acute or chronic diseases.

Tuina is not suitable for the treatment of such intracranial disorders as brain abscess, cerebrovascular disease in its acute period, and intracranial space occupying lesion, brain contusion and traumatic intracranial hematoma in their acute stage. In general, headache due to other diseases may be relieved by *Tuina*, which is especially effective in treating migraine, muscular contraction, common cold and hypertension.

Etiology and Pathology

1. Headache due to Exopathy: Improper work and rest and irregular life provide a chance for the six pathogenic factors to in-

vade the body. They go upward along the channels to disturb the lucid *Yang*, causing headache.

2. Headache due to Internal Injury: It may be resulted from the liver impaired by rage, phlegm produced in the spleen, deficiency of the kidney, and insufficiency of marrow.

Clinical Manifestations

1. Headache due to Exopathy: headache, stiff neck, fever and chills which are worsened by wind, nasal obstruction, running nose and thin and whitish tongue coating, which are the signs due to wind–cold; distending pain and even splitting pain of the head, flushed face, reddened eyes, constipation, deep–colored urine, reddened tongue with yellowish coating, and floating and rapid pulse, which are the signs due to wind–heat.

2. Headache due to Hyperactivity of the Liver–*Yang*: distending pain of the head, vertigo, tinnitus, vexation, irritability, insomnia, dreamfulness, flushed face, bitter taste in the mouth, reddened tongue with thin and yellowish coating, and taut, forceful pulse.

Treatment

1. Therapeutic Method: relieving pain through dispelling wind and removing obstruction in the channels. Headache due to exopathy should be treated through dispelling wind and cold to relieve pain, while headache due to internal injury, through calming the liver to suppress *Yang* hyperactivity, promoting blood circulation to remove blood stasis, and dredging the channels.

2. Manipulation: *Tui*, *Na*, *An* and *Mŏ*.

3. Point Selection: Yintang (EX–HN 3), Touwei (ST 8), Taiyang (EX–HE 5), Yuyao (EX–HN 4), Baihui (DU 20), Fengchi (GB 20), Fengfu(DU 16), Tianzhu (BL 10), Feishu(BL

13), Fengmen (BL 12) and Hegu (LI 4).

4. Operation:

(1) Stand behind the patient in the sitting position and *Tui* Fengchi, Fengfu and Tianzhu for about 5 minutes.

(2) Let the patient take the sitting posture and conduct *Yizhichan Tui* from Yintang and Yuyao to Taiyang for 5 minutes. Then, *An* and *Rou* the points Jiaosun (SJ 20) and Baihui for about 3 minutes.

5. Supplement:

(1) If headache of wind—cold type is treated, *Qia* (nipping) and *Rou* Dazhui (DU 14), Quchi (LI 11) and Hegu.

(2) If headache of wind—heat type is treated, *An* and *Rou* Feishu and Fengmen.

(3) If headache due to hyperactivity of the liver—*Yang* is treated, *Tui* Qiaogong and *Qia* (nipping) and *Rou* Taichong (LR 3).

6. Treatment Course: Treatment is given once daily. 6 times of treatment make 1 course of treatment.

6.3   Insomnia

Being hard to go to sleep, easy to wake, dreamful and even awake all night are characteristic of insomnia.

Etiology and Pathology

1. Over—thinking impairs the heart and spleen. The heart impaired *Yin*—blood will be consumed gradually. The spleen impaired, food essence can not be produced, blood can not be supplemented, and the heart can not be nourished. Under this condition, the mind will be disturbed to cause insomnia.

2. Improper diet hurts the intestines and stomach, leading to retention of food or accumulation of phlegm—heat in the stomach. This will disorder the stomach—*Qi* and disturb the mind, causing insomnia. Generally speaking, insomnia is due to *Yang* in excess, *Yin* in insufficiency and imbalance of *Yin* and *Yang*.

Clinical Manifestations

1. Insomnia due to deficiency of *Qi* and blood in the heart and spleen is marked by dreamfulness, no sound sleep, palpitation, amnesia, pale complexion, acratia of the limbs, emaciation, listlessness, poor appetite, sleeplessness or staying awake all night, pale tongue with thin coating, and thready, weak pulse.

2. Insomnia due to deficiency of *Yin* and hyperactivity of fire is marked by distension of the head, deafness, tinnitus, irritability, sleeplessness, palpitation, restlessness, dizziness and amnesia.

3. Insomnia due to disorder of the stomach—*Qi* is marked by sleeplessness, distension and fullness in the stomach and abdomen, loss of appetite, hiccup, eructation and disturbed sleep.

4. Insomnia due to weakness in the convalescence is marked by weakness of the body, sleeplessness, pale complexion, emaciation, acratia, night sweating, spontaneous sweating and tending to wake after going to sleep.

Treatment

1. Therapeutic Method: Soothing the liver to remove heat and regulating the stomach to calm the mind is applicable to the syndrome of excess type. Strengthening the spleen to replenish *Qi* and tranquilizing the mind is suitable for the syndrome of deficiency type.

2. Manipulation: *Na, Mǒ, An, Rou* and *Cuo*.

3. Point Selection: Fengchi (GB 20), Fengfu (DU 16), Naokong (GB 19), Yintang (EX-HN 3), Jingming (BL 1), Yingxiang (LI 20), Renzhong (DU 26), Chengjiang (RN 24) and Jiaosun (SJ 20).

4. Operation:

(1) Stand behind the patient in the sitting position, prop his / her forehead with one hand, open the five fingers of the other with the middle finger put on the Du Channel of his / her head, the index and ring fingers put on the region which the Bladder Channel of Foot—Taiyang goes through, and *Na* is carried out with the five fingers to and fro 3—5 times from the front hairline to the occipitoposterior portion. Then, *Na* Fengchi and Naokong. Finally, *Mǒ* alternately with the bellies of the two thumbs the sternocleidomastoid muscles on the both sides of the neck from the above to the below and do this 10—20 times.

(2) Stand right before the patient in the sitting position, *Mǒ* with the two thumbs the area from Yintang to Shenting (DU 24), *An* Jingming, *Mǒ* the area from Cuanzhu (BL 2) to Sizhukong (SJ 23), *An* and *Rou* with the thumbs each of all the above points 3—5 times *Tui* rapidly downward from Touwei to Jiaosun alternately with the sides of the thumb—radius of the two thumbs, and, finally, *An* and *Rou* the points Anmian I (Extra) and Anmian II (Extra) each for 1—2 minutes.

(3) Stand at the left or right side of the patient in the sitting position, prop his / her shoulder with one hand, *Ca* his / her chest with the other repeatedly to and fro and up and down, then, *Ca* his / her back with the hand proping the shoulder or with the other hand supporting the shoulder instead. Finally, stand behind

the patient and *Ca* his / her costal regions with the two palms until they feel warm.

(4) Stand before the patient in the sitting position, *Na* Neiguan (PC 6) 50 times and *Dian—rou* Daling (PC 7) 50 times, both with the right thumb.

5. Treatment Course: Treatment is given once daily 12 times make 1 course of treatment.

6.4   Diarrhea

Diarrhea, also called as "loose stools", refers to too many times of defecating with thin or even watery stools, In modern medicine, it includes those due to the functional and organic changes of the stomach, intestines, liver, gallbladder and pancreas, such as acute or chronic enteritis.

Etiology and Pathology

The pathologic change of diarrhea is taken place mainly in the spleen and stomach and the large and small intestines. Its etiology includes two: external and internal. External, the exopathogens invade the body. Internal, improper diet weakens *Zang* and *Fu* so as to cause them to dysfunction. But the direct cause of diarrhea is as follows: The pathogenic dampness attacks the spleen and weakens it, the weakened spleen dysfunctions and it can not turn food into essence, and water and dampness are accumulated in the body with diarrhea caused at last.

Remarkable curative effects are seen when *Tuina* is used to treat prolonged diarrhea due to weakness of *Zang* and *Fu* or decline of the fire from the gate of life.

Clinical Manifestations

1. Diarrhea due to weakness of the spleen and stomach is marked by intermittent and repeated loose stools with indigested food times of defecating increased obviously whenever a little greasy food is eaten, poor appetite, discomfort in the epigastrium occurring after the intake of food, sallow complexion, listlessness, pale tongue with whitish coating, and slow, weak pulse.

2. Diarrhea due to weakness of the kidney—*Yang* is marked by pain around the umbilicus occurring before dawn which is followed by borborygmus and diarrhea, the pain relieved after diarrhea, cold body and limbs, pale tongue with white coating, and deep, thready pulse.

Treatment

1. Therapeutic Method: strengthening the spleen, warming the kidney, removing dampness and relieving diarrhea.

2. Manipulation: *Yizhichan Tui, Mó, An, Rou* and *Na*.

3. Point Selection: Zhongwan (RN 12), Qihai (RN 6), Guanyuan (RN 4), Tianshu (ST 25), Zusanli (ST 36), Pishu (BL 20), Weishu (BL 21) and Dachangshu(BL 25).

4. Operation:

(1) Let the patient in the supine position, conduct gentle and slow *An—rou* along Zhongwan, Shenque (RN 8) and Guanyuan of the Ren Channel to and fro 5—6 times, and then, *Mó* the abdomen counterclockwise for about 3 minutes.

(2) Let the patient in the prone position, undertake *Gun* for about 2 minutes along the Bladder Channel and from the above to the below, and, then, *An—rou* Ganshu (BL 18), Shenshu (BL 23), Pishu, Weishu and Dachangshu until the sensation of soreness and distension takes place.

(3) Let the patient in the supine position with his / her low-

er limbs slightly flexed, *An-rou* Zusanli for about 2 minutes. Then, let the patient in the prone position and undertake *Tui* with one thumb from below the tendo calcaneus to Chengshan (BL 57) where forceful pressing is done as the ending maneuver. Do the above to and fro 7—8 times and conduct such *Tui* in the same way on the other leg. Such *Tui* is especially suitable for the treatment of diarrhea due to simple dyspepsia.

5. Supplement:

(1) If diarrhea is due to improper diet, *Rou* Shangwan (RN 13).

(2) If the hyperactive liver—*Qi* attacks the spleen, *Rou* Ganshu, Qimen (LR 14) and Zhangmen (LR 13).

(3) If there exists *Yang*—deficiency of the spleen and kidney, *An* Jingmen (GB 25) and Guanyuan.

6. Treatment Course: Treatment is carried out 1 time daily and 3 times comprise 1 course of treatment.

6.5　Epigastralgia

Epigastralgia is a syndrome of the digestive system, whose main symptom is pain in the upper abdomen. It includes gastriculcer, acute or chronic gastritis, gastrospasm, gastroneurosis, cholecystitis, pancreatitis and cholelithiasis.

Etiology and Pathology

1. Attack of the stomach by pathogens: Affection of exogenous cold pathogen or over—intake of raw and cold food leads to accumulation of cold in the stomach, causing pain. Improper diet or over—intake of heavy food leads to production of dampness in the interior, also causing hot pain or pain due to

indigested food.

2. Imbalance between *Zang* and *Fu:* Epigastralgia may be caused by the following: dysfunction of the liver due to stagnation of its *Qi,* original weakness of the spleen and stomach, overstrain, and irregular diet.

Clinical Manifestations

1. Attack of the stomach by cold pathogen: sudden pain occurring in the epigastrium which is worsened by cold but relieved by heat, local comfort resulted from heat, absence of thirst and desire for drink, borborygmus followed by watery stools, whitish tongue coating, and tense pulse.

Epigastralgia due to retention of food is marked by distending pain, foul eructation, acid regurgitation, pain relieved after vomiting, inability to defecate smoothly, and thick, greasy tongue coating.

2. Imbalance between *Zang* and *Fu:* Epigastralgia due to insufficiency of the spleen−*Yang* is marked by dull pain in the epigastrium, vomiting clear watery thing, comfort resulted from warmth and pressing, cold hands and feet, loose thin stools, light reddish tongue with thin and white coating, and soft, weak or deep, thready pulse. That due to stagnation of the liver−*Qi* is marked by belching, pain in the hypochondria, and taut pulse.

Treatment

Tuina is effective remarkably in treating epigastralgia, especially in treating that due to imbalance between *Zang* and *Fu*. It may be cured after a period of treatment. Acute stomachache may be relieved by pressing and kneading more forcefully and continuously about for 2 minutes the pressure pain point on the back or the stomach point on the 2nd metacarpal bone. By and large, *Tuina* is clinically used to regulate the flow of *Qi* for the purpose of relieving pain. Yet, the cause of epigastralgia need to be carefully investigated through analysing the symptoms, and the treatment must be based on overall differentiation. For example, epigastralgia due to stagnation of the liver—*Qi* should be treated through soothing the liver and regulating the flow of *Qi;* epigastralgia due to weakness of the spleen and stomach, through warming the middle—*Jiao* to dispel cold; epigastralgia due to retention of blood in the interior, through promoting blood circulation to remove blood stasis. But *Tuina* should not be used to treat gastroduodenal ulcer in its bleeding stage for fear that hematorrhea be led to.

1. Treatment of Sudden Epigastralgia

(1) Point Selection: Ashi (non—fixed point), Ganshu (BL 18), Danshu (BL 19),Pishu (BL 20), Weishu (BL 21), Zusanli (ST 36), Neiguan (PC 6) and the Ashi points around Pishu and Weishu.

(2) Manipulation: *An, Rou, Na* and *Zhen.*

(3) Operation:

A. Stand at the right side of the patient in the prone position, explore with the right thumb along the Bladder Channel of Foot—Taiyang and from the above to the below the pressure pain points around Pishu and Weishu and press them for 1 minute, and *An—rou* either of Pishu and Weishu for 1—2 minutes or until the epigastralgia is relieved.

B. Sit at the right side of the patient in the supine position, *Qia* (nipping) and *Na* with the right thumb and index finger Neiguan and Zusanli on the either side 30—50 times, ending the treatment. If the pain has not be stopped, repeat A. and B. until it is stopped.

(4) Treatment Course: Treatment is given once daily. 3 times of treatment make 1 course.

2. Treatment of Epigastralgia due to Insufficiency of the Spleen—*Yang*

(1) Point Selection: Shangwan (RN 13), Zhongwan (RN 12), Guanyuan (RN 4), Qihai (RN 6), Geshu (BL 17), Ganshu (BL 18), Pishu (BL 20), Weishu (BL 21), Zusanli (ST 36) and Neiting (SI 44).

(2) Manipulation: *Yizhichan Tui, An, Zhen, Mó* and *Na*.

(3) Operation:

A. Sit at the right side of the patient in the supine position. Firstly undertake light rapid and gentle *Yizhichan Tui* repeatedly for 2—3 minutes along Shangwan, Zhongwan, Xiawan (RN 10), Qihai and Guanyuan. Secondly, press Zhongwan with the right middle finger, which moves up and down following the breathing of the patient, and press it gradually harder for about 1 minute. Thirdly *An* Qihai and Guanyuan each for half a minute, and *Mó* Zhongwan for 1 minute. Finally, stand up, put the two middle fingers on the patient's lumbar portion with one on one side, the two thumbs on Tianshu (ST 25) by the umbilicus with one at one side, make the thumb and the middle finger of either hand work together to conduct forceful *Na* 3—5 times, and *Zhen* Zhongwan with the palm for 2 minutes.

B. Take the same posture as above, *Na* with the right thumb and the middle finger either of Zusanli and Neiting 3—5 times or until local soreness appears.

C. Stand at the right side of the patient in the prone position, carry out *Yizhichan Tui* along the Bladder Channel of

Foot−Taiyang on the back and from the above to the below and do this 4−5 times, and, then, *An−rou* with proper pressure Ganshu, Pishu, Weishu and Sanjiaoshu (BL 22) for about 1−2 minutes.

(4) Treatment Course: Treatment is given once daily. 6 times of treatment make 1 course.

3. Treatment of Epigastralgia due to Attack of the Stomach by the hyperactive liver−*Qi*.

(1) Point Selection: Qimen (LR 14), Zhangmen (LR 13), Jiquan (HT 1) and Jianjing (GB 21).

(2) Manipulation: *An, Mó, Na* and *Mo*.

(3) Operation:

A. Sit at the right side of the patient in the supine position, conduct *Mó* for 2−3 minutes along the liver region and from the above to the below, and, then, *An* either of Qimen and Zhangmen for 1 minute.

B. Stand behind the patient who sits upright with his ∕ her head held by his ∕ her own hands, perform *Mǒ* 40−50 times with the two palms from the armpit to the anterior superior iliac spine, *Na* Jiquan 3−5 times, and *Na* Jianjing 3−5 times.

(4) Treatment Course: Treatment is given once daily. 6 times of treatment make 1 course.

6.6　Hemiplegia due to Apoplexy

Marked mainly by hemiparalysis, distortion of the eyes and mouth and dysphasia, hemiplegia is usually due to hypertensive apoplexy, encephalopathy or trauma. *Tuina* is effective in treating hemiplegia to certain extent, for it can promote the recovery of the body's function. If early treatment with *Tuina* is given, more evident will curative effects result.

Etiology and Pathology

Invade of wind—phlegm into the channels and collaterals leads to obstruction of the blood vessels and stagnancy of *Qi* and blood. In this case, the channels and collaterals are blocked, *Qi* fails to flow, blood fails to nourish *Zang* and *Fu*, and hemiplegia results. Damage of the cerebral bone and meninges due to direct or indirect trauma may also lead to stagnancy of blood and obstruction of the channels and collaterals, resulting in hemiplegia.

Clinical Manifestations

Paralysis of the arm and leg of one side of the body, distortion of the eyes and mouth, stiff tongue, dysphasia, etc. In the beginning, the affected limbs become soft and weak with disturbance of perception and motor impairment. Then, they grow stiff and spasmodic. Long—time disease will have the limbs changed or distorted.

Treatment

1. Therapeutic Method: promoting blood circulation to remove blood stasis, activating the flow of *Qi* to relax the muscles and tendons. It is advisable to give treatment two weeks after the onset.

2. Point Selection: Fengchi (GB 20), Jianjing (GB 21), Jianyu (LI 15), Quchi (LI 11), Shousanli (LI 10), Hegu (LI 4), Zusanli (ST 36), Xinshu (BL 15), Ganshu (BL 18), Shenshu (BL 23) and Weizhong (BL 40).

3. Manipulation: *Yizhichan Tui, Gun, An, Dian, Nian* (twisting) and *Yao*.

4. Operation:

(1) Let the patient in the prone position, conduct *Gun* along the Bladder Channel of Foot—Taiyang at the both sides of the spinal column from the above to the below for 2 minutes and undertake *An* mainly on Xinshu, Ganshu, Pishu (BL 20), Feishu (BL 13) and Shenshu. Then, carry out *Gun* on the hip portion, the posterior aspect of the thigh, popliteal fossa and the posterior aspect of the shank and perform *An—rou* mainly on chengfu (BL 36), Yinmen (BL 37), Weizhong, Chengshan (BL 57), Kunlun (BL 60) and Taixi (KI 3). Finally, flex, inward—rotate or outward—rotate the patient's hip, knee, etc. many times.

(2) Stand at one side of the patient in the supine position, conduct *Gun* on the interior aspect of the affected arm, from the above to the below along the forearm and especially around the shoulder, elbow and wrist joints for 3—5 minutes. While doing so, abduct the shoulder joint, flex the elbow joint, and flex, extend, inward—rotate and outward—rotate the wrist joint. Then, perform *Nian* (hold—twisting) with the thumb and the index finger to each finger of the affected arm, especially to the thumb.

5. Treatment Course: Treatment is given every two days. One course involves 15 times.

6.7 Flaccidity Syndrome

Flaccidity syndrome is marked by loosened and weak muscles and tendons which have been unable to move voluntarily for a long—time, myophagism, and loss of control of the hands and feet. Flaccidity of the lower limbs is common in clinical practice. Paralyses due to disorders of the nervous system or the muscles in modern medicine, such as multiple neuritis, myelitis, progressive myatrophy, myasthenia gravis, periodic paralysis, myody-strophia, hysterical paralysis and sequelae of infection of the central nervous system, are all included in the flaccidity syndrome of TCM.

Etiology and Pathology

1. Affection of Wind—heat: Invade of exogenous wind—heat into the lung impairs the body fluid in it, making the muscles and tendons unable to be moistened.

2. Retention of Damp—heat: Retention of damp—heat in the interior exhausts the body fluid, making the joints unable to be lubricated.

3. Deficiency of *Yin* of the Liver and Kidney: General debility and intemperance in sexual life consume the essence of the liver and kidney, making the muscles and tendons unable to be nourished.

Clinical Manifestations

1. Type of the Body Fluid Impaired by the Lung—heat: It appears usually after epidemic febrile diseases, manifested as sudden loss of control of the weak limbs accompanied by vexation, thirst, constipation, deep—colored urine, reddened tongue with yellow coating, and thready, rapid pulse.

2. Type of Deficiency of *Yin* of the Liver and Kidney: It appears usually during a prolonged disease, marked by progressive soft limbs, or loss of control of the lower limb, emaciated muscles, soreness and weakness of the loins and knees, vertigo, and thready, rapid pulse.

3. Type of Weakness of the Spleen and Stomach: It appears after severe or prolonged diseases, marked by gradual loss of control of the weak lower limbs, lassitude, acratia, poor appetite,

loose stools, pale complexion, pale tongue with thin and whitish coating, and soft, thready pulse.

4. Type of Retention of Damp—heat: It is marked by paralysis, slight swelling and numbness of the lower limbs, fullness in the chest and epigastrium, sallow body and face, deep—colored urine, difficulty and hot pain in passing water, reddened tongue with yellow and greasy coating, and soft, rapid pulse.

Treatment

1. Therapeutic Method: nourishing *Yin* to strengthen the stomach and regulating the liver, spleen and kidney.

2. Point Selection: Jianyu (LI 15), Quchi (LI 11), Hegu (LI 4), Yangxi (LI 5), Biguan (ST 31), Futu (ST 32), Liangqiu (ST 34), Zusanli (ST 36) and Jiexi (ST 41).

3. Manipulation: *Gun, An, Rou* and *Dian*.

4. Operation:

(1) Sit at one side of the patient in the supine position, hold the affected limb with the left hand and conduct *Gun* with the right hand for 3—4 minutes along Jianyu, Quchi, Hegu and Yangxi of the Large Intestine Channel of Hand—Yangming. Then, *An—rou* each of the points selected for 1 minute and *Dian* each of them for 30 seconds. Finally, flex and extend the upper limb.

(2) Take the same position as above and carry out *Gun* for 3—4 minutes in the direction of the Stomach Channel in the lower limb and from the above to the below. Then, *An—rou* each of the points Biguan, Liangqiu, Zusanli and Jiexi for about 1—2 minutes. Finally, *Qia* (nipping) the nail root of each toe and the interphalangeal joints of the hand and *Nian* (twisting) each of the fingers from the above to the below, each of all the above maneu-

vers being repeated 7—8 times.

5. Supplement:

(1)*Qia* (nipping) and *Rou* Quchi, Hegu and Sanyinjiao (SP 6) for type of body fluid impaired by the lung—heat.

(2)*Rou* Pishu, Weishu, Shousanli and Zusanli for type of weakness of the spleen and stomach.

(3)*Rou* Ganshu, Shenshu, Xuanzhong (GB 39) and Yanglingquan (GB 34) for type of deficiency of *Yin* of the liver and kidney.

(4)*Rou* Pishu and Fenglong (ST 40) for retention of damp—heat.

6. Treatment Course: Treatment is given every two days and one course consists of 15 times of treatment.

6.8   Arthralgia—syndrome

Arthralgia—syndrome refers to those due to stagnation of *Qi* and blood by pathogens.

Etiology and Pathology

Pathogenic wind, cold and dampness invade the channels and collaterals in the superficies of the body to make the channels and collaterals obstructed, the *Qi* and blood stagnated, resulting in pain, soreness, numbness and heavy sensation in the limbs, joints and muscles and tendons.

Clinical Manifestations

1. Arthralgia due to Wind—cold—dampness: pain in the joints of the four limbs or the lumbodorsal region which is aggravated by movement, no local redness and swelling or aversion to wind, the pain migrating or worsened by cold but relieved by heat, or heavy sensation in the limbs, white and greasy tongue

coating, and tense or taut pulse.

2. Arthralgia due to Wind—damp—heat: redness, swelling and pain of the joints which are relieved by cold but aggravated by pressure, limited movement of the joints, fever, thirst, dry throat, yellow and dry tongue coating, and slippery, rapid pulse.

Treatment

1. Therapeutic Method: Arthralgia due to wind—cold—dampness is treated mainly by way of dispelling wind, cold and dampness. The way of dredging the channels and collaterals is used as an accessory treatment of arthralgia due to wind—damp—heat.

2. Point Selection: Jianjing (GB 21), Quchi (LI 11), Hegu (LI 4), Huantiao (GB 30), Yinlingquan (SP 9), Yanglingquan (GB 34), Heding (EX—LE 2), Kunlun (BL 60), Fengchi (GB 20), Dazhui (DU 14), Feishu (BL 13), Shenshu (BL 23), Dachangshu (BL 25) and Xiaochangshu (BL 27).

3. Manipulation: *Gun, Dian, An, Rou* and *Ca.*

4. Operation:

(1) Manipulations selected according to the affected joints are first carried out, then, conduct *Nian* (twisting) and *Bashen*. Functional movement is suitable for the limited joints.

(2) *Yizhichan Tui* or *Gun* is first undertaken lightly and gently on the points around the affected part for 3—5 minutes. Then, the operation gradually shifts to the affected joints. Finally, *An* Dazhui 20—30 times and *Na* either of Quchi and Hegu 5 times.

5. Supplement:

(1) For arthralgia due to heat, *Qia* (nipping) and *Rou* Dazhui, Quchi and Hegu.

(2) For migrating arthralgia, *An—rou* Baihui (DU 20),

Fengfu (DU 16) and Fengchi.

6. Treatment Course: Treatment is given once daily and 12 times of treatment make 1 course.

6.9 Hypertension

While the organism is calm, if the systolic pressure reaches or exceeds 20 kpa or the diastolic pressure exceeds 12 kpa, hypertension results. Marked mainly by distension in the head and dizziness, it falls into two: primary and secondary.

Etiology and Pathology

Long–time nervousness or vexation and anxiety leads to stagnation of the liever–Qi, long–time stagnation of the liver–Qi results in fire, the fire consumes the liver–Yin, the consumed Yin can not restrict $Yang$, and the liver–$Yang$ acts over–actively. Insufficiency of the kidney–Yin due to senility makes the liver unable to be nourished, causing hyperactivity of the liver–$Yang$. Over–intake of greasy food or alcohol gets phlegm–dampness produced in the interior, long–time accumulation of the phlegm–dampness is responsibe for the formation of heat, the heat burns body fluid into phlegm, the phlegm blocks the channels and collaterals. All the above are the cause of hypertension.

Clinical Manifestations

Dizziness and distending pain in the head which are most seen, tinnitus, blurred vision, irritability, choking sensation in the chest, palpitation, flushed face, reddened eyes, numbness of the fingers, dry mouth and throat, constipation, deep–colored urine, reddened tongue with yellow coating, and taut, rapid pulse.

1. Type of Retention of Phlegm–dampness: headache, diz-

ziness, heavy sensation in the head, full sensation in the chest and epigastrium, tendency of vomiting, evne vomiting of phlegm and saliva, white and greasy tongue coating, and taut, slippery pulse.

2. Type of Hyperactivity of the Liver—*Yang:* dizziness, headache, flushed face, reddened eyes, bitter taste in the mouth, irritability, inclining to be angry.

3. Type of Deficiency of Both *Yin* and *Yang:* vertigo, headache, tinnitus, palpitation, dyspnea due to movement, soreness and weakness of the loins and knees, insomnia, dreamfulness, frequency of micturition at night, pale or reddish tongue with whitish coating, and taut, thready pulse.

Treatment

1. Therapeutic Method: calming the liver and removing phlegm.

2. Point Selection: Baihui (DU 20), Sishencong (EX—HN 1), Fengchi (GB 20), Jianjing (GB 21) and Qiaogong.

3. Manipulation: *An, Rou, Qia* (nipping) and *Na.*

4. Operation:

(1) Let the patient in the sitting position and do this for about 5—6 minutes: *An—rou* Baihui, *Mó* his / her head with the palm, and *An* Sishencong forcefully. Then, *Na* Fengchi with the thumb and the index finger. Finally, *Na* Jianjing several times.

(2) Let the patient in the prone position and conduct *Ca* with the hypothenar dozens of times from the above to the below along the Bladder Channel in the back.

(3) Stand at one side of the patient in the sitting position, hold the patient's head with one hand and undertake one—way *Tui* downward with the index and middle fingers of the other hand over Qiaogong with the trail connecting Yifeng (SJ 17) pos-

terior to the ear and Quepen (ST 12), and do this for about 5 minutes. Then, do the same at the other side.

5. Supplement:

(1) *Qia* (nipping) and *Rou* Xingjian (LR 2), Shenmen (HT 7) and Shaohai (HT 3) for severe headache and dizziness.

(2) *Qia* (nipping) and *Rou* Zusanli (ST 36) and Sanyinjiao (SP 6) for insomnia, lassitude and sallow complexion.

6. Treatment Course: Treatment is given once daily and 15 times of treatment make 1 course.

Points for Attention

When *Tui* is carried out over Qiaogong, performance on the both sides at the same time is strictly forbidden.

6.10   Hiccup

Hiccup is due to going up adversely of *Qi* from below the diaphragm. It is manifested as sudden, sharp, frequent sound in the throat. Its onset is intermittent and uncontrollable.

Etiology and Pathology

Improper diet leads to accumulation of food in the middle—*Jiao*, which impairs the spleen and stomach and causes the stomach—*Qi* not to descend but to ascend adversely. The adverse ascending of the stomach—*Qi* is responsible for hiccup. Vexation and anger hurt the liver. The hurt liver dysfunctions with the flowing of of its *Qi* disordered. In this case, phlegm is produced and the spleen is attacked. Ascending of the phlegm along with the adverse flowing of the liver—*Qi* is responsible for hiccup. Debility due to prolonged disease consumes the stomach—*Yin*. Insufficiency of the stomach—*Yin* makes the stomach unable to be nourished. And this is also responsible for hiccup.

Clinical Manifestations

1. Hiccup due to Deficiency Syndrome: hiccup with low sound, pale complexion, poor appetite, sleepiness, shortness of breath, palpitation, weakened voice, pale tongue with white coating, and deep, thready, weak pulse.

2. Hiccup due to Excess Syndrome: continual and forceful hiccup with loud sound, distending pain in the chest and hypochondria, foul breath, restlessness, thirst, constipation, brown urine, yellow tongue coating, and slippery, rapid pulse.

3. Hiccup due to Cold Syndrome: weak hiccup with low sound accompanied by dyspnea and relieved by heat, poor appetite, absence of thirst, cold limbs which are worsened by cold, white and moist tongue coating, and slow pulse.

4. Hiccup due to Heat Syndrome: loud hiccup, halitosis, restlessness, preference for cold drink, dry mouth and tongue, flushed face, reddened eyes, reddish tongue with yellow coating, and rapid pulse.

Treatment

1. Therapeutic Method: Regulating the stomach to make the adverse flow of *Qi* descend is the main method.

2. Point Selection: Cuanzhu (BL 2), Yuyao (EX−HN 4), Quepen (ST 12), Danzhong (RN 17), Zhongwan (RN 12), Geshu (BL 17), Weishu (BL 21), Dachangshu (BL 25), Zhongkui (EX−UE 4), Zusanli (ST 36), Fenglong (ST 40) and Neiguan (PC 6).

3. Manipulation: *Qia* (nipping), *An, Rou, Mó* and *Yizhichan Tui*.

4. Operation:

(1) Sit at one side of the patient in the supine position, apply *Qia* with the nails of the two thumbs to Cuanzhu at the both sides and Yuyao each for 1 minute. If the hiccup is stopped, conduct light, rapid and gentle *Yizhichan Tui* on Danzhong and Zhongwan for 1-2 minutes each, *Mó* clockwise Zhongwan for 3-5 minutes, and *Na* Zusanli and Fenglong 3-5 times each.

(2) Let the patient in the prone position, apply *Yizhichan Tui* with the right thumb to Geshu and Weishu each for 3-4 minutes, *Dian* the above points forcefully with the middle finger 3-4 times each, and *An-rou* Dachangshu 20-40 times.

(3) Let the patient in the sitting position, hold his / her left hand with the left hand to get his / her middle finger flexed, *Qia* Zhongkui on the radius aspect of the 2nd interphalangeal joint of the flexed middle finger for 1 minute with the thumb nail, then, *Na* Quepen 3-5 times, *Na* Neiguan 3-5 times.

5. Treatment Course: Treatment is given 1 time daily. 1 course of treatment involves 3 days.

6.11　Uroschesis

Uroschesis refers to difficulty in urination or even retention of urine.

Etiology and Pathology

The onset of this disease is mainly related to the abnormal functional activity of the tri-*Jiao* -*Qi* and the dysfunction of the lung, spleen and kidney. Abundant lung-heat, damp-heat in the bladder, insufficiency of the kidney-*Yang,* and *Qi* deficiency of the lung and kidney are all responsible for difficulty in urination. So are traumatic injury and accumulation of blood stasis.

Clinical Manifestations

1. Type of Damp—heat in the Bladder: difficulty in urination, dribbling urine, or scanty, deep—colored urine, burning sensation in urinating, retention of urine, difficult defecation, reddened tongue with yellowish, greasy coating, and soft, rapid pulse.

2. Type of Abundant Lung—heat: difficulty in urination, or dribbling urine, dry mouth and throat, restlessness, thirst with desire for drink, shortness of breath, reddened tongue with yellowish coating, and rapid pulse.

3. Type of Deficiency of the Kidney—*Yang:* dribbling urine, difficult urination and defecation, cold lower abdomen, soreness and weakness of the loins and knees, pale complexion, pale, enlarged and tender tongue with whitish coating, and deep, thready pulse.

Treatment

1. Therapeutic Method: promoting the functional activity of *Qi* to reduce the difficulty in urination.

2. Manipulation: *An, Rou* and *Tui.*

3. Point Selection: the points Liniao, Dantian, Sanyinjiao (SP 6) and Jimen (SP 11).

4. Operation:

(1) Let the patient in the supine position and calm his / her mind, stand at the side of the patient, conduct *An* with the middle finger on the point Liniao at the midpoint of the line connecting the umbilicus and Zhongji (RN 3) with the pressure becoming forceful gradually up to the extent that the patient can endure. If mild or moderate pressure can result in urination, heavy pressure is not needed. After the urination is stopped, take away the mid-

dle finger slowly. If urination refuses to occur, *An* Dantian for 3—5 minutes.

(2) Let the patient in the supine position with the lower limbs stretched straight and a little abducted, powder the interior aspects of the lower limbs with a thin layer of talc powder, undertake *Tui* 1000 times from the interior aspect of the knee via Jimen to the groin. 10 minutes later after doing the above, order the patient to pass water.

(3) *Na* Sanyinjiao 3—5 times and *Yao* each of the ankle joints 5—10 times.

5. Treatment Course: Treatment is given 1 time daily. 1 course of treatment is made up of 3 times.

6.12 Constipation

Constipation refers to difficulty in defecation and prolonged interval between every two times of defecation. It is mainly due to dysfunction of the large intestine, which is responsible for too long retention of feces in the intestine. This long retention gets feces over—dried and hard to discharge.

Etiology and Pathology

General excessive *Yang* and addiction to pungent and greasy food lead to accumulation of heat in the stomach and intestines; heat lingered after febrile disease consumes body fluid; deficiency of *Qi* and blood due to senile infirmity is responsible for dysfunction of the large intestine and scanty of body fluid; all the above are the cause of constipation.

Clinical Manifestations

1. Type of Excess: dry feces, scanty and brown urine,

flushed face, fever, or distending abdomen, dry mouth, restlessness, or frequent belching, fullness in the chest and hypochondria, poor appetite, reddened tongue with yellow, dry coating, and slippery, rapid pulse.

2. Type of Deficiency: constipation or smoothenless defecation, a little dry feces, defecating with effort followed by tiredness and even sweating and shortness of breath, pale complexion, lassitude, pale tongue with thin coating, weak pulse, or clear and abundant urine, cold limbs, cold pain of the loins and knees, or cold pain in the abdomen, etc.

Treatment

1. Therapeutic Method: clearing away heat to moisten the intestines and promoting the flow of *Qi* to remove stagnation for the treatment of constipation of excess type, replenishing *Qi* to nourish blood and relieving constipation through warming for the treatment of constipation of deficiency type.

2. Manipulation: *Mó, An, Rou* and *Ca*.

3. Point Selection: Tianshu (ST 25), Zhongwan (RN 12), Shenque (RN 8), Qihai (RN 6), Pishu (BL 20), Weishu (BL 21), Ganshu (BL 18), Dachangshu (BL 25), Baliao (BL 31-34), Changqiang (DU 1), Zhigou (SJ 6) and Chengshan (BL 57).

4. Operation:

(1) Stand at one side of the patient in the supine position, undertake *Mó* clockwise over the abdomen with the palm for about 5 minutes, and, then, carry out *An-rou* on Tianshu, Zhongwan, Shenque, Qihai for about 2 minutes.

(2) Let the patient in the prone position, perform *Ca* with the hypothenar from the patient's waist to the coccyx for about 2 minutes, and *An-rou* Pishu, Shenshu and Dachangshu several

times each.

(3) Let the patient in the sitting posture, and *Qia* (nipping) and *Rou* Zhigou and Shangjuxu (ST 37) for about 3 minutes.

5. Treatment Course: Treatment is given once daily and 6 times of treatment make 1 course.

6.13 Angina Pectoris

Angina pectoris is mainly manifested as paroxysmal and continuous pain in the precordial region behind the sternum. TCM believes that it is due to obstruction of *Qi* in the chest.

Etiology and Pathology

TCM believes that the onset of this disease has something to do with insufficiency of the kidney—*Qi* due to senile infirmity, impairment of the spleen and stomach due to rich fatty diet or stagnation of *Qi* and blood due to accumulation of the liver—*Qi* resulting from mental disorder.

Clinical Manifestations

1. Type of Obstruction of the Heart—collaterals due to Stagnation of *Qi* and Blood: paroxysmal stabbing pain in the precordial region which refers to the shoulder and back, choking and oppressed sensation in the chest, dyspnea, dark tongue with petechiae on the margins and tip, and deep, uneven or knotted pulse.

2. Type of Deficiency of *Yang—Qi* in the Upper *Jiao*: choking and oppressed sensation in the chest, paroxysmal pain in the heart, palpitation, shortness of breath, dyspnea, pale complexion, lassitude, acratia, chills, cold limbs or spontaneous sweating, disturbed sleep in the night, poor appetite, clear and abundant urine, loose stools, pale, enlarged and tender tongue with whitish, moist

or greasy coating, and deep, slow or knotted, intermittent pulse.

3. Type of Deficiency of both *Yin* and *Yang*: choking sensation in the chest, pain of the heart, waking up in the night due to dyspnea, palpitation, shortness of breath, dizziness, tinnitus, poor appetite, weakness of the limbs, soreness of the loins, cold limbs, fever in the palms, frequent urination, purple—dark tongue with whitish and dry coating, and thready, weak or knotted, intermittent pulse.

Treatment

1. Therapeutic Method: promoting blood circulation to remove blood stasis, activating the flow of *Qi* to dredge the collaterals.

2. Manipulation: *Mó, An, Rou* and *Dian*.

3. Point Selection: Yunmen (LU 2), Zhongfu (LU 1), Rugen (ST 18), Qimen (LR 14), Zhangmen (LR 13), Jiquan (HT 1), Jueyinshu (BL 14), Feishu (BL 13), Xinshu (BL 15), Ganshu (BL 18), Shenshu (BL 23), Mingmen (DU 4), Neiguan (PC 6), Daling (PC 7) and Yongquan (KI 1).

4. Operation

(1) Sit to the left of the patient in the supine position, conduct slow, gentle but steady *Mó* with the right palm from the above to the below on the points Zhongfu, Yunmen, Qimen and Zhangmen for 5 minutes, and, then, *Na* Jiquan 3—5 times gently.

(2) Sit to the left of the patient in the supine position and hold his / her left hand with the left hand, *An—rou* either of Neiguan and Daling 50 times with the thumb. Then, stand at the right side of the patient and *An—rou* either of the right Neiguan and Daling 50 times.

(3) Let the patient in the sitting position or in the lateral po-

sition, stand to one side of his / hers and undertake *Yizhichan Tui* on each of the points Feishu, Jueyinshu, Xinshu, Ganshu and Shenshu 100 times.

5. Supplement:

(1) For type of stagnation of phlegm, *Rou* Zusanli (ST 36) 300 times, either of Pishu and Wishu 300 times.

(2) For type of deficiency of both *Yin* and *Yang*, *Mó* either of Shenshu and Mingmen 300 times, *Cuo* Yongquan (KI 1) 300 times, *Mó* with the palm the left–upper part of the back where Jueyinshu (BL 14) and Xinshu are located for 5 minutes, and *An* either of the above two points gently 3–5 times.

6. Treatment Course: Treatment is given once daily and 15 times of treatment make 1 course.

Points for Attention

Gentle manipulations and non–prone position are suggested lest chest choking and palpitation be aggravated.

6.14   Colicky Pain of the Gall–bladder

Colicky pain of the gall–bladder is a common symptom of diseases of the digestive system, such as acute cholecystitis, cholelithiasis and biliary ascariasis. It is included in the range of hypochondriac pain in TCM.

Etiology and Pathology

Exteriorly–interiorly related to the liver, the gall–bladder has the same function as the liver in dredging, and its *Qi* should be downward–flowing. Stagnation of *Qi* of the liver and gall–bladder due to anxiety and anger or disorder of the gall–bladder–*Qi* due to accumulation of damp–heat in the middle—*Jiao* resulting from dysfunction of the spleen and stomach caused by improper diet will cause pain.

Clinical Manifestations

1. Type of Stagnation of *Qi*: distending, colicky or paroxysmal wandering pain in the hypochondriac regions, bitter taste, dry throat, loss of appetite, slightly reddish tongue tip, thin, whitish or slightly yellow tongue coating, and taut, tense pulse.

2. Type of Damp—heat: continuous distending pain accompanied by paroxysmal pain sometimes in the hypochondriac regions, bitter taste, dizziness, alternate attack of chills and fever, sallow eyes and body, yellow, turbid or brown urine, difficult urination, constipation, poor appetite, burning sensation in the epigastric part, belching and indigestion.

Treatment

1. Therapeutic Method: soothing the liver to regulate the circulation of *Qi*, promoting blood circulation to remove blood stasis.

2. Manipulation: *An* and *Rou*.

3. Point Selection: Geshu (BL 17), Ganshu (BL 18), Danshu (BL 19), Jiuwei (RN 15), Zhangmen (LR 13), Dannang (EX—LE 6) and non—fixed points along the Bladder Channel in the back.

4. Operation:

(1) Stand at one side of the patient in the prone position, seek for the pressure pain points carefully along the Bladder Channel of Foot—Taiyang in the back and press them gently with the right middle finger. At the same time, put the left middle finger on Jiuwei and do upward—*An* for 2—3 minutes. When the pain is stopped, *An* each of Geshu, Danshu and Ganshu gently 3—5 times.

(2) Sit at one side of the patient in the supine position, carry out *An* with the right middle finger on Zhangmen and Qimen (LR 14) for about 2—3 minutes up to the extent that mild soreness occurs.

(3) Let the patient in the supine position, and conduct powerful *An* on either of the two points Dannang at the two sides with the surfaces of the two thumbs 50 times.

5. Supplement:

(1) In case of nausea and inclining to vomit, *Rou* Neiguan (PC 6) and Zhongwan (RN 12).

(2) In case of radiating pain in the back and the scapular region, *Rou* Jianzhen (SI 9), Bingfeng (SI 12) and Jianjing (GB 21).

(3) In case of constipation, *Rou* Tianshu (ST 25) and Shenque (RN 8).

6. Treatment Course: Treatment is given once daily and 6 times of treatment make 1 course.

Points for Attention

1. Persuade the patient to rest calmly and keep happy.

2. Pay attention to the change of the patient's body temperature. When the disease condition grows worse, drugs should be given timely.

6. 15 Mastitis

Mastitis is common in the postpartum lactation. Most subjects are primiparae.

Etiology and Pathology

Mastitis is due to the following three factors:

1. stagnancy of the liver—*Qi*,

2. accumulation of the abundant stomach—heat,

3. The noxious—fire takes the chance of papillary destruction, crater nipple and galactostasis to invade the breasts so as to obstruct the papillary channels and collaterals.

The above three contribute to stagnation of both Qi and blood and cause this disease.

Clinical Manifestations

1. Type of Stagnation of the liver—Qi: distending pain in the breast with tender mass but without red skin, perhaps accompanied by irritability, bitter taste and poor appetite, thin and white tongue coating, and taut pulse.

2. Type of Stomach—heat: red, swollen, burning and painful mammary mass which may lead to mammary swelling and masthelcosis; fever, aversion to cold, dry mouth and tongue, constipation, yellow tongue coating, and taut, rapid or slippery pulse.

Treatment

Different treatment is given in its three different stages: initial stage, suppurative stage and ulcerative stage. *Tuina* is usually given in the initial stage.

1. Therapeutic Method: soothing the liver to regulate the flow of Qi, relieving swelling to dredging the collaterals.

2. Manipulations: *Mó, Mǒ* and *Nieji* (pinching and squeezing).

3. Point Selection: Rugen (ST 18), Ruzhong (ST 17), Qimen (LR 14), Danzhong (RN 17), Shaoze (SI 11), Hegu(LI 4), Ganshu (BL 18), Pishu (BL 20) and Weishu (BL 21).

4. Operation:

(1) Sit at the affected side of the patient in the supine position, conduct *Rou* with the thenar of one hand rapidly and moderately around the mass for 5 minutes, undertake gentle *Nie*

(pinching) and *Rou* around the mass with the thumbs and the index fingers of the two hands, and carry out *Rou* with the middle finger on Rugen, Ruzhong and Qimen for 1 minute each.

(2) Sit face to face with the patient in the sitting position, spread talc powder on the affected part, prop the breast with the left hand, do light, gentle, skilled and rhythmic *Nie—ji* (pinching and squeezing) toward the nipple for 2 minutes with the thumb and index finger of the right hand, expelling the stagnated milk until yellowish milk is seen.

(3) Stand at one side of the patient in the prone position, perform *Tui* with the surface of the thumb on each of Ganshu, Pishu and Weishu for 1 minute,and conduct *An—rou* with the surface of the thumb on each of the above points 3—5 times.

5. Treatment Course: Treatment is given once daily and 3 times of treatment make 1 course.

Points for Attention

1. Keep happy and be careful about the clean of the nipples.

2. Lactation should be on time in the breast feeding period, the mouth cavity of the infant should be got clean, and timely treatment should be given to cracked nipple.

3. *Tuina* is not used in the suppurative and ulcerative stages.

6.16   Dysmenorrhea

Dysmenorrhea is characterized by such symptoms as distending pain of the lower abdomen and soreness and weakness of the loins and knees which appear before, after or in the menstrual period. Severe cases disturb work and lift.

Etiology and Pathology

Mental disorders, attack of exogenous cold pathogens and cold diet may lead to stagnation of *Qi* and blood, causing dysmenorrhea.

Clinical Manifestations

1. Type of *Qi* Stagnancy: tender and distending lower abdomen before or in the menstrual period, scanty menstruation or difficulty in menstruation, distending pain in the breasts, headache or migraine, reddened tongue, and deep, uneven pulse.

2. Type of Cold—dampness: cold pain in the lower abdomen occurring before or in the menstrual period which is aggravated by coldness, scanty, pale or dark—red menstruation with blood lumps, white, moist and greasy tongue coating, and deep, tense pulse.

3. Type of Deficiency of Both *Qi* and Blood: dull pain relieved by pressing in the lower abdomen after the menstrual period, scanty, pale and thin menstruation, lassitude, acratia, pale complexion, pale tongue with white coating, and deep, thready and weak pulse.

Treatment

1. Therapeutic Method: activating the flow of *Qi* to remove blood stasis, warming the channels to dispel cold, and replenishing *Qi* to nourish blood.

2. Manipulation: *Yizhichan Tui, An, Mó* and *Ca.*

3. Point Selection: Suliao (DU 25), Guanyuan (RN 4), Qihai (RN 6), Shenshu (BL 23), Baliao (BL 31—34), Hegu (LI 4) and Sanyinjiao (SP 6).

4. Operation:

(1) Let the patient in the supine position, conduct *Mó* with the palm on the lower abdomen for about 7—8 minutes up to the

extent that the patient has hot sensation, then, *An—rou* either of Qihai and Guanyuan 3—5 times, finally, *Rou* Suliao at the tip of the nose for 1 minute.

(2) Let the patient in the prone position, *Dian—An* (digital—pressing) Baliao with the two hands for about 3 minutes, then, *Ca* the part where Baliao are located with the hypothenar, finally, *An* Shenshu.

(3)*Qia* (nipping) either of Hegu and Sanyinjiao for about 2 minutes.

5. Supplement:

(1) In case of deficiency of *Qi*, *Mó* the abdomen counterclockwise, in case of stagnation of *Qi*, the *Mó* is conducted clockwise.

(2) In case of nausea with tendency of vomiting, *Tui* Zhongwan (RN 12), Neiguan (PC 6) and Danzhong (RN 17).

(3) In case of stagnation of the liver—*Qi*, *An—rou* Ganshu (BL 18) and Qimen (LR 14).

6. Treatment Course Treatment is given once daily and 6 times of treatment make 1 course.

6.17 Postpartum General Aching

Soreness and numbness of the limbs after giving birth is called postpartum general aching.

Etiology and Pathology

Inability of blood to nourish the muscles and tendons due to postpartum deficiency of *Qi* and blood is combined with invasion of wind—cold—dampness into the body to obstruct the channels and cause pain.

Clinical Manifestations

1. Type of Weakness of *Qi* and Blood: soreness and numbness of the limbs, pale complexion, pale tongue with little coating, and thready, weak pulse.

2. Type of Affection of Exogenous Wind—cold—dampness: limbs with migrating pain or heavy sensation and swelling, pale tongue with thin and white coating, and thready, rapid pulse.

Treatment

1. Therapeutic Method: nourishing *Qi* and blood, warming the channels, and dispelling cold.

2. Manipulation: *An, Rou, Qia* (nipping) and *Na*.

3. Point Selection: Jianjing (GB 21), Pishu (BL 20), Weishu (BL 21), Shenshu (BL 23), Shousanli (LI 10), Neiguan (PC 6), Waiguan (SJ 5), Hegu (LI 4), Quchi (LI 11), Zusanli (ST 36) and Chengshan (BL 57).

4. Operation:

(1) Let the patient in the prone position, *An—rou* Pishu, Weishu and Shenshu for about 3 minutes, conduct gentle *Gun* on the lower limbs from the above to the below for 2—3 minutes, *An* Zusanli 3—5 times, and *Na* Chengshan 3—5 times.

(2) Let the patient in the sitting position, *Qia* (nipping) and *Rou* Shousanli, Quchi, Neiguan, Waiguan, Hegu and Jianjing for about 5 minutes, and *Na* Jianjing 2—3 times.

5. Treatment Course: Treatment is given 1 time daily, 1 course of treatment consists of 5 times.

6.18 Postpartum Tormina

Pain of the lower abdomen occurring after giving birth is called postpartum tormina.

Etiology and Pathology

It is due to blood stasis resulting from the weakened *Qi* and blood in the Chong and Ren Channels or due to stagnated blood resulting from the invasion of pathogenic cold and from the weakened *Qi* and blood. .

Clinical Manifestations

1. Type of Deficiency of Blood: dull pain relieved by pressing in the lower abdomen, little and pale lochia, dizziness, blurred vision, pale nails, pale complexion, constipation, lassitude, acratia, pale tongue with thin coating, and deficient, thready and weak pulse.

2. Type of Blood Stasis: pain relieved by warmth but aggravated by pressing in the lower abdomen, cold limbs, little lochia with blood stasis, dark–purple tongue with white, slippery coating, and deep, uneven pulse.

3. Type of Accumulation of Cold: cold pain relieved by either pressing or warmth, cold limbs, little lochia, dark, pale tongue with white, slippery coating, and deep, tense pulse.

Treatment

1. Therapeutic Method: strengthening *Qi* and blood, promoting blood circulation to remove blood stasis, and warming up the channels to dispel cold.

2. Manipulation: *Mó, An, Rou* and *Ca*.

3. Point Selection: Guanyuan (RN 4), Shimen (RN 5), Sanyinjiao (SP 6), Dahe (KI 12), Pishu (BL 20), Shenshu (BL 23), Mingmen (DU 4), Baliao (BL 31−34) and Shiqizhui (EX−B 8).

4. Operation:

(1) Let the patient in the supine position, conduct *Mó* over

the lower abdomen of the patient for about 5 minutes, and, then, *An* Guanyuan, Shimen, Sanyinjiao and Dahe for 2 minutes.

(2) Let the patient in the prone position, carry out *Rou* with the fingers on Pishu, Shenshu, Mingmen, Baliao and Shiqizhui for about 5 minutes, and, then, perform *Ca* with the palms on Baliao until hot sensation is felt.

5. Treatment Course: Treatment is given 1 time daily, and 1 course of treatment consists of 7 times.

6.19　Toothache

Toothache is a symptom. Modern medicine believes that it is due to dental caries, pulpitis and periodontitis.

Etiology and Pathology

TCM believes that over—intake of pungent and greasy food leads to production of stomach—heat, long—time accumulated stomach—heat turns into fire, and fire tends to go up to cause swelling and pain of the gum. In addition, flaring—up of fire of deficiency type due to insufficiency of the kidney—*Yin* can do the same thing, too.

Clinical Manifestations

1. Type of Stomach—fire: severe toothache, foul breath, constipation, yellow and greasy tongue coating, and rapid, forceful pulse.

2. Type of Wind—fire: severe pain with swelling, cold limbs, and floating pulse.

3. Type of Deficiency of the Kidney—*Yin:* intermittent dull pain, loose teeth, and thready pulse.

Treatment

1. Therapeutic Method: removing heat from the stomach to clear up fire, expelling wind to dispel heat, and nourishing *Yin* to sweep away fire.

2. Manipulation: *An, Rou, Qia* (nipping), *Nie* (pinching) and *Na*.

3. Point Selection: Jiache (ST 6), Xiaguan (ST 7), Neiting (SI 44), Hegu (LI 4), Waiguan (SJ 5), Fengchi (GB 20), Taixi (KI 3) and Xingjian (LR 2).

4. Operation:

(1) Stand at one side of the patient in the sitting position, fix his / her head with the left hand, *An* Jiache and Xiaguan with the right hand for 2—3 minutes, and, then, *Rou* is performed on them for 2—3 minutes.

(2) Stand to the side of the patient in the sitting position and *Na* Hegu with the right hand for 1—2 minutes with the pain relieved right away. If pain of the right side is severe, Hegu of the right side is first treated.

(3) Let the patient sit with the lower limbs stretched out and *Qia* (nipping) Neiting, Taixi or Xingjian.

5. Treatment Course: Treatment is given once daily, and 1 course of treatment consists of 3 times.

6.20 Pharyngitis

Dry throat, pharyngolynia and pharyngeal paraesthesia are characteristic of pharyngitis.

Etiology and Pathology

Exogenous wind—heat burns the lung or stomach system and goes up along the two channels to cause throat pain of excess type. Flaring—up of fire of deficiency type due to deficiency of *Yin* of the kidney may lead to throat pain of deficiency type.

Clinical Manifestations

1. Type of Excess Heat: sore throat, dry mouth with desire for drink, foul breath, swollen gum, burning—pain in epigastric region, deep—red tongue with yellow, greasy coating, and slippery, rapid pulse.

2. Type of *Yin*—deficiency: dry and itching throat, low and hoarse voice, thirst with desire for drink, cough without or with little sputum, reddened tongue with little or without coating, and thready, rapid pulse.

Treatment

1. Theerapeutic Method: clearing away heat to relieve sore throat, nourishing *Yin* to expel fire.

2. Manipulation: *Na, Rou* and *Qia* (nipping).

3. Point Selection: Fengchi (GB 20), Tianzhu (BL 10), Renying (ST 9), Lianquan(RN 23), Quchi (LI 11), Hegu (LI 4), Shaoshang(LU 11) and Shangyang (LI 1).

4. Operation:

(1) Stand behind the patient in the sitting position, support his / her forehead with the left hand and *Na* Fengchi and Tianzhu with the thumb and the index ginger of the right hand for about 4—5 minutes until the patient feels the increasing of secretion in the mouth. Then, *Rou* gently Renying and Lianquan for about 2 minutes.

(2) Stand behind the patient in the sitting position and *Qia—rou* Quchi, Hegu, Shaoshang and shangyang for about 5 minutes.

5. Supplement:

(1) *Qia—rou* Taixi (KI 3) and Zhaohai (LI 6) to treat tooth-ache due to deficiency of the kidney.

(2) *Qia—rou* Fenglong (ST 40) and Zhigou (SJ 6) to treat constipation due to abundant heat in the lung and stomach.

6. Treatment course: Treatment is given once daily, and 1 course of treatment consists of 3 times.

6.21 Dislocation of Tendon of Long Head of Biceps Brachii

The long tendon of the brachial biceps starts from the superior node of the pelvis of scapula, goes downward to pass over the head of humerus and through the superior transverse liga- ment of scapula and the stretching portion of the tendon sheath of the brachial biceps. and enters the osseofibrous canal of intertubercular sulcus. Under normal condi- tion, the movement of the shoulder joint on- ly brings this long tendon of the brachial bi- ceps to slide longitudianlly but not to shift right or left.

Etiology and Pathology

If the arm is over—abducted or outward—rotated when there exist either flaccid superior transverse ligament of scapula, flaccid or prolonged long—tendon of the biceps and shallowed bed of the bot-

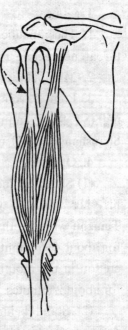

Fig.81

tom of the intertubercular sulcus all of which are due to congenital maldevelopment of the microjoints, lessened slope of the medial wall of the intertubercular sulcus, local retrograde affection and hyperosteogeny, or there exist laceration of the superior transverse ligament of scapula and acute or chronic laceration or dislocation of the terminal of the greater pectoral muscle or the subscapular muscle both of which are due to trauma of the shoulder joint, there will occur laceration and dislocation of the soft tissues protecting the long—tendon of the biceps. This will cause this tendon to shift into the medial side of, or out of, the intertubercular sulcus (Fig.81), or to be set into the tendon canal together with the thicker part around the muscular junction, leading to this disorder.

Clinical Manifestations

Dislocation of tendon of long head of biceps brachii falls into two in clinical practice: habitual and traumatic. The former is chronic, but it is usually due to mild trauma and easy to relapse. Acute dislocation of tendon of long head of biceps brachii due to trauma is marked by the following abrupt symptoms and signs: pain in the anterior of the shoulder, inward—rotated humerus, dysfunction of the joint in abduction, adduction, outward—rotation and intorsion, and the arm failing to swing forward and backward so that the patient has to prop it with the hand of the other arm while walking in order to lessen the pain due to the arm's movement and weight.

Treatment

Tuina is effective in treating both habitual and traumatic dislocation of tendon of long head of biceps brachii. But the former tends to relapse, even if treated with *Tuina*. Therefore, suture, if necessary, should be performed. Ideal effect will be attained when the latter is treated with *Tuina*. However, if it is due to disloction of the shoulder joint or fracture of humeral neck, orthopedic taxis is needed instead of *Tuina*.

1. Therapeutic Method: restoring and treating injured soft tissues, dredging the channels and promoting blood circulation.

2. Manipulation: *Yizhichan Tui, Rou, Cuo* and *Bashen*.

3. Point Selection: Jianyu (LI 15), Jianjing (GB 21), Binao (LI 14), Quchi (LI 11), Shousanli (LI 10), Waiguan (SJ 5), Hegu (LI 4) and so on.

4. Operation:

(1) Stand in front of the patient sitting upright, put the four fingers of the right hand on the affected shoulder of the patient with the palm downward and the thumb on the midpoint of the anterior border of the deltoid muscle where the tendon of long head of biceps brachii is located and support the humeral neck with effort, hold with the left hand the wrist of the affected arm with the palm got forward, the shoulder 60 ° abducted and 40 ° forward−flexed.

(2) While doing countertraction with the two hands, rotate the forearm of the patient progressively backward with the shoulder returned to the position of 40 ° abduction and the low-ered forearm rotated as backward as possible. Meanwhile, push the right thumb out−upward with effort to press the dislocated tendon of long head of the biceps brachii and rotate the affected arm rapidly forward with the left hand (Fig.82).

(3)Push and knead gently with the thumb the tendon of long head of biceps brachii for 3−5 minutes, and, then, conduct gentle *Cuo* and *Rou* around the shoulder with the two palms.

If necessary, keep the affected arm in the position of

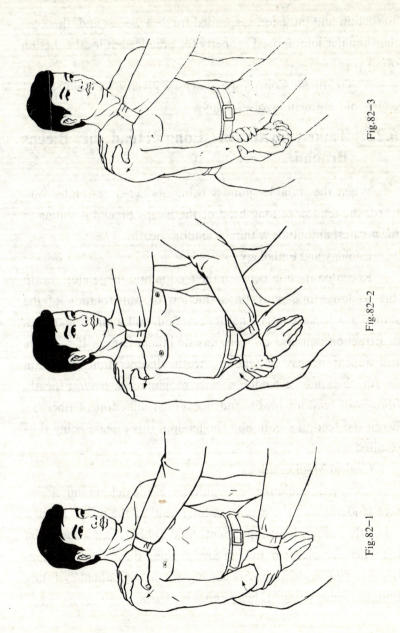

Fig.82-1　　　　　Fig.82-2　　　　　Fig.82-3

adduction and intorsion suspended for 2–4 weeks, and, then, get the shoulder joint moved properly for practice lest local adhesion occur.

5. Treatment Course: Treatment is given once daily, and 1 course of treatment involves 3 days.

6.22 Tenosynovitis of Long Head of Biceps Brachii

When the shoulder joint is being abducted or rotated outward, the tendon of long head of the biceps brachii is sliding in the greatest amplitude within its tendon sheath.

Etiology and Pathology

Repeated friction between the tendon and the tendon sheath due to long–time powerful abduction or out–rotation of the shoulder will cause inflammatory reaction, and injury due to sudden traction will also cause traumatic inflammation. If so, there will appear dropsy of tendon sheath, degeneration of tendon sheath, thickness of tendon sheath, roughness of tendon sheath, fibrosis of tendon sheath, and occasional adhesion of fiber between the tendon sheath and the tendon, this disease being thus resulted in.

Clinical Manifestations

Local pain radiating to the inferior of the deltoid muscle, severe tenderness in the tendon of long head of the biceps brachii, evidently limited joint movement, mild rubbing sensation often felt when the biceps muscle of arm is being diastolized and contracted, and evident pain occurring when the patient is lifting things or contracting his biceps muscle of arm.

Pain pressure point limited to the intertubercular sulcus in the cases due to chronic strain, and pain occurring only when the shoulder joint is being abducted and backward—extended (usually not when movement in other direction is being done).

Treatment

Rapid and remarkable curative effects will be attained when *Tuina* is used to treat the cases due to acute trauma. Longer course of treatment is needed when *Tuina* is used to treat the cases due to chronic strain. During the treatment, it is advisable to reduce the movement of the affected shoulder, especially the active abduction.

1. Therapeutic Method: relaxing the tendon, dredging the collaterals, removing blood stasis, and relieving pain.

2. Manipulation: *Yizhichan Tui, Tanbo* (plucking and poking), *Rou, Ca, Yao* and *Dou*.

3. Point Selection: Jianneiling, Jianyu (LI 15), Jianjing (GB 21), Binao (LI 14) and so on.

4. Operation:

(1) Stand or sit to the affected side ot the patient in the sitting position and conduct with the edge or belly of the thumb *Yizhichan Tui* for about 3—5 minutes from the tendon of long head of the biceps brachii to the intertubercular sulcus where the point Jianneiling is located.

(2) Conduct *Tanbo* gently with the thumb on the tendon of long head of the biceps brachii 20—30 times and, then, carry out gentle *Na* downward along the deltoid muscle up to the elbow.

(3) Put the two palms at the affected shoulder with one at the anterior and the other at the posterior, and perform *Cuo* in the opposite directions for about 1—2 minutes. Then, rotate the

shoulder joint clockwise for 3 circles and counterclockwise for 3 circles as well. Finally, *Dou* the upper limb.

Or, apply Chinese ilex ointment to the shoulder and conduct *Ca* in the direction towards the intertubercular sulcus with the hypothenar up to the extent that the heat produced goes deep. If hot compress is added, better effect will be achieved.

5. Treatment Course: Treatment is given once daily, and 1 course of treatment involves 5 days.

6.23　Tendinitis of Supraspinatus Muscle

Supraspinous muscle, part of rotator cuff, starts from the supraspinous fossa of scapula. Its tendon goes from under acromial tendon of coracoid process and subacromial bura and above the narrow space superior to shoulder joint capsule, and terminates at the superior of the greater tuberosity of humerus, connecting closely with the joint capsule to increase its stability. Supraspinous muscle functions mainly in causing the upper arm to abduct.

Etiology and Pathology

Long–time repeated abduction of the arm tends to injure the tendon of supraspinous muscle or to lead to chronic strain and retrograde degneration of the tendon, causing this disorder, an aseptic inflammation.

Clinical manifestations

With pain, limited abduction and tenderness as the main symptoms, this disorder is marked by the pain at the lateral aspect of the shoulder spreading to the point of attachment of the deltoid muscle, sometimes radiates up to the neck and down to the elbow, forearm and fingers; evident tenderness at the greater tubercle where the tendon of supraspinous muscle terminates, usually-free extension and flexion of the shoulder joint, severe pain occurring when the shoulder is 60° —120° abducted which even limits the movement of the shoulder, and muscular atrophy may be seen in prolonged cases.

Treatment

Tuina is more effective in treating this disease. If it is in the acute stage, the manipulations applied should be gentle and slow, and the movement of the shoulder joint should be restricted properly. If it is in the chronic stage, the manipulations should have the effect of deep-going. While treatment with manipulation is carried out, proper functional exercises should be added. Meanwhile, keep the shoulder warm and protect it from being attacked by cold.

1. Therapeutic Method: promoting blood circulation to remove blood stasis, expelling obstruction in the channels and collaterals.

2. Manipulation: *Yizhichan Tui, An, Rou, Na, Pingtui* (flat-pushing), *Yao* and *Dou.*

3. Point Selection: Jianjing (GB 21), Bingfeng (SI 12), Quyuan (SI 13), Tianzong(SI 11), Jianwaishu (SI 14), Naoshu (SI 10) and Binao (LI 14).

4. Operation:

(1) Stand to the affected side of the patient in the sitting position, have the affected arm passively abducted to 30 degrees with the muscles relaxed, prop the elbow of the patient with one hand and carry out *Yizhichan Tui* to and fro at the top of the subacromial greater tuberosity of humerus and along the suprospinous muscle for 3-5 minutes.

(2) Conduct *Tanbo* (flicking–poking) and *An–rou* alternately with the thumb over the affected portion for 3–5 minutes.

(3) Apply some ointment made from Chinese holly leaf or some of other *Tuina* media to the part where the supraspinous muscle of scapula is located and *Pingtui* is performed with the palm root or hypothenar. Meanwhile, *Dian–an* with the tip of the middle or index finger is conducted on the points Bingfeng, Quyuan, Jianwaishu and Jianliao (SJ 14). *Pingtui* should be done to the extent that hot sensation is deep–going, while *Dian–an* soreness and distension occur.

(4)*Nie–na* (nipping–grasping) Jianjing and the deltoid muscle 3–5 times.

(5)Rotate the shoulder joint in a circle clockwise 3 times and counterclockwise 3 times as well, *Cuo–rou* the affected arm 3–5 times to and fro from the shoulder to the wrist, and, finally, *Doula* (shake–pull) the affected arm.

Local hot compress may be added during the treatment.

5. Treatment Course: Treatment is given once daily, and 1 course of treatment consists of 3 times.

6.24　Sub–acromial Bursitis

There are many synovial bursae around the shoulder joint, of which the bigest ones are the subacromial bursa and the subdeltoid bursa. The former is below the acromion and the latter is on the deep aspect of the deltoid muscle. They function mainly in preventing friction occurring between the greater tuberosity of humerus and the acromial process.

Etiology and Pathology

Acute traumatic subacromial bursitis is caused by injury of

the synovial bursae in the deep layer of the deltoid muscle due to direct or indirect trauma of the shoulder, while the chronic one is due to degeneration of the synovial bursae. In addition, retrograde degneration of the subcromial bursa due to long–time repeated strain of the shoulder will lead to aseptic inflammation marked by bursal edema and thickness, or cause adhesion of bursal walls so as to limit abduction and rotation of the arm and normal function of the shoulder.

Clinical Manifestations

Pain on the lateral aspect of the shoulder which usually refers to the end of the deltoid muscle and becomes severe when the arm is abducted or outward–rotated, evident tenterness in the subacromial region, round mass on the anterior border of the deltoid muscle appearing in the acute stage due to bursal tympany, slightly restricted movement of the shoulder in the beginning which becomes greatly limited because of adhesion of rotator cuff as the time passes by, and atrophy of the supraspinous and infraspinous muscles followed by that of the deltoid muscle.

Treatment

Treatment in the acute stage is carried out with gentle manipulations and be sure not to press the affected part hard lest the injury of the bursa be worsened. Manipulations used in the chronic stage may grow powerful appropriately. There is no need for the patient to limit the movement of his ∕ her shoulder too much and proper gentle movement is suggested in the acute stage. In the chronic stage, appropriate functional exercises should be undertaken. In addition, the affected part should be kept warm.

1. Therapeutic Method: removing blood stasis to relieve

pain in the acute stage, promoting blood circulation to remove blood stasis and lubriating the joint in the chronic stage.

2. Manipulations: *Yizhichan Tui, Rou, Cuo, Pingtui* (flat—pushing), *Dou* and *Yao*.

3. Point Selection: Jianyu (LI 15), Binao (LI 14), Jianneiling, Tianzong (SI 11) and Quchi (LI 11).

4. Operation:

(1) Stand to the affected side of the patient in the sitting position and conduct *Yizhichan Tui* to and fro on the portion around the deltoid muscle for about 3—5 minutes.

(2) Apply some ointment of Chinese holly leaf or some oil of safflower to the lateral, anterior and posterior aspects of the arm, where *Pingtui* is carried out until the heat produced has gone deep. Then, hold the arm with the two hands and perform *Cuo—rou* (foulage—kneading) with the two palms to and fro along the upper arm and forearm 3—5 times.

(3) Undertake *An—rou* with the tip of the thumb or the middle finger on the points Tianzong, Jianyu, Quchi, Shousanli (LI 10) and Hegu (LI 4) until the patient feels sore and distending.

(4) *Yao* the affected arm gently in a circle and conduct gentle *Dou—la* (shake—pulling) of the affected arm as the last procedure of the treatment.

Hot compress may be added locally after the treatment with manipulations in order to promote the absorption of inflammation.

5. Treatment Course: Treatment is given once daily, and 1 course of treatment consists of 5 times.

6.25　External Humeral Epicondylitis

Common in the middle–aged, this disorder is also called as syndrome of external humeral epicondyle, tennis elbow or humeroradial bursitis.

Etiology and Pathology

External humeral epicondyle is the place which the brachioradial muscle and the general tendon of the forearm extensor are fixed on. If the wrist joint is often dorsiextended when the forearm is in the pronator position, the soft tissues near the point of attachment will be injured due to pulling, causing local bleeding, adhesion and even pain due to invasion of the joint synovium into the humeroradial articulattion. Usually without the history of evident trauma, its onset is due to either acute sprain or chronic strain. It is common in the middle–aged who have to keep their forearms rotating and their wrists stretching strenuously. The right arm is often affected.

Clinical Manifestations

Soreness on the lateral aspect of the posterior of the elbow which becomes worse when rotate–dorsiextending, lifting, pulling, levelly–holding or pushing is being done and radiates downward along the extensor muscle of wrist; local mild swelling, difficulty in rotating the forearm and holding things, and positive results of the tests of tensions of the extensor muscle and tennis elbow.

Treatment

Better results may be attained if it is treated with *Tuina*, Even better curative effects will be achieved if local block therapy is added if the cases with short disease duration are treated with

Tuina. When the cases with longer disease duration fail to respond to conservative treatment, operation should be considered.

1. Therapeutic Method: relaxing the muscles and tendons, removing obstruction from the channels, promoting blood circulation to eliminate blood stasis.

2. Manipulations: *Yizhichan Tui, Rou, Tanbo* (flicking and poking), and *Ca*.

3. Point Selection: Quchi (LI 11), humeroradial articulattion space, Shousanli (LI 10), Waiguan (SJ 5) and Hegu (LI 4).

4. Operation:

(1) Sit to the affected side of the patient in the sitting position, carry out *Yizhichan Tui* to and fro from the external humeral epicondyle to the forearm for 3—5 minutes, and, then, undertake local *Tanbo* 5—10 times.

(2) Take *Tui* conducted on the right for example. Hold the wrist of the patient with the right hand and get his / her right forearm rotated to the supinator position, press the anterior of the external humeral epicondyle with the flexed left thumb with the other four fingers put on the medial aspect of the elbow joint, flex with the right hand the elbow joint of the patient gradually to the maximum, press hard with the left thumb the anterior of the external humeral epicondyle of the patient, straighten the bent elbow joint and, meanwhile, shift the left thumb to the anterior and superior of the head of radius of the affected arm and conduct backward—*Tanbo* on the origin of the wrist extensor muscle along the anterior—lateral border of the head of radius.

(3) Apply Chinese holly leaf ointment or safflower oil to the lateral aspect of the elbow and carry out *Pingtui* on the external humeral epicondyle and the group of extensor muscles of the

forearm until the heat produced has gone deep, hold the far end of the humerus with the left hand and the four fingers (except for the thumb) with the right hand, and *Dou* the forearm and the elbow joint as the last procedure of the treatment.

5. Treatment Course: Treatment is given once daily, and 1 course of treatment consists of 7 times.

6.26   Medial Humeral Epicondylitis

Medial humeral epicondylitis is also called "student elbow", for it is common in youth and young children.

Etiology and Pathology

Medial humeral epicondyle is where the general tendon of forearm flexor is attached. Over-traction of the group of forearm wrist-flexor due to long-time repeated wrist-flexion, wrist-extension and forearm pronation results in accumulating strain of the attachment point of tendon of medial humeral epicondyle, leading to chronic aseptic inflammation. Or, acute laceration occurring at the attachment point of tendon due to traumatic injury, dorsoextension of the wrist joint, and abduction and pronation of the forearm brings about hematoma and fibrosis, causing this disorder.

Clinical Manifestations

soreness in and around the medial humeral epicondyle which becomes more evident when the forearm is being pronated or the wrist is being actively flexed, and, meanwhile, radiates downward along the ulnar wrist-flexor; difficulty in flexing the wrist, evident tenderness in the medial humeral epicondyle, extensive tenderness in the ulnar wrist-flexor and the superficial flexor of finger, and positive results of resistive test of wrist flexion.

Treatment

1. Therapeutic Method: relaxing muscles and tendons, eliminating obstruction from channels, promoting blood circulation to remove blood stasis.

2. Manipulation: *An, Rou, Tanbo* (flick—poking), *Na* and *Cuorou* (foulage—kneading).

3. Point Selection: Shaohai (HT 3), Xiaohai (SI 8) and Waiguan (SJ 5).

4. Operation:

(1) Let the patient in the sitting position, conduct gentle *Anrou* with the thumb from the medial humeral epicondyle to the wrist along the ulnar wrist flexor, and, meanwhile, extend and flex the wrist to relax the tense wrist flexors.

(2) Carry out *Tanbo* at the pain pressure point in the medial humeral epicondyle and in the region around the point for 2—3 minutes, and undertake gentle and rapid *Na* to and fro along the wrist flexor several times.

(3)Get the two palms working together to *Cuorou* the patient's elbow and the forearm, and, then, *Doula* (shake—pulling) his / her forearm and elbow as the last procedure of the treatment. Instead, apply Chinese holly leaf ointment to the medial humeral epicondyle and conduct local *Ca* and *Mó* until the heat produced has gone deep.

5. Treatment Course: Treatment is given once daily, 1 course of treatment consists of 7 times.

6.27 Sprain of the Wrist Joint

Including radiocarpal articulation and intercarpal joint, the wrist joint may be flexed, extended, adducted, abducted and circled. Sprain is easy to happen to it because of its broad and frequent movement.

Etiology and Pathology

Injury of the soft tissues around the wrist joint due to direct or indirect voilence, over-strain due to overload or long-time repeated over-working of the wrist joint are responsible for this disorder.

Clinical Manifestations

Sprain of the wrist joint may or may not have evident trauma history.

The symptoms of the acute sprain are: swelling and pain in the wrist, limited functional activity of the joint, pain becoming severe when the wrist joint is moving, and evident local tenderness, while the symptoms of the chronic one are: mild pain in the wrist joint, no evident swelling and distending, pain in the injured point occurring when the joint is moving in large range, and acratia and stiffness sensation often existing in the wrist.

Pain on the dorsum found in examination when the wrist joint is being palm-flexed indicates an injury of the dorsal carpal ligament and extensor digitorum. Otherwise, the pain indicates an injury of the ligamentum carpivolare or the tendon of flexor. Pain occurring in whatever direction the obviously-limited wrist joint is moving indicates a compound injury of the ligament and the tendon.

Clinical Manifestations:

Better curative effects will be attained if *Tuina* is used to treat sprain of the wrist joint. However, there are many wrist disorders because of the complicated anatomic structure of the wrist. In clinical practice, sprain of the wrist joint must be distinguished from the following disorders: fracture of the distal end of radius and ulna, fracture of scaphoid, fracture or dislocation of lunate bone, avulsion fracture of the dorsal aspect of triangular bone, and aseptic necrosis of scaphoid and lunate bone, any of which should be treated through orthopedic reduction or operation.

1. Therapeutic Method: relaxing muscles and tendons, promoting blood circulation, removing blood stasis and relieving pain.

2. Manipulation: *Yizhichan Tui, Dian, Rou Yao, Na, Ca* and *Bashen.*

3. Point Selection: Shaohai (HT 3), Tongli (HT 5), Shenmen (HT 7), Chize (LU 57), Lieque (LU 7), Taiyuan (LU 9), Hegu (LI 4), Yangxi (LI 5) and Quchi (LI 11).

4. Operation:

(1) Gentle and slow manipulations should be used to treat acute injury with more evident pain and swelling. But what should be done first is to select proper points around the injury and along the corresponding channels. For example, points along the Heart Channel of Hand—Shaoyin such as Shaohai, Tongli and Shenmen may be selected on the ulnar palmar surface; points along the Lung Channel of Hand—Taiyin such as Chize, Lieque and Taiyuan may be selected on the radial palmar surface; points along the Large Intestine Channel of Hand—Yangming such as Hegu, Yangxi and Quchi may be selected on the radial dorsal surface. The way to select points in other region is the same as the above. Points selected, conduct *Dian, An* and *Rou* with the thumb until *Qi,* i.e., a sensation of soreness and distension, is got, and, then, continue the manipulations for about 1 minute so as to promote the flowing of *Qi* and blood through the channels and

collaterals.

(2) Carry out *Yizhichan Tui* upward, downward, leftward and rightward around the injury for about 3—5 minutes so as to promote blood circulation, remove blood stasis and improve the blood circulation around the injury, and, meanwhile, add the manipulations *Na* and *Tanjin* (flicking tendons) to relieve spasm.

(3) Conduct *Yao* together with *Bashen* to get the wrist circled, dorsiflexed, palmar—flexed and laterally—bent so as to restore its normal function of activity.

(4) Apply safflower oil on the wrist and undertake *Ca* on it until the heat produced has gone deep.

Following the treatment with manipulations, hot compress with herbal medicine may be given to the cases with distinct swelling.

There are only slight pain and swelling in the later stage of acute sprain or in chronic strain. When they are treated with the above manipulations, the strength should be added correspondingly and the amplitude should be enlarged gradually in order that the spasm can be relieved, the adhesion can be released, and the joint's function of activity can be improved.

5. Treatment Course: Treatment is given once daily, 1 course of treatment consists of 3 times.

6.28　Carpal Tunnel Syndrome

Carpal tunnel syndrome refers to nervous symptoms, such as numbness of finger, due to the median nerve pressed within the carpal canal.

Etiology and Pathology

Transverse palmar ligaments and carpal bone form a carpal

canal with the former on the palmar surface and the latter in the posterior. Besides the median nerve, in the carpal canal, there are also 4 tendons of superficial flexor muscle of fingers, 4 tendons of deep flexor muscle of fingers and 1 tendon of long flexor muscle of thumb. As the volume of the content in the carpal canal is enlarged, the volume of the canal is reduced. If this occurs, the tendons and median nerve will be pressed with nervous symptoms appearing. The disorders getting the volume of carpal canal decreased are as follows: (1) hyperplasia, fracture and dislocation of carpal bone, (2) pachynsis of interosseous intercarpal ligaments, (3) swelling and distension of the content(tendons) in carpal canal.

Clinical Manifestations

In the initial stage: numbness and stabbing pain of fingers which often disturb sleep suddenly but become relieved as soon as the affected hand is waved; the numbness and pain mainly involving the index finger, secondly the middle and ring fingers and the thumb but not the little finger; and burning pain of the small finger in few cases.

In the later stage: atrophy, numbness and myodynamic attenuation of muscles of thenar eminence (short abductor muscle of thumb and opposing muscle of thumb), and semi-radial anesthesia of the thumb, the index, middle and ring fingers.

Myophagism usually appearing gradually 4 months later after the onset whose seriousness is closely related to the disease course, hypoesthesia or anesthesia of the fingers with the symptoms found in examination, pain sense remaining in the palm, and the symptoms aggravated if the point Daling (PC 7)on the affected limb is pressed.

Treatment

Tuina is only suitable for the type due to tumefaction of the tendons in the carpal canal resulting from injury or diseases. Operation is applicable to the other two.

1. Therapeutic Method: relaxing muscles and tendons, eliminating obstruction from the channels and collaterals, promoting blood circulation to remove blood stasis.

2. Manipulation: *Yizhichan Tui, An, Rou, Yao* and *Ca*.

3. Point Selection: Quze (PC 3), Neiguan (PC 6) and Daling (PC 7).

4. Operation:

(1) Sit and let the patient sit upright, extend his / her hand with the palm upward, prop the dorsum of his / her wrist with one hand and conduct *An–rou* with the other hand on the points Quze, Neiguan, Daling and Yuji (LU 10).

(2) Conduct first gentle and then gradually forceful *Yizhichan Tui* to and fro from the forearm to the hand along the Pericardium Channel of Hand–Jueyin for 3–5 minutes with the carpal canal and the thenar eminence as the main manipulated portion, *Yao–rou* the wrist joint and the interphalangeal articulations of hand, and, then, *Ca* carpometacarpus to reach the purpose of relaxing muscles and tendons, eliminating obstruction from the channels and collaterals, and promoting blood circulation to remove blood stasis.

(3) *Niewan* (wrist–pinching): Take operation on the right wrist for example. Let the patient sit upright and get his / her forearm in the pronator position with the dorsum of the hand upward. Hold the patient's palm with the two hands, with the right hand in the radial aspect, the left hand in the ulnar aspect,

the thumbs got flat on the dorsum of the wrist joint, and the tips of the thumbs pressed into the space on the dorsal aspect of the wrist joint. *Yao* the wrist joint while *Bashen* is being undertaken. Then, dorsiextend the wrist pressed by the thumbs to the maximum, flex it and circle it clockwise 2—3 times and counterclockwise 2—3 times as well (Fig.83)

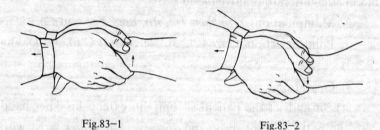

Fig.83—1   Fig.83—2

Following the treatment with manipulations, apply ointment with the action of warming the channels and dredging the collaterals to the wrist and fix the wrist in the rest position. fumigating and washing with the decoction of herbal medicines may be conducted after the synptoms are relieved.

5. Treatment Course: Treatment is given once daily, 1 course of treatment is made up of 10 times.

6.29 Injury of Medial Collateral Ligament of Kee Joint

In the shape of triangle, medial accessory ligament connects the medial condyle of femur and the medial condyle of tibia like a bridge, with its medial aspect closely attached to the lateral border of the medial and posterior portion of medial semilunar plate. While the knee joint is being extended and flexed, the ligament is sliding forward and backward on the medial condyle of femur.

When the knee joint is extended straight or flexed completely, the ligament is kept tense. When the knee joint is in the semiflexion position, the ligament is loosened, this getting the joint unstable and easy to injure. Lateral accessory ligament starts from external epicondyle of femur and terminates at head of fibula, and it has nothing to do with semilunar plate, for it is isolated by loose connective tissues. When the knee is being flexed, this ligament is loosened. When the knee is extened to 150 degrees, the ligament becomes tense. When the knee is extended straight, the ligament is most tense.

Etiology and Pathology

When the knee joint is slightly flexed, both the medial and external accessory ligaments are more loosened and the knee joint is less stable. In this case, sudden stress of inversion or eversion tends to injure the medial or external accessory ligament, leading to the onset of this disorder.

Clinical Manifestations

Sprain or partial laceration of medial accessory ligament: usual evident history of trauma, pain and tenderness on the medial aspect of the knee joint which become severe when the shank is passively abducted, local edema on the medial aspect of the knee, ecchymoses and hematocele within the knee joint maybe appearing within 2—3 days after the onset.

Complete rupture of medial accessory ligament: touchable space of the broken ligament, positive results of test of the lateral knee joint, over—joint outward—turning activity of the knee joint, obviously—widened medial space (compared with the normal side) seen in the X—ray orthophoric roentgenogram, avulsion of little selerite seen in avulsion of the ligament end, and positive results of drawer—test seen in avulsion of the combined cruclate ligament.

Treatment

Tuina is usually suitable for the treatment of sprain and partial laceration of ligament. To treat complete rupture of ligament, operative suture or neoplasty should be given as soon as possible.

1. Therapeutic Method: Promoting blood circulation to remove blood stasis, relieving swelling and alleviating pain.

2. Manipulation: *Dian, An, Yizhichan Tui, Rou, Mó* and *Pingtui* (flat—pushing).

3. Point Selection: Ashi points around the injury, Xuehai (SP 10), Sanyinjiao (SP 6), Yinlingquan (SP 9), Xiguan (LR 7) and Ququan (LR 8).

4. Operation:

(1) Let the patient in the supine position with his / her injured limb straightened and outward—rotated, and conduct *Dian—an* on the points Xuehai, Yinlingquan and Sanyinjiao in order to promote flowing of *Qi* and blood through the channels and collaterals and relieve pain.

(2) Undertake local gentle *Rou* with the palm or thenar eminence for 3—5 minutes, afterwards, conduct first gentle and then gradually—forceful *Yizhichan Tui* with the thumb up and down along the medial accessory ligament for 3—5 minutes.

(3) Coat the manipulated part with Chinese holly leaf ointment or saffower oil and carry out *Pingtui* until the heat produced has gone deep.

Fresh injury with evident pain should be treated with gentle manipulations, while old injury, with more strong ones.

Rare in clinical pracitice, injury of lateral accessory ligament is manifested and treated in the similar way to that of medial accessory ligament.

5. Treatment Course: Treatment is given once daily, 3 times of treatment make 1 course of treatment.

6.30　Sprain of the Ankle Joint

The ankle joint is a hinge joint made up of the lower ends of the tibia and fibula and the talus. Its capsule is lax in the anterior and posterior but tense on the both sides, has thinner and weaker ligaments in the anterior and posterior but stronger collateral ligaments on the medial and lateral sides.

Etiology and Pathology

When the metatarsus is flexed, the posterior portion of talus enters the ankle joint, getting it in an unsteady state. At this time, if the foot turns inward or outward suddenly, a strong stress will be given to either the lateral collateral ligament of ankle or the medial collateral ligament of ankle, causing sprain of the ankle joint.

Clinical Manifestations

History of acute sprain, evident swelling and pain in the ankle which becomes too serious when the patient stands with the foot, tenderness in the anteroinferior of both the medial and lateral malleoli with purple skin; sprain of lateral malleolus marked by pain in the lateral ankle which becomes aggravated when the ankle joint turns inward; swelling and distension mainly seen in the lateral joint and the anteroinferior of lateral malleolus when lateral joint capsule and anterior fibula ligament are injured; fracture of lateral malleolus perhaps following sprain of medial malleolus which, if ever, leads to swelling and pain in both the medial and lateral malleoli.

Treatment

Better effects will be attained if *Tuina* manipulations are used to treat simple sprain of ligament or laceration of partial ligamentous fibrae. If they are accompanied by fracture or dislocation, orthopedic operation or manual reduction should be carried out as early as possible.

1. Therapeutic Method: promoting blood circulation to remove blood stasis, relieving swelling and alleviating pain.

2. Manipulation: *Dian, An, Yizhichan Tui, Rou, Bashen* and *Yao*.

3. Point Selection: Ashi points around the ankle joint, Zusanli (ST 36), Yanglingquan (GB 34), Taixi (KI 3), Kunlun (BL 60), Qiuxu (GB 40), Xuanzhong (GB 39), Jiexi (ST 41) and Taichong (LR 3).

4. Operation:

(1) Let the patient in the supine position and *Dian—an* (digital—pressing) the points Zusanli, Taixi, Kunlun, Qiuxu, Xuanzhong, Jiexi and Taichong so as to remove obstruction from the channels and collaterals and relieve pain.

(2) Conduct local *Rou* with the thenar for 3—5 minutes, and, then, undertake *Tui* with the thumb from the above to the below over the shank and around the ankle joint so as to promote blood circulation, remove blood stasis, relieve swelling and alleviate pain.

(3) Take operation on the right ankle of the patient for example. Let the patient in the supine position, hold the right big toe of the patient tightly and pull it upward, turn the ankle outward to enlarge its medial space and press the left index finger into the space, turn the ankle inward while the traction is kept to enlarge its lateral space and press the left thumb into the space,

hold the ankle joint with the thumb and index finger, pull–shake gently the affected foot and turn it inward 1–2 times with the right hand, get the foot dorsiflexed and plantar–flexed, and push down and pull up both the medial and lateral malleoli with the thumb and index finger holding the ankle joint with the pushing–down following the dorsiflexion and the pulling–up following plantar flexion (Fig.84).

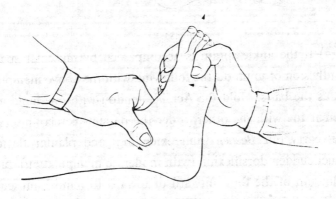

Fig.84–1

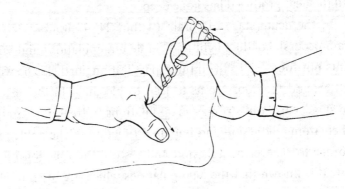

Fig.84–2

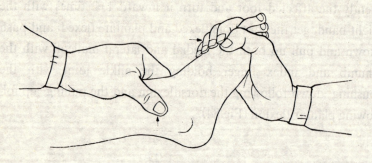

Fig.84—3

(4) If the ankle sprain is accompanied by muscular spasm and adhesion of joint, do the following with the above manipulations as the basis. Hold the Achilles tendon with one hand and the great toe with the other, order the patient to relax his / her ankle, carry out *Bashen* (pull—extending) and plantar flexion, conduct sudden dorsiflexion (with moderate manipulation), turn, the dorsum of the foot outward or inward to remove muscular spasm, and, finally, undertake local gentle *Mó*, *Rou* and *Pingtui* until the heat produced has gone deep.

In the acute stage of sprain (within 24—48 hours after the sprain occurs), conduct light and gentle manipulations and select points not too near to the infured part lest angiorrhexis be worsened around the injury so as to lead to bleeding. In the restoration stage, carry out stronger manipulations to treat organization of hematoma, adhesion and impaired function of the ankle joint in order to relieve the adhesion and restore the function of the joint. It is known that the manipulations which are often used to cause the ankle joint to do passive activity are *Qianyinyaobai* (pulling and swinging), *Yaohuang* (shaking) and *Qushen* (flex—extending).

Fumigating and washing with hot decoction of herbal medicines may be added.

5. Treatment Course: Treatment is given once daily, 3 times of treatment make 1 course of treatment.

6.31 Tarsal Tunnel Syndrome

Tarsal tunnel, located on the medial aspect of the ankle joint, is a canal enclosed with osseofibrous tissue of the posterior shank and the areolar tissue space of deep sole. Through it, there are tendons, blood vessels and nerve.

Etiology and Pathology

Sudden increase of movement of the foot or repeated sprain of the ankle joint gives rise to friction of the tendons within the tarsal tunnel, the friction leads to tenosynovitis and thecal cyst, which are responsible for the enlargement of the content within the tarsal tunnel. But the tarsal tunnel is an osseofibrous canal which is less flexible. And it cannot be enlarged as the content within it is being enlarged. Therefore, the enlargement of the content is, in fact, to narrow the tunnel and raise the pressure within it, resulting in symptoms due to pressure of the posterior tibial nerve. On the other hand, the tunnel may be narrowed due to the degeneration and thickness of division ligament, calcaneal spur formation within the tarsal tunnel or fracture so that the nerve and blood vessels are pressed and this disorder results.

Clinical Manifestations

Discomfort appearing in the posterior medial malleolus due to walking or long—standing in the early stage which may be relieved right away after rest but will appear repeatedly and last a longer time as the disease becomes severe, numbness or formication in the medial calcaneus and sole, dry and bright skin of the toes with trichomadesis and myophagism of the foot in severe cases, exacerbation of prickle in the foot occurring when slight tapping is done on the posterior medial malleolus in examination, and exacerbation of pain in the posterior medial malleolus and the sole appearing when the foot is extremely dorsiflexed.

Treatment

Better curative effects will be attained when *Tuina* is used to treat tarsal tunnel syndrome due to tenosynovitis and thecal cyst within the tarsal tunnel. But better curative effects can not be ensured when *Tuina* is used to treat tarsal tunnel syndrome due to degeneration and thickness of division ligament, calcaneal spur formation within the tarsal tunnel or fracture, and operation is suggested in this case.

1. Therapeutic Method: relaxing muscles and tendons, promoting blood circulation, removing blood stasis and relieving pain.

2. Manipulation: *Yizhichan Tui, Rou, Tanbo* (flicking and poking) and *Ca*.

3. Point Selection: Yinlingquan (SP 9), Sanyinjiao (SP 6), Taixi(KI 3), Zhaohai (KI 6) and Jinmen (BL 63).

4. Operation:

(1) Let the patient in the supine position with his / her affected leg out−rotated, conduct *Dian−an* (digital−pressing) on all the points selected, and carry out *Yizhichan Tui* on the posteromedial aspect of the shank for 5−10 minutes, do it from

the above to the below and up to the ankle with the stress on the local portion where the tarsal tunnel is located and vertically along the longitudinal tarsal tunnel.

(2) Undertake local *Tanbo* on the part where the tarsal tunnel is located for 3—5 minutes.

(3) Perform *Ca* along the tendon until the heat produced has gone deep.

Fumigating and washing with hot decoction of herbal medicines may be added in the course of treatment.

5. Treatment Course: Treatment is given once daily, 10 times make 1 course of treatment.

6.32   Sprain of Achilles Tendon

There is a kind of tissue between the Achilles tendon and its superficial deep fascia. It has 7—8 layers with its structure similar to that of synovium. Every two layers are connected by connective tissue without adhesion. This tissue functions in lubricating the ankle joint while it is being flexed and extended.

Etiology and Pathology

Acute injury or long—time repeated strain causes laceration, oozing of blood or degeneration and necrosis to occur in that synovium—like tissue, leading to adhesion among the layers and between the layers and the Achilles tendon.

Clinical Manifestations

The main clinical manifestation is pain in the Achilles tendon. In the initial stage, the pain usually occurs right when movement starts. After the movement starts, the pain begins to be relieved, but it may be worsened by violent running or jumping.

With the development of this disease, the pain is aroused whenever the Achilles tendon is involved, such as going upstairs or downstairs and walking. There is superficial tenderness, which is especially evident when the superficial Achilles tendon is twisted. In the later stage, there may appear degeneration of the tendon, on which there may be palpable geloses. When they are twisted, a cracking sound may be heard. The Achilles tendon loses tenacity and elasticity and is locally thickened into fusiform. Kicking the ground with toe tips arouses resistive pain.

Treatment

1. Therapeutic Method: promoting blood circulation, removing blood stasis, relaxing muscles and tendons, and eliminating obstruction from the channels and collaterals.

2. Manipulation: *Yizhichan Tui, Nie, Rou, Na, Pingtui* (flat-pushing) and *Yao*.

3. Point Selection: Taixi (KI 3), Fuliu (KI 7), Chengshan (BL 57), Yangjiao (GB 35) and Ashi point around the Achilles tendon.

4. Operation:

(1) Let the patient in the prone position with his / her shank, foot and ankle under a soft cushion, sit by the affected foot of the patient, conduct *Yizhichan Tui* to and fro from the Achilles tendon to the popliteal fossa along the gastrocnemius muscle for 3—5 minutes, carry out gradually—forceful *Nie* and *Na* on the Achilles tendon and the gastrocnemius muscle until there appears sensation of soreness and distension and do it to and fro from the below to the above 5—10 times.

(2) Coat the part where there are the Achilles tendon and the belly of gastrocnemius muscle with Chinese holly leaf ointment or

massage emulsion and conduct *Pingtui* on it until the heat produced has gone deep.

(3) *Tui* and *Rou* the portion of Achilles tendon with the thumb for 3—5 minutes and *Nie* the synovium—like tissue with geloses gently with the thumb and the index finger.

(4) Let the patient flex his / her knee to 90 degrees and do plantar flexion of his / her ankle as well so as to have his / her Achilles tendon fully relaxed, hold the patient's dorsum of foot with one hand and conduct light, quick, gentle *Nie—na* on the posterior aspect of the shank with the other hand, and, then, *Yao* the ankle joint with the hand holding the foot dorsum with the amplitude gradually widened and the ankle joint dorsifiexed.

After the treatment with the above manipulations, hot compress, fumigating and washing with hot decoction of herbal medicines may be added.

5. Treatment Course: Treatment is given once daily, 3 times make 1 course of treatment.

6.33 Scapulohumeral Periarthritis

Common in the middle—aged and the aged, it usually attacks one shoulder with pain and abnormal function of the shoulder joint as the main symptoms.

Etiology and Pathology

It is generally thought that this disease is due to insufficiency of *Qi* and blood, irregular nutrition, attack of the shoulder by wind—cold, or trauma and strain. Experimental observation has found out that it is related to the level of sexual hormones.

Clinical Manifestations

There appear gradually soreness, weakness and disorder of movement in the shoulder usually not due to any special reason. Generally speaking, the pain, as the main symptom and manifested usually as soreness, takes place throughout the shoulder. Being more evident on the anterior aspect of the shoulder Joint, it, sometimes, radiates to the forearm. In the day, it is relieved, but in the night, it is so aggravated that the patient cannot lie in the affected lateral position. The patient has to have his / her shoulder in the fixed posture, because terrible pain will be aroused if the shoulder is touched or the shoulder joint is made to move. Up to the advanced stage, the pain has been gradually relieved but the disorder of movement in the shoulder has been worsened day by day. Abduction and extorsion and lifting are especially difficult and adduction and procurvation are also disturbed. When the shoulder is abducted, there will appear the typical posture—"shoulder —pole— carrying" (Fig.85). And it is difficult for the patient to comb his / her hair or to dress and undress himself / herself. In the severe cases, the elbow is involved to the extent that the hand can not reach the shoulder even if the elbow is bent, and atrophy of the deltoid muscle of different degrees occurs.

Treatment

In the initial stage, the pain is severe, and gentle manipulations are used locally and repeatedly for the purpose of removing obstruction from the channels and collaterals, promoting blood circulation, relieving pain and strengthening the function of local muscles, tendons and ligaments. In the advanced stage, more forceful manipulations such as *Ban, Bashen* and *Yao* may be used together with other kinds of shoulder movement to release adhesion, lubricate the joint and restore the function of the joint gradually.

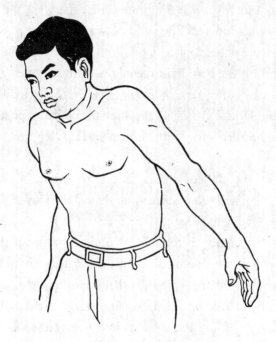

Fig.85

1. Therapeutic Method: relaxing muscles and tendons, dredging the collaterals, releasing adhesion, promoting blood circulation and relieving pain.

2. Manipulation: *Yizhichan Tui, Dian, An, Na, Ban, Bashen, Yao* and *Dou*.

3. Point Selection: Jianneiling, Jianyu (LI 15), Jianliao (SJ 14), Naoshu (SI 10), Tianzong (SI 11), Jianjing (GB 21), Quchi(LI 11) and Hegu (LI 4).

4. Operation:

(1) Stand or sit to the affected side of the patient in the su-

pine or sitting position, conduct *Yizhichan Tui* on the anterior aspect of the shoulder (Jianneiling) and the medial aspect of the upper arm to and fro for 3—5 minutes, and, then, get the affected arm abducted, adducted, lifted and outward—rotated passively.

(2) Let the patient in the lateral recumbent position with the healthy arm on the bed, hold the elbow of the affected arm with one hand, carry out *Yizhichan Tui, Rou* or *Gun* with the other hand on the lateral aspect of the shoulder and the posterior aspect of the armpit, and get the affected arm lifted and adducted passively.

(3) Let the patient in the sitting position, *Na* and *Nie* Jianjing, *Dian* and *Rou* Tianzong, Naoshu, Jianyu, Jianliao, Jianneiling, Quchi and Hegu.

(4) Stand slightly before the affected arm; grasp the disordered shoulder with one hand; hold the wrist, or support the elbow, of the affected arm with the other hand; rotate the arm with the shoulder joint as the axis in small to large circles; adduct the affected arm by lifting the forearm and flexing the elbow to get the hand to reach the healthy shoulder, go over the head and return to the disordered shoulder; repeat the rotation 5—10 times; and, meanwhile, conduct *Nie—na* on the disordered shoulder with the hand grasping it.

(5) Stand slightly before the affected side of the patient, grasp the wrist of the disordered shoulder with one hand, prop the anterior of the disordered shoulder with your own shoulder, pull the affected arm with the hand grasping the wrist from the front to the back of the patient and get it extended as backward as possible with an increasing force (Fig.86), and repeat the above 3—5 times.

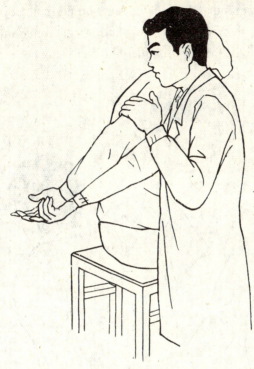

Fig.86

(6) Stand slightly behind the healthy side of the patient, support the healthy shoulder with one hand, grasp the wrist of the affected side with the other hand and pull the affected arm to the healthy side via the back of the patient, do the above with an increasing force and in a widening range as long as the patient can stand (Fig.87).

(7) Stand laterally to the disordered shoulder of the patient, hold with the two hands the slightly anterior portion of the wrist of the affected arm, lift the affected arm as *Dou* is being done until the arm has been pulled obliquely—upward. While the above is being done, the manipulations should be gentle and slow. To an-

swer to the manipulations, the patient should first drop his / her shoulder and flex his / her elbow, and, then, stretch and abduct the elbow and lift the arm obliquely—upward (Fig.88).

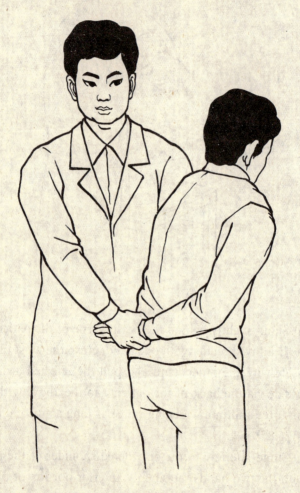

Fig.87

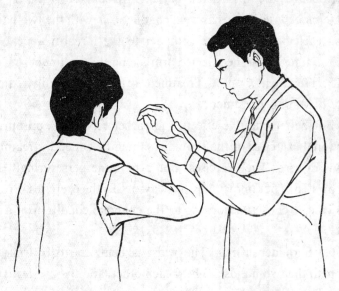

Fig.88-1

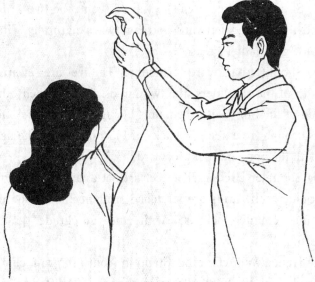

Fig.88-2

(8)Circle the disordered shoulder clockwise 3 times and counterclockwise 3 times as well, conduct *Cuo* with the two hands facing each other from the shoulder to the forearm, repeat the *Cuo* 3—5 times, *Dou* the affected arm to end the treatment.

5. Treatment Course: Treatment is given once daily, 7 times make 1 course of treatment.

For better curative effects and earlier recovery, appropriate functional exercises of the shoulder should be added in treatment of this disease. The exercises should be done perseveringly and step by step. The following is the ways to do the exercises. Proper ones can be chosen according to the concrete condition of a patient.

(1) Shoulder lifting: The waist is bent, the two arms are dropped, the two hands are held each other, and the two arms are swung forward with the amplitude gradually increased.

(2) Shoulder abducting: The waist is bent, the two arms are dropped and swung leftward and rightward naturally with the amplitude gradually increased.

(3) Shoulder backward—extending: The feet are set apart at the width of the shoulders, the two hands are held each other at the back of the body with the palms facing outward, the affected hand is brought to extend as backward as possible by the healthy hand with the body not bent forward.

(4) Shoulder circling: The feet are set apart at the width of the shoulders, the arms are stretched straight and circled clockwise and counterclockwise with the amplitude gradually increased.

(5) Hands wall—climbing: Stand in front of a wall, climb the wall slowly with the two hands until the arms are lifted as high as

possible, and do it again and again.

(6) Shoulder adducting—abducting: Cross the two hands at the back of the neck and adduct and abduct the shoulder joint as far as possible, do the above again and again.

6.34   Disturbance of Costovertebral Joints

Disturbance of costovertebral joints is an acute disorder with sudden onset. It is usually due to improper torsion of the body or unlucky coughing and sneezing.

Etiology and Pathology

Synovial incarceration or mild transposition of the costovertebral joints are the cause of this disease.

Clinical Manifestations

The typical symptom of this disease is sudden pain in one sternocostal part which becomes severe when the patient coughs, sneezes or takes deep breath. Examination may find out that the patient has the chest harbored, the back flexed, and the breath superficial and short; that the tenderness part is in the shape of small tracts around the involved costovertebral joints; and that traction of the affected arm often causes pain.

Treatment

Instant results may be got if this disease is treated with *Tuina*, and best curative effects results if the treatment is given just after the onset. If the disorder has last a longer time, inflammatory reaction usually takes place in and around the dislocated joints. If so, recovery will come after several times of treatment.

1. Therapeutic Method: reducing to stop pain, regulating the flow of *Qi* to promoting blood circulation.

2. Manipulation: *An–rou, Bashen, Yao* and *Dou.*

3. Point Selection: the place where the injured joints are located, Yanglingquan (GB 34) and Chengshan (BL 57).

4. Operation:

(1) Manipulation for relaxation before reduction: Let the patient in the prone position, conduct *An–rou* with the thumb first on Yanglingquan and then on Chengshan for about 5 minutes to gradually relieve the costodorsal pain and the muscular tension, and, then, carry out gentle *Rou* and *Mó* on the local part for about 5 minutes to further relieve the pain and muscular spasm.

(2) Manipulation for reduction:

A. Propping the back to expand the chest: Let the patient in the sitting position with his / her two hands crossed at the back of the neck, stand to the back of the patient and hold his / her two elbows with the two hands, bend the knee of one leg and prop with it the place where the involved costovertebral joints are located, pull gently backward the patient's two elbows with your two hands to expand his / her chest while pushing your bent knee forward and ordering the patient to take deep breath, and do the above 2–3 times. Be sure to coordinate the pulling–back and pushing–forward with gentle and slow strength.

B. Palm–tapping: Let the patient in the sitting position, stand lateral–anteriorly to the patient, insert your forearm from the front into the patient's armpit and exert force to raise the affected shoulder, order the patient to take deep breath and tap the affected part with the palm root of the other hand before the patient is ready for it, and repeat the above 1–2 times.

C. Pull–extending: Stand before the affected side of the patient sitting on a low stool, hold with your two hands the fingers of the affected hand with its palm inward, tightly grasp the hand and rotate it in a circle from the below to the above by way of the inside with the amplitude moderate, and exert force suddenly to pull the affected arm up when the muscles of the affected arm are relaxed and there is no difficulty in the circle—rotating.

(3) Ending—manipulation: Stand to the lateral—front side of the patient in the sitting position, order the patient to stretch straight his / her affected arm, hold the wrist and rotate continuously the affected arm from the below via the front and to the back for 10 circles or so. In the course of doing the above, order the patient to inhale while the affected arm is lifted but to exhale while it is dropped, and, then, grasp the wrist and pull and shake the affected arm to end the treatment.

5. Treatment Course: Treatment is given one time. If cure refuses to come, continue the treatment.

6.35 Cervical Spondylopathy

Hyperplasia of cervical vertebrae leads to inflammatory stimulation, which compresses cervical nerve root, spinal cord in the neck, vertebral artery or sympathetic nerve, bringing about a syndrome. This syndrome is called cervical spondylopathy or cervical spondylotic syndrome. It is common in the middle—aged and the aged.

Etiology and Pathology

Different—degree injuries of cervical intervertebral discs, ligaments and posterior joint capsules due to various acute and chronic trauma decrease the stability of spine and cause compensatory hyperplasia of cervical vertebrae. Hyperplastic things compress nerves and blood vessels directly or indirectly to result in symptoms. The main cause of this disease is degeneration of intervertebral discs.

Hyperplasia of cervical vertebra may occur at the posterior joint, uncinate vertebral joint and vertebral body. Different sites of hyperplasia determine different symptoms. For example, there is no symptom due to hyperplasia on the anterior border of vertebral body; narrowing of the anteroposterior diameter of vertebral canal due to hyperplasia on the posterior border of vertebral body is marked by spinal compression, which is called cervical spondylopathy of myeloid form; compression of vertebral artery due to hyperplasia lateral to uncinate vertebral joint is known as cervical spondylopathy of vertebral—artery type; narrowing of intervertebral foramen due to hyperplasia on the lateroposterior of vertebral body, on the anterior border of posterior joint or on the posterior of uncinate vertebral joint may be marked by compression of the nerves of cervical or brachial plexus, which is called cervical spondylopathy of nerve—root type; hyperplasia of posterior joint accompanied by semidislocation or stimuli to vertebral artery may arouse sympathetic nerve symptoms, which is known as cervical spondylopathy of sympathetic nerve type.

The symptoms of hyperplasia of cervical vertebrae are produced in two ways: direct and indirect. Direct, the hyperplastic things compress nerves and blood vessels directly, causing the symptoms. Indirect, local traumatic inflammation and inflammatory congestive edema due to over—stimulation of the hyperplastic things to their peripheral soft tissues compress nerves and blood vessels, causing the symptoms.

Clinical Manifestations

1. Cervical Sponsylopathy of Nerve—root Type: Symptoms due to stimulation or compression of nerve root, which is resulted from retroplasia of the intervertebral facet joints or uncinate vertebral joints, are as follows: pain in the neck and shoulder or in the neck and occiput; sensory disturbance of the occiput; or stiffness of the neck; radiating pain in the neck, shoulder and arm (one side or both sides) which is accompanied by numbness of the fingers, cold limbs, heavy and weak upper limbs, difficulty of the hand / hands in holding things; unsymmetrical limitation of cervical movement, pain aggravated by backward—extending or turning—to—the —affected—side of the neck; positive results of spurling test, traction test, brachial plexus pulling test, head hypsokinesis test done while spinous processes are being pressed by the fingers, and test of head—turning and force—adding; as well as reflex pain and secondary tenderness points on the interior border of the scapula, in the scapular region or in the shoulder.

2. Cervical Spondylopathy of Myeloid Form: Invasion of the protruded intervertebral discs and the posterior longitudinal ligament or the thickened yellow ligament into the vertebral canal due to hyperplasia on the posterior border of vertebral body gets the spinal cord compressed to give rise to the following symptoms: numbness, soreness and weakness of the upper or lower limbs or one or two sides of the body; quivering neck and trembling arms; and incomplete spasmatic paralysis in different degree marked by limited movement, awkward gait, staggering walking, even keeping the bed and dyspnea, hypermyotonia of limbs, tendon hyperreflexia, weakened or lost superficial reflex, clonus of the patella and ankle, and positive Babinski' s sign.

Usually, there is no neckache and dyskinesia. Incomplete obstruction is often found in dynamic test of cerebrospinal fluid.

3. Cervical Spondylopathy of Vertebral Artery Type: Torsion, spasm or compression of the artery due to degeneration and hyperplasia of the cervical vertebrae lead to poor blood supply of the vertebral artery. Therefore, this type is also called ischemia form. It is marked by pain in the neck and shoulder or in the neck and occiput, dizziness, nausea, vomiting, positional vertigo, cataplexy, tinnitus, deafness, and blurred vision. All the above symptoms are due to ischemia in the inner ear and brain and evoked or worsened by turning of the neck or lateral-flexing of it to certain extent.

4. Cervical Spondylopathy of Sympathetic Nerve Type: The symptoms due to stimulated sympathetic nerve are as follows: pain in the occiput, heaviness sensation in the head, dizziness or migraine, palpitation, choking sensation in the chest, cold limbs, decreased skin temperature or feverish sensation in the hands and feet, soreness and distension of the extremities, seldom seen radiating pain and numbness sensation in the arm, and such symptoms perhaps seen in few patients as retrobulbar pain, blurring of vision, photophobia, lacrimation, rhinorrhea, sensation of foreign body in the throat, precordialgia, and facial sweating.

5. Cervical Spondylopathy of Anterior Scalene Muscle Type: Protruded hyperplastic thing stimulates the 4th and 5th cervical nerve roots, causing spasm of the anterior scalene muscle. The spasmatic muscle compresses the brachial plexus, leading to symptoms due to scalenus syndrome and the involved 4th and 5th cervical nerve roots.

6. Cervical Spondylopathy of Intervertebral Discs: Degener-

ation and atrophy of the intervertebral discs stimulate the endings of meningeal branch, causing reflex pain in the neck, scapular region, back and shoulder not accompanied by the symptoms due to involved nerve roots.

7. Cervical Spondylopathy of Mixed Type: Two or more types of the above are mixed into this type. It has the symptoms of two or more types introduced in the above.

Cervical X−ray film reveals the following abnormalities: disappearance or reverse of physiological lordosis of cervical vertebra, lateral curvature of cervical vertebra, narrowing of intervertebral space, sclerosis of the intervertebral facet joints, uncinate vertebral joints and the edge of vertebral body, narrowing of intervertebral facet joint space, and posteroinferior sliding of inferior articular process. X−ray film of cervical anteflexion and posteroextension indicates abnormal sliding of vertebral bodies of the diseased part. Vertebral arteriography is helpful to the diagnosis of cervical spondylopathy of vertebral artery type. Contrast examination may find incomplete or complete obstruction of the diseased space of subarachnoid cavity in the patients with cervical spondylopathy of spinal cord type.

Treatment

Certain curative effects can be ensured if *Tuina* is used to treat this disease except the type due to direct osseous compression. It is especially effective in treating the types of nerve root, vertebral artery, sympathetic nerve, anterior scalene muscle and intervertebral discs. At the present, *Tuina* is still the therapeutic method of choice for treating cervical spondylopathy. Yet, reduction through turning cervical vertebrae is not suggested for cervical spondylopathy of spinal cord type or the patients with hypertension and severe arteriosclerosis. If this reduction is applied to other types, the operation should be gentle, not violent.

1. Therapeutic Method: relaxing muscles and tendons, promoting blood circulation, restoring and treating injured soft tissues, and conducting reduction.

2. Manipulation: *Yizhichan Tui, An, Rou, Na, Bashen, Bashenxuanzhuan* (pulling, extending and rotating), *Cuo, Pingtui* (flat—pushing), *Yao* and *Dou*.

3. Point Selection: Fengchi (GB 20), Tianzhu (BL 10), Dazhui (DU 14), Dazhu (BL 11), Jianjing (GB 21), Tianzong (SI 11), Quchi (LI 11) and Waiguan (SJ 5).

4. Operation:

(1) Stand behind the patient sitting upright, conduct *Yizhichan Tui* with the thumb from Fengchi along the sides of the spinous processes of cervical vertebrae down to Dazhu, and do this to and fro 5—7 times with the both sides manipulated alternately.

(2) *Nie* and *Na* the neck with the stress on the pressure pain point and rotate gently the neck for 2—3 minutes.

(3) Carry out *An—rou* with the thumb or the index and middle fingers on Tianzong, Bingfeng (SI 12), Quepen (ST 12), and Jianwaishu (SI 14), *Na* with the two hands on Jianjing, *Tanbo* with the index, middle and ring fingers on the area of the upper 1 / 3 of the medial aspect of the upper arm, and *An—rou* with the thumb on Quchi (LI 11), Shousanli (LI 10) and Waiguan. Then, rotate the shoulder joint in a circle and shake the arm.

(4) Three methods for pulling and extending the neck:

A. Let the patient in the supine position with the lower limbs stretched straight and the upper limbs put flat along the sides of the body. Sit right to the top of the patient's head with the knees against the bed legs. Hold the patient's lower jaw with one hand and prop the portion where his / her external occipital protuberance is located with the other hand. Move the waist and the upper body backward to give a pulling force to the neck to do *Bashen* and repeat this for 2–3 minutes, and shake the cervical vertebrae gently and turn the head left and right softly while *Bashen* is being done. While this is being carried out, there may appear a "crack".

B. Stand behind the patient in the sitting position. Put the ulnar sides of the two forearms on the two shoulders of the patient and press them downward. Prop the area above Fengchi respectively with the two thumbs (Violent force is avoided lest the patient feel discomfortable such as dizzy.) with the patient's lower jaw held by the rest fingers and the palms, all of which exert upward–force. Get the forearms pressed downward and the hands lifted upward to widen the cervical vertebral spaces. While this is being done, bend the head and neck of the patient forward and backward and turn them left and right.

C. Stand to the affected side of the patient sitting on a low stool, flex your elbow joint and hold with it the patient's lower jaw with the hand placed on the healthy temporo–occipital part of the patient, pull the head slowly upward and, meanwhile, turn it left and right. While doing this, conduct *An–rou* on the pressure pain point with the thumb of the other hand placed on the corresponding spinous process of the affected part.

To treat cases with the symptoms of headache and dizziness, in addition to the above manipulations, the following is added: *Fenmŏ* (wiping–rubbing) the forehead and the two superciliare arches, *Dian* Jingming (BL 1), *Fenmǒ* Yingxiang (LI 20), Renzhong (DU 26) and Chengjiang (RN 24), and undertake *Saosan* (sweeping—rubbing) on the tempora and from the temporo—occipital area to the back of the neck.

5. Treatment Course: Treatment is given once every two days. 10 times of treatment make 1 course.

6. Functional Exercises of the Neck: In the course of being treated with *Tuina* manipulations, the patient should do the following functional exercises of the neck.

(1) Stand with the two arms naturally dropped or sit with the two hands placed respectively on the two thighs, relax the whole body, bend the head and neck slowly forward up to the maximum and repeat this 20—30 times.

(2) Sit or stand, bend the head and neck laterally and slowly first to the healthy side up to the maximum and then to the affected side to the maximum and repeat this 20—30 times.

(3) Sit or stand, rotate the head slowly from the median position to the healthy side, the back side, the affected side and the original median position, forming a circular movement, and do this 20—30 times. Then, do this in the opposite direction, also 20—30 times.

(4)Hold the lower jaw and the occipital part with a self—made traction support to pull the neck like this. Sit on a stool with the head neither forward—flexed, nor backward—extended nor left / rightward—bent but kept in the median position. The traction weight is 3—5 kg. The traction time is half an hour each time. The traction is carried out 1—2 times daily.

6.36 Stiffneck

With the onset usually in the morning, stiffneck is clinically marked mainly by acute muscular spasm, aching, distension, pain and motor impairment of the neck.

Etiology and Pathology

Improper height of the pillow, improper sleeping posture or exposure of the neck and shoulder to wind, any of which, if ever, exists in the course of sleeping, keeps the muscle group of one side in the over-extension state for a longer time and causes myospasm or myofibrositis, leading to this disease. It is rarely due to sudden improper turning of the neck or due to spasm and sprain of certain muscles occurring when one is carrying heavy things on the shoulder.

Clinical Manifestations

The main manifestations are spasm, stiffness and pain of sternocleidomastoid muscle and trapezius muscle of one side of the neck. The head is distorted towards the affected side with the jaw turned to the normal side. The movement of the neck is obviously limited. In severe cases, the pain may refer to the head, the upper back and the upper arm. In the affected area, there is evident tenderness.

Treatment

Better curative effects may be attained when *Tuina* is used to treat stiffneck. By and large, cure comes after 1—2 times of treatment. The shorter the disease course, the better the curative effects.

1. Therapeutic Method: relaxing muscles and tendons, promoting blood circulation, removing obstruction from channels

and collaterals, and stopping pain.

2. Manipulation: *Yizhichan Tui, An, Rou, Yao* and *Na*.

3. Point Selection: Ashi point, Fengchi (GB 20), Fengfu (DU 16), Jianjing (GB 21) and Tianzong (SI 11).

4. Operation:

(1) Stand behind the affected side of the patient in the sitting position, conduct gentle *Yizhichan Tui* on the neck and shoulder of the affected side, and, at the same time, support the lower jaw of the patient and push—shake it gently with the other hand.

(2) When the cervical muscles are relaxed and the neck can be turned to larger extent, bend the neck a little forward and turn it rapidly with the hand supporting the lower jaw to the affected side in larger amplitude (5 degrees beyond those of the functional position). At the same time, push gently the corresponding spinous processes of cervical vertebrae towards the normal side with the other hand. To carry out the above manipulations, the two hands should be coordinated to get the manipulations gentle, soft and flexible. As for the amplitude of turning, it should be within the range that the patient can stand.

(3) Finally, *Na* Fengchi, Fengfu, Jianjing; *An—rou* Tianzong; and *Pingtui* the shoulder up to the extent that heat has been produced, with the treatment coming to an end.

5. Treatment Course: Treatment is given once daily and 3 times of treatment make 1 course.

6.37　Disturbance of Lumbar Vertebral Facet Joints

Etiology and Pathology

This disorder is caused by anatomic malposition of lumbar

vertebral facet joints—dislocation of joints or incarceration of synovium due to knock of external force or improper movement of the waist.

Clinical Manipulations

Absence of history of obvious trauma; pain that is suddenly felt when the waist is being bent forward, leftward or rightward or rotated and that is followed by inability to move, the pain aggravated by coughing and sneezing, no radiating pain in the lower limbs; onset sometimes due to coughing and sneezing; evident and fixed tenderness point, obviously—limited waist, muscular tension and spasm at the affected side; local percussion pain, no evident tenderness in the lower limbs which are not limited; and no abnormal changes of the bones or the intervertebral space found in roentgenogram.

Treatment

Once *Tuina* is used, the cure comes. If treatment is given just after the onset, 1 time of treatment is enough.

1. Therapeutic Method: restoring and treating the injured soft tissues, conducting reduction, promoting the flowing of *Qi*, and stopping pain.

2. Manipulation: *An, Rou, Xieban* (obliquely—pulling) and *Bashen*.

3. Point Selection: Weizhong (BL 40), Chengshan (BL 57) and Ashi point in the waist.

4. Operation:

(1) Stand or sit to the affected side of the patient in the prone position, *An—rou* gently the pain point with the thumb of one hand to relax the muscles, and, at the same time, *An—rou* Chengshan and Weizhong of the affected side with the thumb of

the other hand to relieve spasm, relieve pain and promote the flowing of *Qi* and blood.

(2) Let the patient in the recumbent position with his / her involved leg stretched straight in the below and the other leg flexed in the above, and conduct *Xieban* (obliquely—pulling) like this. Press the patient's hip anteroinferiorly with one elbow, his / her shoulder posteroinferiorly with the other elbow, and the corresponding spinous process where there is pain with a thumb, and, then, exert forces in opposite directions with the elbows to undertake *Xieban* with a "crack" maybe heard. Order the patient to stretch his / her leg with effort and pull his / her foot and ankle while the patient is doing so, and do this 3 times. Up to this time, the patient has felt that the waist is relaxed and the pain is driven away. Finally, conduct gentle *Rou* on the original pain point for 2—3 minutes to end the treatment.

5. Treatment Course: Treatment is given 1 time. If cure fails to come, continue the treatment.

6.38 Acute Lumbar Sprain

The waist is the pivotal part to dominate the activity of the whole body and transmit the weight of the upper body. It is one of the parts of the body to act most in daily life and work. Loaded with weight and kept acting, it is easy to injure by the muscles.

Etiology and Pathology

Over—backward—extension or forward—flexion, torsion or bending beyond normal range, over—loading or over—exertion, improper posture, fall or direct violent attack will get the muscles of the loins rotated and pulled violently so that the muscles are suddenly injured and this disorder results.

Clinical Manifestations

There is the history of distinct sprain in most cases. In the severe ones, serious pain in the loins appears just after the injury, movement of the waist is limited so that there occurs difficulty in sitting, lying and walking, and coughing and sneezing as well as deep—breathing will worsen the pain. In the mild cases, pain in the loins is mild just after the injury occurs, but several hours or 1—2 days later, it gradually becomes so serious that the waist can not act. Examination may find evident local pressure pain point usually in fresh injury, absence of radiating tenderness and percussion pain in the lower limbs, distinct muscular tension and spasm in the injured region, and lateral curvature of spine in the lumbar portion.

Treatment

Remarkable curative effects will be seen when this disease is treated with *Tuina*. In the course of treatment, bed rest is suggested so as to keep off resprain. For cases with serious pain, hot compress may be added. When undertaking manipulations, select the position in which the patient can feel comfortable and get his / her limbs relaxed, and be sure not make his / her muscles tense owing to the stress of some position, otherwise, resprain may occur.

1. Therapeutic Method: promoting blood circulation to remove blood stasis, eliminating obstruction in the channels and collaterals to stop pain.

2. Manipulation: *Rou*, *Pingtui* (flat—pushing), *Gun* and *Dian—an* (digital—pressing).

3. Point Selection: Ashi point, Shenshu (BL 23), Weizhong

(BL 40) and Chengshan (BL 57).

4. Operation:

(1)Stand to the affected side of the patient in the prone position, *An—rou* the pressure pain point gently with one, thumb and, meanwhile, *Dian—an* the point Chengshan at the same side with the other thumb up to the extent that the lumbar muscles are slightly relaxed, finally, conduct *Gun* on the lumbar muscles at the both sides with the manipulation gradually becoming forceful up to the extent that the pain can not be worsened.

(2) Coat the areas where the lumbar muscles of the both sides are located with Chinese holly leaf ointment and carry out *Pingtui* there until the heat produced has gone deep into the muscles, with the stress put on the affected side.

(3) Let the patient in the supine position with his / her knees and hips flexed, hold the knees of the patient with the two hands and rotate them gently to bring his / her waist and hips into action with the treatment thus ended.

5. Treatment Course: Treatment is given once every two days, 3 times of treatment make 1 course.

6.39 Syndrome of the Third Lumbar Vertebral Transverse Process

The third lumbar vertebra is located at the apex of the physiological lordosis of the lumbar vertebrae. It is the pivot that the movement of lumbar vertebrae depends on. Having longer transverse process than all the others, it acts in a broader range, touches the deep layers of lumbodorsal fasciae more often and bears stronger acting—force of lever. As a result, the muscles attached to it tend to be rubbed and pulled to lead to injury.

Etiology and Pathology

Injury of the muscles and fasciae attached to the 3rd lumbar vertebral transverse process due to over-loading, improper twisting of the waist or long-time repeated lumbar bending will cause tension or spasm of the lumbodorsal muscles, stimulating or compressing the lateral branch of the posterior branch of the spinal nerve to lead to waist pain, and this disease results.

Clinical Manifestations

Lumbogluteal pain at one side of the body of the patient who usually has a history of different-degree lumbar sprain or strain, the pain radiating along the thigh to the superior of the knee and aggravated while the waist is being bent or twisted; evident tenderness at the ends of the 3rd lumbar vertebral transverse process and palpable thick, hard and cordlike mass both of which are found out in examination, and mild atrophy of lumbar muscles maybe seen in the advanced stage.

Treatment

Satisfactory curative effects may be ensured if this disease is treated with *Tuina*. But in the initial stage of the disease, the manipulations used should be gentle. Violent or too powerful manipulations, if used at this time, may lead to new injury, so, they must be avoided. In the course of treatment, the patient should avoid or decrease lumbar extension, flexion and rotation.

1. Therapeutic Method: Relaxing muscles and tendons, promoting blood circulation to remove blood stasis, and subduing swelling to stop pain.

2. Manipulation: *Yizhichan Tui, Ca, Tanbo* (flicking and poking) and *An-rou*.

3. Point Selection: Ashi point at the ends of the 3rd lumbar vertebral transverse process of the affected side, Chengshan (BL 57) and Yanglingquan (GB 34).

4. Operation:

(1) Stand to the affected side of the patient in the prone position, *An—rou* with the thumb Chengshan and Yanglingquan of the affected limb with strength that the patient can stand in order to remove obstruction in the channels and collaterals, relieve spasm and pain, and, then, conduct gentle *Yizhichan Tui* on the affected area where the 3rd lumbar vertebral transverse process is located for 3—5 minutes.

(2) Carry out vertical *Tanbo* on the cordlike hard mass with the strength becoming gradually strong up to the extent that the patient can stand.

(3) Coat the manipulated part with Chinese holly leaf ointment or other lubricating medium and undertake *Ca* on it until the heat produced has gone deep.

(4) Perform *Houshenban* (backward—extending—pulling) and *Jiance Xieban* (obliquely—pulling of the normal side) as the last procedure of the treatment.

Hot compress on the loins may be used in combination with the manipulations.

5. Treatment Course: Treatment is given once every two days, 3 times of treatment make 1 course.

6.40   Chronic Strain of Lumbar Muscle

Etiology and Pathology
This disorder is due to long—time repeated lumbar strain, de-

layed or mal–treated acute injury of lumbar muscle, repeated injury of the lumbar or chronic muscular fibrositis of the lumbus caused by cold and dampness.

Clinical Manifestations

A history of repeated–occurring lumbago manifested usually as lumbar aching which relapses or becomes severe due to strain, pain appearing in the loins when the patient sits or stands for a longer time, extensive tenderness in the loins which has no fixed pressure pain point, palpable tendor hard knot in the severe cases with prolonged pain, no marked motor impairment in the waist and legs, various symptoms all worsened due to acute attack and perhaps accompanied by muscular spasm, lateral curvature of the lumbar vertebrae and pain referring to the lower limbs.

Treatment

1. Therapeutic Method: relaxing muscles and tendons, activating collaterals, warming up channels, and promoting blood circulation.

2. Manipulation: *Gun, Rou, Dian–an, Ca* and *Paiji* (Pat–hitting).

3. Point Selection: Shenshu (BL 23), Mingmen (DU 4), Dachangshu (BL 25) and Weizhong (BL 40).

4. Operation:

(1) Stand or sit at the side of the patient in the prone position, conduct *Gun* over the lumbar muscles of the both sides of the patient's body for about 5 minutes, and, then, carry out *An–rou* with the thumb or the palm root of one hand on the sacrospinal muscles of the two sides from the above to the below and do this 5–10 times with the stress on the points Shenshu, Dachangshu and Zhibian (BL 54), and, at the same time, under-

take *Dian—an* Weizhong and Chengshan with the thumb of the other hand.

(2) Apply massage emulsion or Chinese holly leaf ointment to the two sides of lumbar vertebrae and perform *Ca* until the heat produced has gone deep.

(3) *Paiji* the sacrospinal muscles of the lumbodorsal sides to end the treatment.

5. Treatment Course: Treatment is given once daily, 7 times of treatment make 1 course.

6.41 Prolapse of Lumbar Intervertebral Disc

Also called rupture syndrome of the fibrous rings of the lumbar intervertebral disc, it is common in the young and usually due to the prolapse of the 4th and 5th lumbar intervertebral discs and the 5th lumbosacral intervertebral disc.

Etiology and Pathology

Retrograde affection or aplasia of lumbar intervertebral disc and sudden attack of the loins by external force or long—time repeated strain of the waist get the pulpiform nucleus to break through the fibrous ring and protrude backward, leading to the compression of the nerve root or the spinal cord. Attach of cold—dampness on the loins is responsible for further injury.

Clinical Manifestations

1. Symptoms

(1) Lumbocrural pain: A history of long—time recurrent lumbago in most cases, the pain gradually radiating to one leg (two legs seldom seen), the radiating pain aggravated by coughing

and sneezing, pain or numbness on the lateral or posterior aspect of one shank which gradually shifts to the loins in some cases, and tending to lie on the normal side with the affected leg flexed in the above seen in most cases.

(2) Motor impairment of the loins: Movement of the waist in all directions evidently disturbed in the acute stage, the range of waist movement gradually enlarged with the alleviation of the disease.

(3) Subjective numbness: Subjective numbness often seen in the cases with longer disease duration, the numbness usually localized on the lateral aspect of the shank and the dorsum, heel or great toe of the foot, and numbness in the sella area perhaps seen in the protrusion of pulpiform nucleus of the central form.

(4) Cold affected limbs: Coldness in the affected limbs complained by most patients, skin temperature of the affected limbs lower than that of the normal ones.

2. Signs

(1) Lateral curvature of the spine, decrease or disappearance and even backward-protrusion of the physiological lordosis of the lumbar vertebrae.

(2) Tenderness and percussion pain in the loins which radiate to the affected lower limb and sole, and evident tenderness along the region where the sciatic nerve of the affected side is located.

(3) Positive results of straight-leg-lifting test and dorsiflexion-strengthening test.

(4) Decreased myodynamia of dorsiflexion of the great toe and plantar flexion.

(5) Positive results of supine abdomen—straightening test or neck—flexing test.

(6) Positive results of posteroextension of the lower limbs.

(7) Decreased knee reflex and Achilles jerk, hypoesthesia of the skin of the posterolateral aspect of the shank and the dorsum of the foot.

(8) Disappearance of the physiological radian of lumbar vertebrae, lateral curvature of lumbar vertebrae and narrowing of the intervertebral spaces not accompanied by other vertebral and joint lesions, which are found through X—ray examination.

(9) Protrusion or bulge of the intervertebral discs in different directions found on CT examination.

Treatment

For the present, among the non—operative therapeutic methods, *Tuina* is the most effective one in treating prolapse of lumbar intervertebral disc.

In the course of attack and treatment of this disease, patients should confine themselves to plank beds for rest with their waists kept warm. When the symptoms and signs are relieved, they should do proper functional exercises of the waist.

1. Therapeutic Method: reducing and repositing, releasing adhesion, promoting the circulation of *Qi* and blood, eliminating obstruction in the channels, removing blood stasis, and stopping pain.

2. Manipulation: *Qianla* (pulling), *Xieban* (obliquely—pulling), *Xuanzhuan* (rotating) and *An—rou*.

3. Point Selection: Ashi point in the lumbar region, Zhibian (BL 54), Huantiao (GB 30), Yinmen (BL 37),

Weizhong (BL 40), Chengshan (BL 57), Yanglingquan (GB 34) and Jiexi (ST 41).

4. Operation:

(1) Stand to the affected side of the patient in the prone position, conduct *An—rou* with the thumb on the pressure pain point by the spinous process for 2—3 minutes with the strength gradually becoming forceful, and, at the same time, carry out *Dian—an* on Weizhong or Chengshan and Yanglingquan of the affected side until the lumbar muscles are slightly relaxed, order the patient to lie on the affected side with his / her normal side in the above and perform *Xieban* by pressing the deviated spinous process with the thumb with a "crack" maybe heard.

(2) Let the patient in the supine position, hold the affected foot and ankle with the two hands and *Doula* (shake and pull) the affected lower limb 3 times.

After *An—rou* on the spinous process and the points Weizhong and Chengshan is done, rotating—reposition of lumbar vertebrae may be carried out in order to regulate the posterior joints of lumbar vertebrae, pull the nerve roots and enlarge the nerve root canals and the intervertebral spaces.

Manual countertraction or mechanical traction with a traction table may be conducted with the traction weight 10 kg more than the body weight of the patient. At the same time as traction is being done, press the area around the spinous process so as to reposit the pulpiform nucleus.

If a case with long disease duration fails to respond well to many kinds of manipulations, traction and *Tuina* may be undertaken after medicines are injected into the sacral hiatus or the intervertebral foramen. That is, countertraction and reposition by pressing are performed after 20 ml of 1% lidocaine and 10 mg of dexamethasone are injected into the corresponding intervertebral foramen or sacral hiatus.

5. Treatment Course: Treatment is given once every two days, 7 times of treatment make 1 course.

7　Adult *Tuina* for Health−care

Tuina performed with one's own hands and simple manipulations, on the channels and points or some specialized parts of one's own body surface and for the purpose of health−protection or health−preserving and self−treatment of some diseases is called "health−care *Tuina*". Since health−care *Tuina* is carried out mainly by self−rubbing and self−pinching for the sake of self−treatment, it is also called "self−*Tuina*". Health−care *Tuina* works mainly due to the curative effects attained by activating one's own system of channel and point with one's own manipulations. In addition, the duration of self−manipulating is also the duration of active exercising. As a result, as long as self−*Tuina* is conducted according to one's own concrete condition, on the selected manipulated parts, channels and points, step by step, and perseveringly, ideal effects of health−protection, health−preserving and self−treatment of diseases are bound to gain. The following is the introduction to the methods for health−care *Tuina* commonly used on various parts of the body and their effects.

7.1　Health−care of the Head, Face and the Five Sense Organs

1.　Health−care of the Head and Face

Operation

(1) Performing *Tui* on either side of the forehead

Bend the two index fingers like bows and conduct *Tui* with the interior aspects of the 2nd knuckles from the midline of the forehead, which runs from the point Yintang (EX–HN 3) to the midpoint of the anterior hairline, respectively toward the left and right Sizhukong (SJ 23), Taiyang (EX–HE 5) and Touwei (ST 8), and do this 40–60 times or so (Fig. 89).

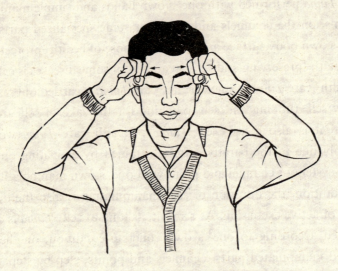

Fig. 89

(2) Performing *Mǒ* on the both temples

Put the whorled surfaces of the two thumbs tightly and respectively on the hairlines around the temples and conduct backward, repeated and forceful *Tui* and *Mǒ*, and do this about 30 times until a sensation of soreness and distension comes (Fig.90).

(3) Performing *An–rou* on the back of the head

Put the whorled surfaces or the tips of the two thumbs tightly and respectively on the two points Fengchi (GB 20), and first conduct forceful *An–ya*(pressing) 10 times, then rotative *An–rou*(press–kneading), and finally *An–rou* on the point

Naokong (GB 19) 30 times or so until a sensation of soreness and distension comes (Fig.91).

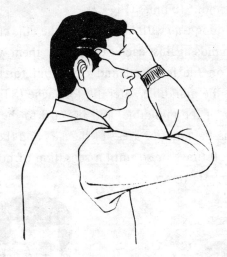

Fig. 90

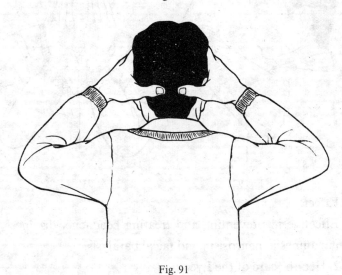

Fig. 91

(4) Performing *Paiji* (tapping) on the vertex

Sit upright, open the eyes and look straight forward, clench the teeth, and undertake rhythmic *Paiji* with the palm on the point Xinmen about 10 times (Fig.92).

(5) Performing *Cuo* with hands to °bathe′ the cheeks

Rub the hands against each other to get them warm, put the palms tightly on the forehead and carry out forceful *Ca* with them down to the mandible, laterally to Jiache (ST 6) along the inferior border of the mandible, and upward to the midpoint of the forehead via the anterior areas of the ears and the temples, do this about 20−30 times or so until a sensation of hotness on the face comes (Fig.93).

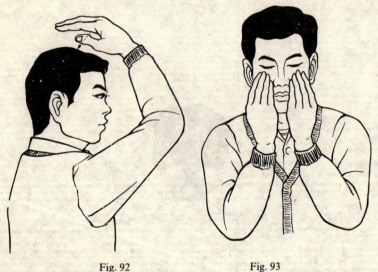

Fig. 92　　　　　　　Fig. 93

Effect

Effective in preventing and treating headache, dizziness, insomnia, amnesia, neurosism and facial paralysis.

2. Health—care of the Eye

Operation

(1) Performing *Rou* on Cuanzhu (BL 2)

Put the whorled surfaces of the two thumbs respectively on the points Cuanzhu (BL 2) in the depressions proximal to the medial ends of the eyebrows and conduct first gentle then forceful *Rou* about 20 times or so until a sensation of soreness and distension comes (Fig.94).

(2) Performing *Rou* on Jingming (BL 1)

Put the whorled surfaces of the thumb and the index finger of the right hand on the points Jingming (BL 1) in the depression 0.1 *Cun* superior to the inner canthus and conduct downward−pressing and upward−squeezing−pinching, repeat the above about 20−30 times or so (Fig.95).

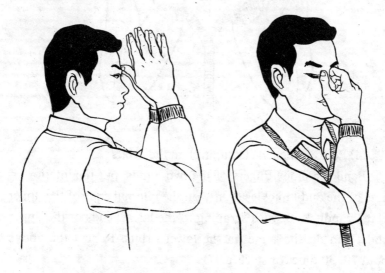

Fig. 94   Fig. 95

(3) Performing *An−rou* on Sibai (ST 2)

Put the whorled surfaces of the index fingers of the two hands respectively on the points of Sibai (ST 2), either of which is

1 *Cun* inferior to the midpoint of the lower orbit, and undertake *An—rou* 20 times or so until a sensation of soreness and distension comes (Fig.96).

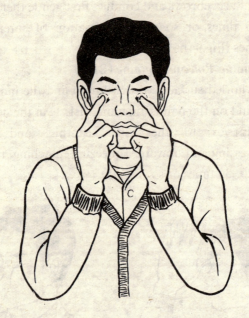

Fig. 96

(4) Performing *Gua* (scraping) on the orbits

Bend the index fingers of the two hands, put the interior aspects of the 2nd knuckles tightly on the internal ends of the upper orbits, conduct outward scraping to the lateral ends of the upper orbits, and do the same on the lower orbits. Repeat the above about 20—30 times or so (Fig.97).

(5) Performing *Yun* (ironing) on the eye

Close the eyes gently, rub the hands to get them warm, press their palm roots slightly on the eyes to iron them for 30 seconds, and, then, undertake gentle *Rou* more than 10 times (Fig.98).

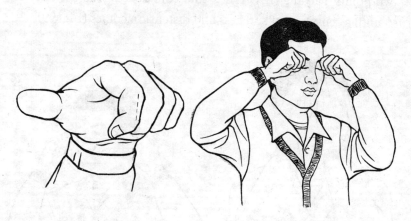

Fig. 97−1　　　　　　Fig. 97−2

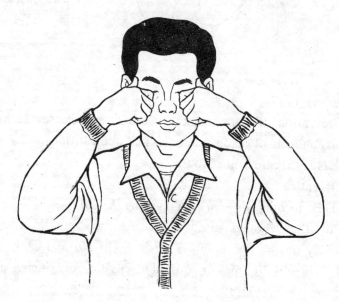

Fig.97−3

(6) Performing *Rou* on Taiyang (EX−HE 5)

Put the whorled surfaces of the two thumbs tightly on the

two points Taiyang (EX—HE 5) and conduct *An—rou* 30 times or so until a sensation of soreness and distension comes (Fig. 99).

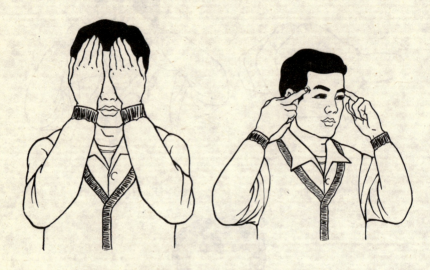

Fig. 98   Fig. 99

Effect

Prevention and treatment of various eye dieases such as myopia, blurring of vision, glaucoma and optic atrophy.

3. Health—care of the Nose

Operation

(1) Performing *An—rou* on Yingxiang (LI 20)

Put the whorled surfaces of the two middle fingers repectively on the two points Yingxiang (LI 20) and carry out forceful *An—rou* 30 times or so until a sensation of soreness and distension comes (Fig. 100).

(2) Performing *Cuo* and *Ca* on the sides of the nose

Rub the bellies of the two index or middle fingers, immediately put them on the nasolabial grooves lateral to the wings of the nose, and conduct *Cuo* and *Ca* up and down 30 times or so until heat is produced (Fig. 101).

Effect

Effective in preventing and treating common cold, stuffy and running nose, allergic rhinitis, chronic rhinitis and paranasosinusitis.

4. Health—care of the Ear

Operation

(1) Performing *An—rou* on the points around the ear

Undertake *An—rou* with the tips of the two thumbs or the two middle fingers repectively on Ermen (SJ 21), Tinggong (SI 19), Tinghui (GB 2) and Yifeng (SJ 17) around the ears with each point pressed and kneaded 20 times or so until a sensation of soreness and distension comes (Fig.102).

(2) Performing *Mó* and *Ca* on the helix

Get the whorled surface of the thumb and the radial aspect of the index finger flexed like a bow, of either of the two hands to work together to pinch the helixes of the two ears, and conduct *Mó* and *Ca* up and down 20—30 times or so (Fig. 103).

(3) Performing *Tanji* (flick—hitting) to produce boom in the ear (*Ming Tiangu*)

Cover the two ears with the two palms with the palm roots forward and the fingers backward, put either of the index fingers on either of the middle fingers, and conduct *Tanji*(flick—hitting) with the index fingers sliding down from the middle ones on either of the external occipital protuberances. Do this 20 times or so to get boom produced in the ears (Fig. 104).

(4) Performing *Cuo* and *Ca* in front of the ear

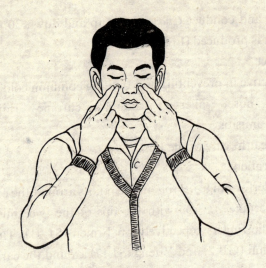

Fig. 100

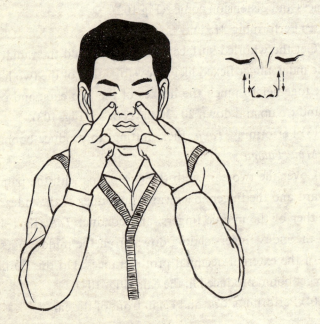

Fig. 101

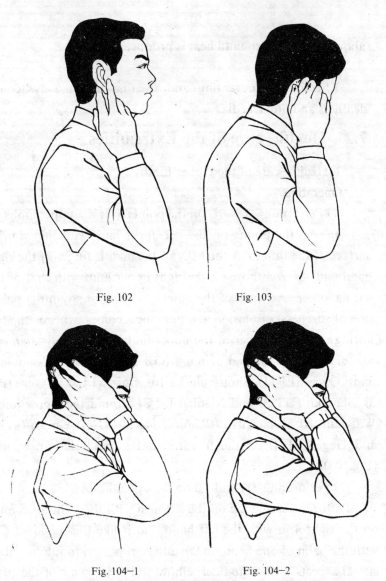

Fig. 102　　　　　Fig. 103

Fig. 104-1　　　　Fig. 104-2

Put the radial aspects of the two thumbs or the bellies of the two index fingers tightly on the anterior areas of the ears and conduct *Cuo* and *Ca* down and up and up and down. Do this about 30 times or so until heat is produced.

Effect

Effective in preventing and treating tinnitus, dysacousis, deafness and otitis media.

7.2   Health–care of the Extremities

1. Health–care of the Upper Limbs

Operation

(1) Performing *An–rou* on the points over the upper limbs

An–rou the points on the left upper limb with the whorled surface of the thumb or the belly of the middle finger of the right hand and *An–rou* those on the right upper limb with that of the left hand. *An–rou* each of the points 20 times or so until a sensation of soreness, distension and numbness comes. *An–rou* the following points on either of the upper limbs successively: Jianneiling, Jianyu (LI 15) and Jianjing (GB 21) around the shoulder joint; Quchi (LI 11), Shousanli (LI 10), Chize (LU 57), Quze (PC 3), Shaohai (UT 3) and Xiaohai (SI 8) around the elbow joint; Waiguan (SJ 5), Neiguan (PC 6), Yangchi (SJ 4), Yangxi (LI 5) and Hegu (LI 4) on the forearm and around the wrist joint (Fig.105).

(2) Performing *Tui* and *Ca* on the upper limbs

Perform *Tui* and *Ca* on the left arm with the right hand and on the right arm with the left hand. Do it like this: conduct *Ca* with the palm of one hand on the anterior, posterior, interior and lateral aspects of the shoulder, elbow and wrist joints of the corresponding arm with every aspect rubbed 10–20 times or so until heat is produced. Then, carry out *Ca* again with the same palm along the channels on the same arm and do it like this: undertake

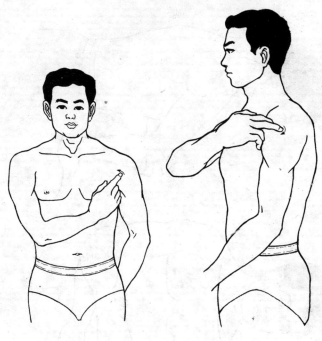

Fig.105-1   Fig. 105-2

Ca from the dorsal carpal cross striation, along the lateral aspect of the arm, straight up to the point Jianyu at the lateral aspect of the shoulder, via the anterior aspect of the shoulder, along the medial aspect of the arm, and straight down to the intracarpal cross striation, and repeat this 30 times or so to get a warm sensation in the arm (Fig. 106).

(3) Performing *Ca* and *Nian* on the knuckles

Perform *Ca* with the major thenar eminence of one hand on the dorsum of the other hand to get the intermetacarpal muscles warm, and conduct *Rou* and *Nian* (kneading and twisting) with the thumb and the index finger of the same hand on the

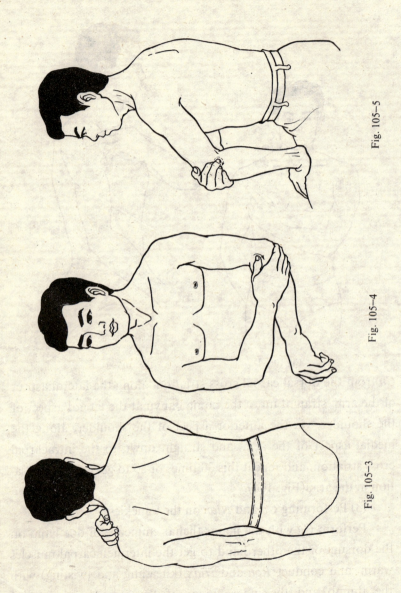

Fig. 105-5

Fig. 105-4

Fig. 105-3

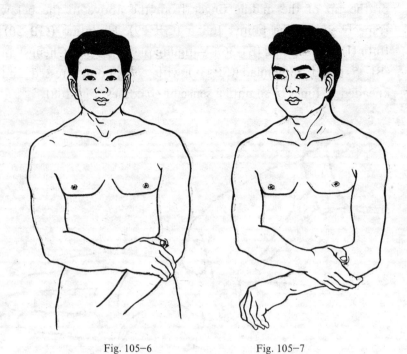

Fig. 105—6   Fig. 105—7

interphalangeal joints of the manipulated hand with one joint kneaded and twisted after another (Fig. 107).

Effect

Effective in preventing and treating scapulohumeral periarthritis, subacromial bursitis, tennis elbow and carpal tenosynovitis, in relaxing the muscles of the upper limbs, in relieving fatigue, in improving the motor function of the joints of the upper limbs and in preventing occupational strain.

2. Health—care of the Lower Limbs

Operation

(1) Performing *An—rou* on the points over the lower limbs Conduct *An—rou* with the whorled surface or the tip of the thumb

or the tip of the middle finger from the above to the below respectively on the points Juliao (GB 29), Huantiao (GB 30), Futu (LI 18), Zusanli (ST 36), Yanglingquan (GB 34), Chengshan (BL 57) and Sanyinjiao (SP 36) with each point pressed and kneaded 20 times or so until a sense of *Qi* comes (Fig. 108).

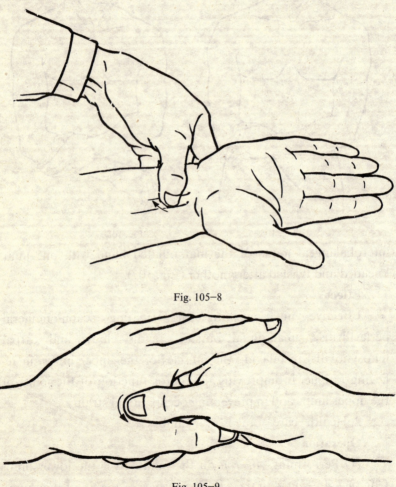

Fig. 105—8

Fig. 105—9

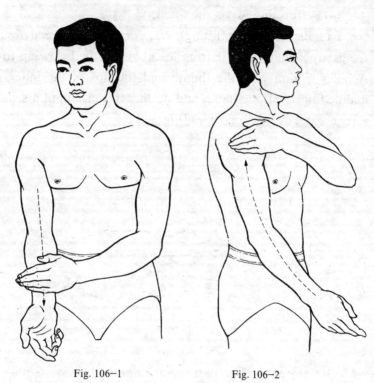

Fig. 106—1   Fig. 106—2

(2) Performing *An—rou* on the thigh

Carry out strong *An—rou* with the two palm roots from the above to the below respectively on the lateral, medial and anterior muscles of the thigh, and do this 3—5 times until a sensation of soreness and distension comes (Fig. 109)

(3) Performing *An—rou* on the knee—cap

Stretch the lower limbs naturally with the muscles relaxed, conduct   *Na—nie*   (grasping—pinching)   and   *An—rou* (pressing—kneading) on the knee—caps with the belly of the thumb and the radial aspect, bent like a bow, of the index finger of one hand (Fig. 110)

(4) Performing *Na* on the shank

Conduct gentle *Ti* (lifting), *Na, Nie* (pinching) and *Rou* on the gastrocnemius muscle from the above to the below up to the Achilles tendon with the thumb and the tips of the index and middle fingers of one hand, and do this 10 times until a sense of soreness and distension comes (Fig. 111).

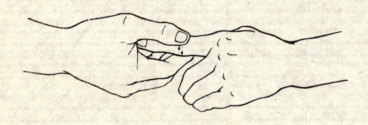

Fig. 107

(5) Performing *Paiji* (patting—hitting) on the lower limbs

Get the centres or roots of the two palms to exert forces in the opposite directions to conduct *Paiji* on the leg from the upper part of the thigh down to the lower part of the shank, and do this about 10—15 times or so (Fig. 112).

(6) Performing *Ca* on Yongquan (KI 1)

Carry out rapid and strong *Ca* on Yongquan (KI 1) at the sole 30 times or so with the hypothenar of one hand until heat is produced. Rub the left foot with the right hand, the right foot with the left hand, with one foot rubbed after the other (Fig. 113).

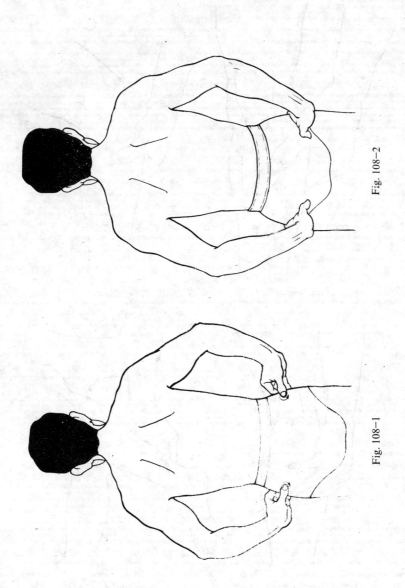

Fig. 108-2

Fig. 108-1

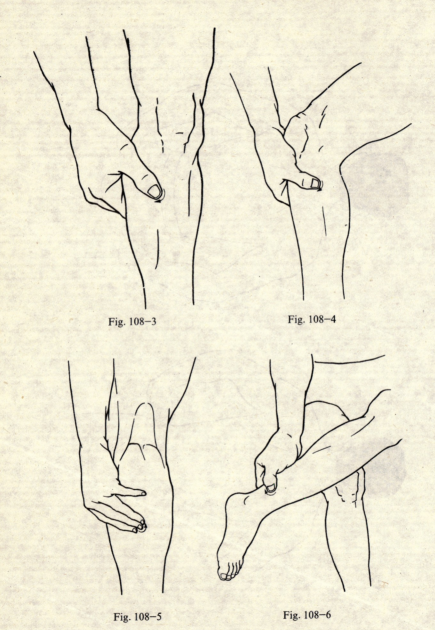

Fig. 108-3

Fig. 108-4

Fig. 108-5

Fig. 108-6

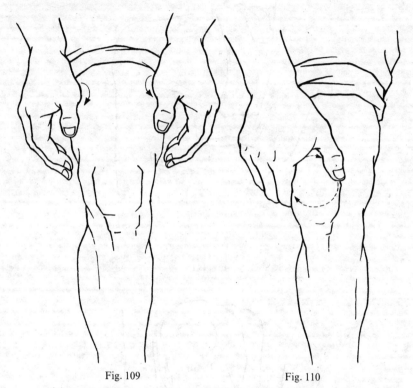

Fig. 109   Fig. 110

(7) Performing *Yao* on the ankle joint

Sit upright with the shank of one leg on the knee of the other leg, hold the superior malleolar portion of the supported shank with one hand and its metatarsophalangeal part with the other hand, rotate the ankle joint clockwise and counterclockwise each about 20 times or so (Fig. 114)

Effect

Effective in treating in jury of the superior clunial nerves, strain of the gluteal fasciae, swelling and pain in the knee joint,

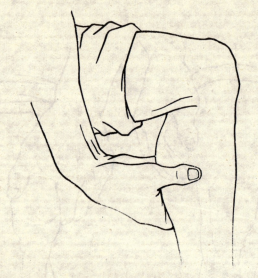

Fig. 111

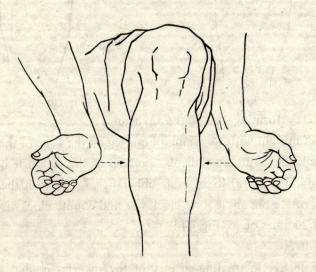

Fig. 112

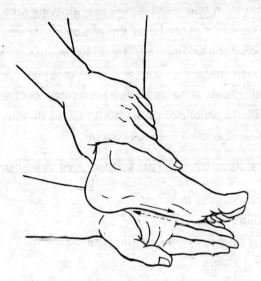

Fig. 113

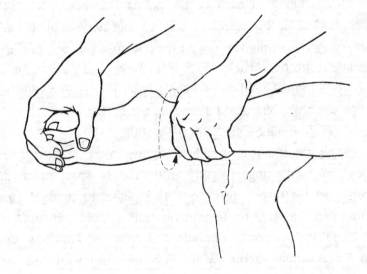

Fig. 114

systremma and injury of the ankle joint, in relaxing the muscles of the lower limbs, in relieving fatigue, in improving motor function of the various joints of the lower limbs, and in preventing various kinds of occupational injuries. In addition, the manipulations *An—rou* Zusanli and Sanyinjiao and *Ca* Yongquan used together with the self—*Tuina* manipulations performed on the abdomen and the head are beneficial to the health of the digestive, urinary, reproductive and central nervous systems.

7.3 Health—care of the Chest and Abdomen

1. Health—care of the chest

Operation

(1) Performing *An—rou* on the points over the chest and on the intercostal spaces

Conduct *An—rou* with the whorled surface of the middle finger of one hand on each of the points Danzhong (RN 17), Zhongfu (LU 1), Rugen (ST 18) and Rupang 20 times or so, and, then, carry out strong *An—rou* on the intercostal spaces from the one inferior to the clavicle down to the below and from the interior aspect to the lateral one with each space pressed and kneaded until a sense of soreness and distension comes (Fig. 115).

(2) Performing *Na* on the muscles of thorax

Apply the thumb of one hand tightly to the chest with the index and middle fingers tightly on the lateral aspect under the armpit, get the three fingers to work together to conduct *Tina* (lifting and grasping) on the anterior axillary fold consisting of the lateral greater pectoral muscle, and carry out *Ti* (lifting—up) and *Na* (grasping) alternately and in combination with slow and gentle *Nie* (pinching) and *Rou* (kneading). Repeat the above 5 times or so (Fig. 116).

(3) Performing *Pai* (tapping) on the chest

Cup the hand and tap the chest from the above to the below, do this along the thoracic median line 10 times or so and along either of the two breast median lines 10 times or so as well. Be sure not to hold the breath while tapping (Fig.117)

(4) Performing *Ca* on the chest

Put the major thenar eminence or the whole palm of one hand tightly on the surface of the chest and conduct powerful transverse *Ca* (rubbing) to and fro 20 times or so until heat is produced (Fig. 118).

Effect

Preventing and treating pain occurring in the chest due to breathing, chest pain, choking sensation in the chest, cough, asthma, disorders of the functional activity of *Qi*, and palpitation.

2. Health−care of the Abdomen

Operation

(1) Performing *An−rou* on the points over the abdomen

Conduct *An−rou* with the tip of the middle finger, the major thenar eminence or the palm root of one hand on each of the points Zhongwan (RN 12), Zhangmen (LR 13), Tianshu (ST 25), Qihai (RN 6), Guanyuan (RN 4) and Zhongji (RN 3) 20−30 times or so until a sense of *Qi* comes (Fig. 119,120).

(2) Performing *Mo* on the abdomen

Put one palm around each of the points Zhongwan (RN 12), Shenque (RN 8) and Guanyuan (RN 4) and conduct circular *Mó* on each of them first clockwise 30−50 times or so then counterclockwise also 30−50 times or so (Fig. 121).

(3) Performing *Ca* on the lower abdomen

Put the two hypothenars of the two hands tightly on the

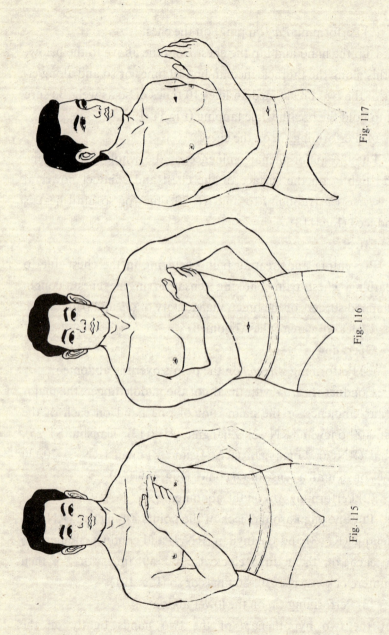

Fig. 115

Fig. 116

Fig. 117

points Tianshu (ST 25) 2 *Cun* beside the navel and conduct *Ca* up and down 30 times or so (Fig. 122)

(4) Performing *Dian* on Qihai (RN 6), Guanyuan (RN 4) and Zhongji (RN 3)

Conduct *Dian* on each of the points Qihai (RN 6), Guanyuan (RN 4) and Zhongji (RN 3) 30—50 times or so until a sensation of distension and numbness radiating to the external genital organs comes.

Effect

Effective in preventing and treating discomfort in the epigastrium, indigestion, constipation, abdominal pain, irregular menstruation and impotence.

7.4 Health—care of the Neck, Back and Waist

1. Health—care of the Neck and Back

Operation

(1) Performing *An—rou* on the neck and back

First, conduct *An—rou* with the tips of the index, middle and ring fingers of either of the hands along Fengchi (GB 20) on the both routes via Tianzhu (BL 10) to the root of the neck and do this 5—10 times or so, second, carry out *An—rou* with the tips of the index, middle and ring fingers of one hand along the line from Fengfu (DU 16) to Dazhui (DU 14) with each of the points on the line pressed and kneaded about 20—30 times and do the above 5—10 times, finally, extend one hand to the back of the other side and undertake *An—rou* with the middle finger on each of the points Dazhui (DU 14), Dazhu (BL 11), Shenzhu (DU 12), Fengmen (BL 12) and Feishu (BL 13) 30 times or so until a sense of soreness and distension comes and, then, do the same with the

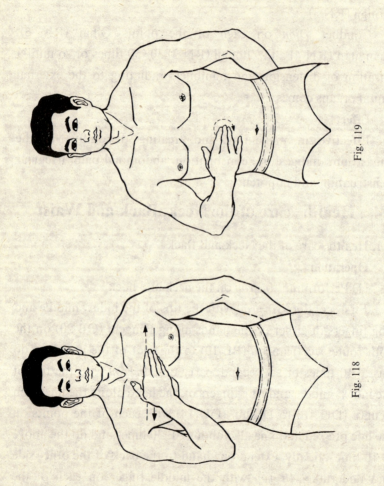

Fig. 119

Fig. 118

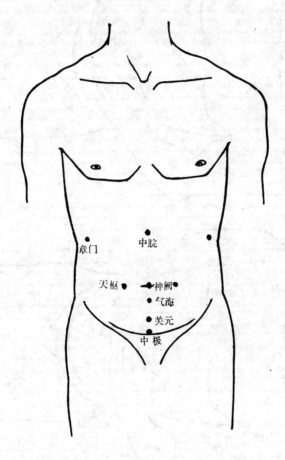

Fig. 120

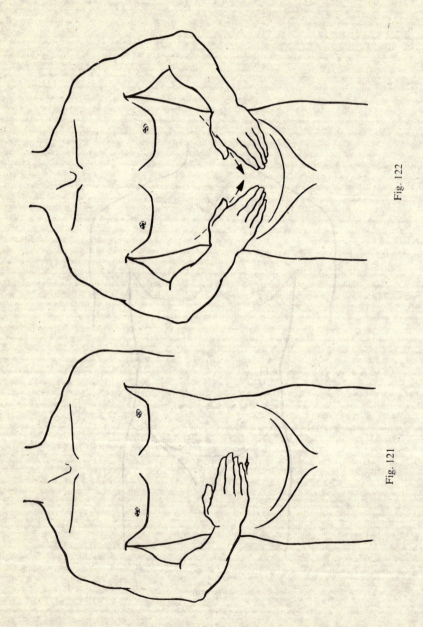

Fig. 122

Fig. 121

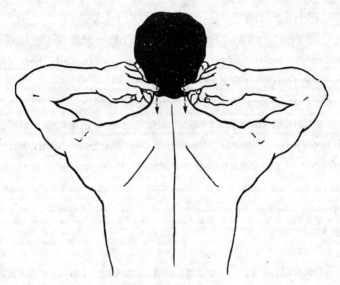

Fig. 123—1

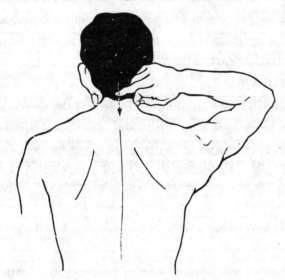

Fig. 123—2

other hand (Fig. 123).

(2) Performing *Pai* (tapping) on the back

Cup one hand and extend it to the other side of the back and conduct *Pai* on the upper back 10 times or so, and, then, do the same with the other hand (Fig. 124)

(3) Performing *Mó* on Gaohuang (BL 43)

Straighten the upper body with the two arms 90 ° abducted and the elbows flexed, rotate the two shoulder joints with the amplitude of the backward—movement being as large as possible so as to stimulate through the rotative movement of the scapulae the points such as Gaohuang located in the interscapular region (Fig. 125).

Effect

Effective in preventing and treating pain, aching and distension in the back, cervical spondylopathy, stiffneck, cough, asthma, accumulation of phlegm, consumptive disease, choking sensation in the chest, chest pain, palpitation and angina pectoris.

2. Health—care of the Waist

Operation

(1) Performing *Rou* on the points over the loins

Conduct *An—rou* with the protruded parts of the metacarpophalangeal joints of the two fists on each of the points Shenshu (BL 23), Zhishi (BL 52) and Yaoyan (EX—B7) 30 times or so until a sensation of soreness and distension comes (Fig. 126).

(2) Performing *Chuizhen* (pound—vibrating) on the lumbar region

Carry out tapping, pounding and vibrating with the ulnar aspects of the two fists from the above to the below along the three lines on the lumbar region: the line from Shenshu (BL 23) to

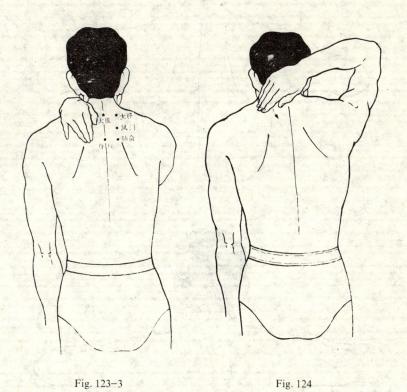

大椎　　大杼
風門
肺俞
身柱

Fig. 123-3　　　　　　　Fig. 124

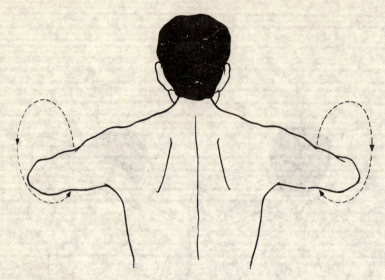

Fig. 125—1

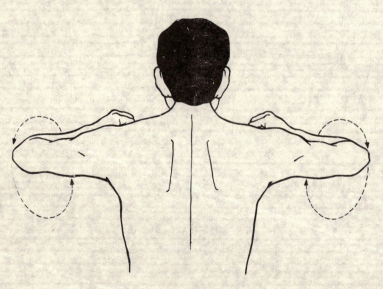

Fig. 125—2

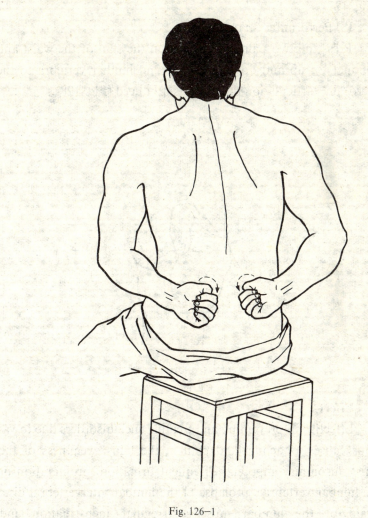

Fig. 126—1

Pangguangshu (BL 28), the line from Zhishi (BL 52)via Yaoyan (EX—B7) to Baohuang (BL 53) and the line from Mingmen (DU 4) to the lumbosacral joint, and do this along each line 5—10 times (Fig. 127).

(3) Performing *Ca* on the loins

Press the two palm roots hard on the skin of the waist and conduct *Ca* up and down from the 2nd lumbar vertebra to the sacro—iliac articulation until heat is produced (Fig. 128).

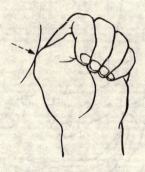

Fig. 126—2

Effect

Effective in preventing and treating such disorders due to various causes as aching and pain in the loins, weakness of the waist, insomnia, impotence, frequent urination, proliferation of the lumbar vertebrae, prolapse of the lumbar intervertebral disc, strain of the lumbar muscles, irregular menstruation and diarrhea, in relaxing the lumbar muscles, in relieving fatigue, and

· 330 ·

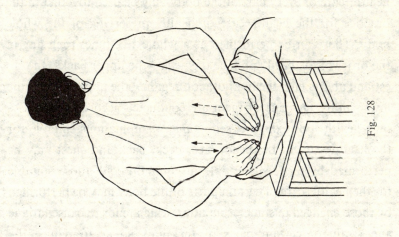

Fig. 128

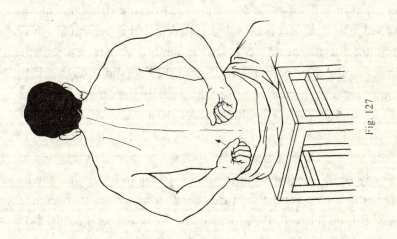

Fig. 127

in improving the motor functional activity of the waist.

The above self—*Tuina* manipulations suitable for the health—care of every part of the body may be used together in the practice for the health—care or health—preserving of the whole body. They can be performed as a whole 1—2 times each day in the order of the head and face the neck→the upper back→the chest and abdomen→the lumbosacral region→the upper limbs→the lower limbs. Or, part of them are conducted according to one's own health. For example, self—*Tuina* manipulations suitable for the health—care of the head, face, neck, back and chest may be performed by those susceptible to common cold; those suitable for the health—care of certain parts of the body may be performed by those engaged in some occupation which tends to cause fatigue and strain of certain parts of the body so as to reduce the workers' efficiency and by those who tend to be attacked by occupational diseases, in so doing, the working efficiency may be raised and the occupational diseases may be prevented; those suitable for the health—care of the lumbosacral region and the lower limbs may be performed daily before and after work by long—distance runners or those who work in the standing posture; those suitable for the health—care of the head, face, neck, back, waist and upper limbs may be performed during the intervals of work or after going home from work by mental workers who usually bend over their desks while working in order that the fatigue due to long—time forward—bending of the waist, back and neck can be relieved, the efficiency of the brain can be raised. In addition, health—care *Tuina* may be used by the middle—aged and the aged as methods for self—treatment of many common chronic diseases and self—restoration. When ever it is applied, do the following: select self−*Tuina* manipulations suitable for the health−care of the related parts of the body according to the disease to be treated so as to make up a self−*Tuina* prescription and perform the manipulations according to the prescription every day. For instance, those suffering from chronic diarrhea may carry out self−*Tuina* according to the following prescription: *An−rou* Baihui (DU 20) 50 times, *Mó* the area around the navel 50 times, *Mó* Guanyuan (RN 4) 50 times, *Ca* the lower abdomen 30 times, *An−rou* Shenshu (BL 23) 30 times, *Mó−ca* the areas where the kidneys are located 50 times, *Dian* Guanyuan (RN 4) 30 times, *An−rou* Zusanli (ST 36) 30 times, *An−rou* Sanyinjiao (SP 6) 20 times. Take the prescription for treating diabetes for another example. it is : *An−rou* either of Zhongwan (RN 12) and Guanyuan (RN 4) 50 times, *Mó* either of Zhongwan (RN 12) and Shenque (RN 8) clockwise 30 times and counterclockwise 30 times, *Chuizhen* (pound and vibrate) the kidney areas 30 times, *Mó−ca* the lumbar region 30 times, *An−rou* Zusanli (ST 36) 30 times.

Part Two: Infant *Tuina*

8 Brief Introduction to Infant *Tuina*

8.1 An Outline of Infant *Tuina*

As an important component of TCM, infant *Tuina* is a clinical medical subject in which manipulations are performed on the specialized parts or certain points of the surface of an infant's body to treat some diseases.

Simple and convenient in performing and bringing no sufferings to infants, infant *Tuina* is highly effective in treating certain diseases without any side effects. Not only can it be used to treat various common and difficult diseases but also to prevent diseases. Therefore, it is a medical means with brilliant future.

8.2 Relevant Knowledge of Infant *Tuina*

1. Characteristics of Infant *Tuina*

(1) Concept of Wholism and Treatment Based on Differentiation

Guided by the theories of *Yin* and *Yang*, *Wuxing*, *Zang* and *Fu*, *Jingluo*, *Ying* and *Wei*, and *Qi* and *Xue* of TCM, infant *Tuina* takes the concept of wholism as its base. Directed by the principle of "treatment based on the differentiation of symptoms and signs and other factors", it is carried out through performing manipulations on the body surface of an infant patient to regulate *Zang* and *Fu, Ying* and *Wei*, and *Qi* and *Xue* and treat diseases.

(2) Theory of Channels and Collaterals

It is through the function of channels and collaterals to promote the circulation of *Qi* and blood and balance *Yin* and *Yang* that infant *Tuina* works in regulating *Zang* and *Fu*, and *Ying* and *Wei*. That is to say, it is by way of channels and collaterals that infant *Tuina* plays its part in regulating the physiological function of the organism.

2. Reinforcement and Reduction of Manipulations of Infant *Tuina*

Manipulations performed in the way that the functional activity of the body may be improved, the *Qi* and blood may be supplemented, the *Yin* and *Yang* may be invigorated, and various syndromes of deficiency type may be treated are called reinforcing method, while manipulations performed in the way that various syndromes of excess type may be treated, the retended food, dry feces and other harmful substances in the intestines may be removed through defecation, and the noxious heat within the body may be reduced through induced diarrhea are called reducing method.

Owing to the infants' physiological and pathological characteristics, the two methods should be used in point, either of them should be stopped as soon as the purpose is reached, and either of over—reduction and over—reinforcement is strictly forbidden.

The times and force of a manipulation being performed are as important as the dosage of a drug. A manipulation performed gently and for a longer time may play a reinforcing part, while a manipulation performed forcefully and for a shorter time may play a reducing part. Long—time performing means more times of manipulating.

The direction of the acting of a manipulation is related to *Bu* or *Xie* (reinforcement or reduction). Towards the heart is *Bu* (reinforcement), while from it, *Xie* (reduction). But for some points, towards the heart is *Xie*, while from it, *Bu*. The same manipulation performed in different directions has different actions. This shows that a point manipulated will have a two—way regulating effect. So, the purpose of supplementing deficiency or reducing excess can be reached only when a manipulation is performed in the right direction on a specific point.

The times of each manipulation involved in this chapter are suitable for a one—year infant. The young the infant, the less the times of a manipulation performed on it, and the lighter the manipulation. On the contrary, the older the infant, the stronger its constitution, the more excessive the pathogenic factor, the more the times of a manipulation performed, and the heavier the manipulation. Generally, each of gentle *Tui*, *Rou* and *Mó* performed on a point of a one—year infant is 300 times, while each of more powerful *Qia*, *An*, *Na* and *Yao*, 3—5 times. As for the duration of treatment, 15—20 minutes or so is suitable for infants of 1—3 years old, 5—10 minutes or so, for infants of 6 months —1year old, and 3—5 minutes, for newborns.

The course of treatment is determined according to disease condition. When prolonged or chronic diseases are treated such as anorexia, asthma, enuresis and paralysis, 1 course may involve 15 times of treatment, if cure does not come after one course of treatment, another 1—2 courses may be added. When diseases with short duration or common or frequently—encountered diseases are treated, 1 course usually involves 3–6 times of treatment, if cure refuses to come after one course of treatment, another may be added. Between the 2nd–3rd course of treatment, if chronic diseases are treated, there may be an interval of 10–15 days.

3. Specific Points for Infant *Tuina*

In addition to the points on the fourteen regular channels and the extra–ordinary points, there are also many specific points used in infant *Tuina*. They are in point form, linear form or regional form and usually located below the elbows and knees. The effects of infant *Tuina* in treating diseases, especially diseases of *Zang* and *Fu*, owe a great deal to them.

4. Other Points for Attention

(1) Procedure of infant *Tuina*

Manipulations are usually performed first on the arms, second on the head and face, then on the chest, back, waist and spine, and finally on the legs. Whether the infant is a boy or girl, his / her left arm is usually manipulated rather than the right one, but sometimes, the right arm may be manipulated instead. In practice, the order may also depend on the disease condition and the affected part of the body of an infant patient. Yes, it all depends.

(2) Composition of prescriptions in infant *Tuina*

In one prescription, there may well be many points, one or some of them is the principal, the others are the coordinating. To select the principal point or points and the coordinating ones to compose a sound prescription is closely related to the clinical curative effects. And this has to be known by the learners of *Tuina*.

(3) Medium used in infant *Tuina*

Medium commonly—used in infant *Tuina* includes Chinese onion juice, ginger juice, sesame oil, Chinese chives, garlic, white mustard seed, borneol and musk. They function in lubricating, dredging the channels and activating the flow of *Qi*, restoring consciousness and inducing resuscitation.

5. Physiological and Pathological Features of Infants

(1) Physiological feature

The main features are as follows: *Zang* and *Fu* are delicate, the body is just developing, and the *Qi* is weak. The younger the infant, the more remarkable the above features.

The lung governs the *Qi* of the whole body, but it is called a delicate organ, for it tends to be attacked by pathogenic factors and has no the ability to tolerate cold and heat. Frequent insufficiency of the spleen tends to weaken the lung—*Qi*, leading to frequent insufficiency of the lung.

The spleen is the source of growth and development, but the ever—developing of the infant body needs more nutrients, which overloads the spleen and worsens the frequent insufficiency of it.

An infant's development and ability of resisting disease are related to the kidney. The *Yin* of each *Zang* is nourished by the kidney —*Yin*, while the *Yang* of each *Zang* is warmed up by the kidney—*Yang*. Therefore, whether an infant is healthy or not depends greatly on its kidney. By and large, the function of an infant's kidney is weak, which is called "frequent insufficiency of the kidney".

In short, an infant is far from developed either in its body structures or in the functional activities of its body. This is one of the physiological features of an infant.

However, an infant has another physiological feature opposite to the above one. That is, it is full of vitality and develops rapidly. Its physique, intelligence and *Zang—fu* function are kept in the course of ever—improving and developing. The younger the infant, the more rapidly its growth, just as the morning sun is rising or the plant is budding.

(2) Pathological feature

"Frequent insufficiency of the lung" of an infant weakens the defensive function of its body, pathogenic factors tend to take this chance to invade the lung system through the superficies of the body, easily causing seasonal epidemic disease, cough and common cold.

" Frequent insufficiency of the spleen" of an infant is often aggravated by food—intake, easily causing diarrhea, vomiting, retension of food in the stomach and infantile malnutrition.

The other *Zang* fails to be strengthened due to "frequent insufficiency of the kidney" and the kidney essence fails to be nourished due to "frequent insufficiency of the spleen", easily affecting the development of an infant and causing hypoevolutism. The syndromes such as coldness, heat, deficiency and excess change obviously and shift rapidly after an infant falls into a disease. This is because its *Zang* and *Fu* are delicate, its physique is not developed and its body function is weak.

Rapid development, plenty of vitality, clear *Qi* of *Zang* and simple cause of a disease (less accomanied by the disorders of the seven emotions) provide the ground for easy recovery. This is also a pathological feature of an infant.

9 Manipulations for Infant *Tuina*

9.1 *Tui*(push / pushing)

Explanation: *Tui* means pushing straight in one dirction on the manipulated part of the body surface of an infant patient with the whorled surface or the radial aspect of the thumb or the whorled surfaces of the closed index and middle fingers.

Essentials

Relax the arm, flex the elbow naturally, direct the finger or fingers right to the manipulated surface, exert even gentle light and rapid strength, flex and extend the wrist joint in a small amplitude when *Tui* is conducted with the whorled surface or radial aspect of the thumb (Fig. 129–1), abduct and adduct the wrist joint in a small amplitude when *Tui* is conducted with the closed index and middle fingers so as to coordinate, and deepen the effect of , the manipulation (Fig. 129–2). Keep pushing mainly forward and in a straight line, make the manipulating finger or fingers leave the manipulated surface a little when backward—pushing is being done, and ensure a frequency of 240 times per minute.

Application

Having the effect of dispelling wind, dispersing cold. clearing away heat, stopping pain, and clearing and activating the channels and collaterals, it is applied extensively to the points on the head, face, arms, chest, abdomen, waist, back and legs. Clinically, it is used for both *Xie* (reduction) and *Bu* (reinforement). For example, when it is conducted on the point Dachang, pushing from the finger root to the tip is *Xie* while from the tip of the finger to the root, *Bu*.

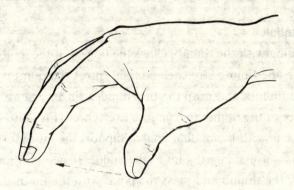

Fig. 129–1

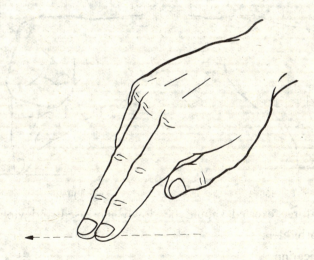

Fig. 129–2

9.2 *An* (press / pressing)

Explanation: Pressing with the tip of the thumb or the middle finger certain part or point of an infant patient's body is called *An*.

Essentials

Pressing with the thumb: Close the fingers of the left or right hand with the thumb stretched straight, press the point with the tip of the thumb, and prop the flexed index finger against the inner surface of the thumb to help it to exert force (Fig. 130—1).

Pressing with the middle finger: Support the inner surface of the distal interphalangeal joint of the middle finger with the inner surface of the thumb and press the point with the tip of the middle finger (Fig. 130—2).

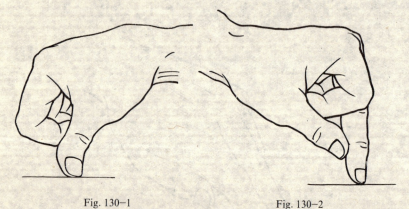

Fig. 130—1   Fig. 130—2

The force exerted should be slowly increased and violent force is forbidden.

Application

Performed on all parts of the body, this manipulation will produce the effect of clearing and activating the channels and collaterals, removing obstructions, dispersing cold and relieving pain.

9.3 *Mó* (rub / rubbing)

Explanation: Rubbing certain part of an infant patient's body with the fingers or palm is called *Mó*.

Essentials

Relax the shoulder and elbow, flex the wrist joint slightly, stretch the fingers and palm naturally straight and cover the manipulated part, and do rotary rubbing with the hand working together along with the wrist joint and the forearm.

Rubbing with the fingers: Do continuous rotary rubbing on the point with the bellies of the index, middle and ring fingers (Fig. 131-1).

Rubbing with the palm: Do rotary rubbing on the manipulated part with the palm (Fig. 131-2).

The force should be harmnious and gentle. The frequency is determined according to disease condition. Usually, rubbing with the fingers is conducted 80 times per minute, while rubbing with the palm, 60-80 times.

Application

Performing this manipulation may gain the effect of promoting the circulation of *Qi* and blood, subduing swelling, abating fever, removing food stagnation, warming the middle—*Jiao* to strengthen the spleen. In general, rubbing with the fingers is applicable to smaller parts of the body such as the head and face, while rubbing with the palm, to the chest, abdomen and hypochondriac retion. It is said, clinically, that rubbing counterclockwise is *Bu* (reinforcement), while clockwise, *Xie* (reduction); rubbing with the palm is *Bu*, while with the fingers, *Xie*; slow rubbing is *Bu*, while rapid, *Xie*. *Mó* is most effective in treating gastrointestinal disorders.

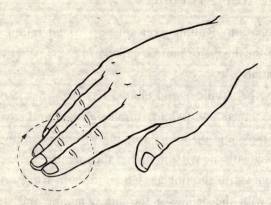

Fig. 131—1

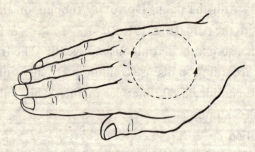

Fig. 131—2

9.4 *Qia* (nip / nipping)

Explanation: Doing deep and intermittent nipping and pressing with the nail on certain part or point of an infant patient's body is called *Qia*.

Essentials

Cup the hand with the thumb stretched straight or bent

slightly and the other four fingers closed and propped against the thumb, direct the tip of the thumb to the manipulated part and do nipping and pressing (Fig. 132). Be sure to exert slow force to get the tip of the thumb to nip in and not to exert sudden force. As for the force volume and the operating time, they depend on the disease condition and the patient's response. *Qia* is usually the last procedure (except in treating emergency cases).

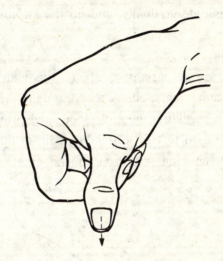

Fig. 132

Application

Performed on the points over the head, face, hands and feet, this manipulation will play a part in arresting convulsion, restoring conciousness and inducing resuscitation. It may be used to treat emergency cases of infant or infantile convulsion.

9.5 *Rou* (knead / kneading)

Explanation: Kneading conducted on the body of an infant

patient with the finger surface (the thumb or the middle finger), the palm root or the major thenar is called *Rou*.

Essentials

Relax the shoulder and the wrist, attach the finger surface, the palm root or the major thenar to the affected part, rotate the wrist joint and the forearm to conduct kneading (Fig. 133), fix the manipulating part on the skin of the manipulated part to get the subcutaneous tissue moved along with the manipulating part, increase the amplitude gradually, and do the kneading 160 times per minute.

Application

Performed on all parts of the body, this manipulation will play a part in subduing swelling, relieving pain, dispelling wind, dispersing heat, regulating *Qi* and blood, and promoting digestion. It may be used to treat distending pain in the epigastrium and abdomen, choking sensation in the chest, pain in the

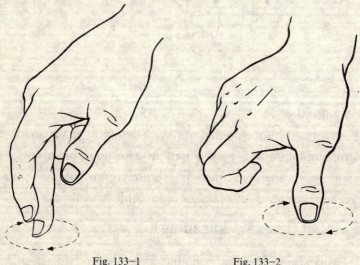

Fig. 133—1   Fig. 133—2

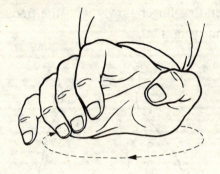

Fig. 133—3

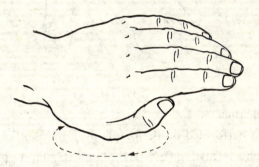

Fig. 133—4

hypochondriac region, constipation and diarrhea. It is especially effective in treating acute injury of soft tissues.

9.6 *Yun* (arc–push / pushing)

Explanation: Conducting continuous arc / circling–movements on the selected part of an infant patient's body with the palmar surface of the thumb or the index and middle finger is called *Yun*.

Essentials

Apply the surface of the finger tightly to the operated part with gentle force, make the effect act only on the superficial layers of the body but usually not on the subcutaneous tissues, and move the operating finger slowly with the frequency being 160 times per minute (Fig. 134).

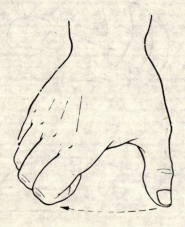

Fig. 134

Application

Often performed on the points over an infant's temples and hands such as Taiyang (EX−HE 5) and Bagua, it gives the effect of regulating *Qi* and blood, relaxing muscles and tendons, and activating the channels and collaterals.

9.7 *Nie* (pinch / pinching)

Explanation: Taking certain part of an infant patient's body where points are located with the hand to conduct pinching−squeezing or lifting / grasping−pinching is called *Nie*. It falls into two according to the different manipulated parts.

1. Pinch on the spine: Flex the index finger, prop the skin of the infant with the radial border of the middle knuckle of the in-

dex finger, press the tip of the thumb laterally, get the thumb and the index finger to work together to pinch up the skin and to lift it with strength, and do this with the two hands alternately (Fig. 135). This manipulation is only suitable for the operation on the spine and back. That is why it is called *Nie Ji* (pinch on the spine).

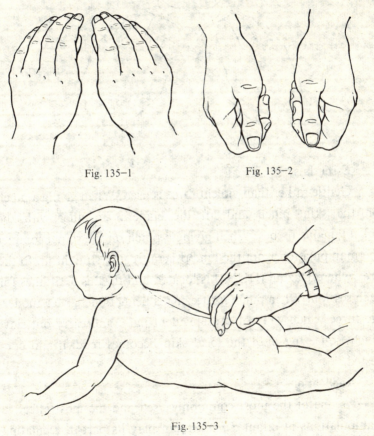

Fig. 135—1   Fig. 135—2

Fig. 135—3

2. Pinch–squeezing: This is a manipulation conducted by pinch–squeezing from around the point or the manipulated part to its centre with the tips of the thumbs and the tips of the index,

middle and ring fingers of the two hands (Fig. 136).

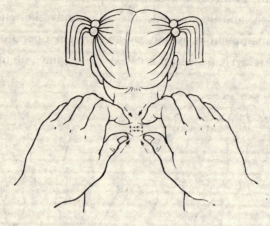

Fig. 136

Essentials

Gentle rather than violent force is used. When giving a pinch on the skin, pinch and lift the epiderm together with the subcutaneous tissues. When giving a pinch on the spine, conduct the manipulation from the lumbosacral region straight up to the area where Dazhui (DU 14) is located and do this 3—5 times for each session. When pinch—squeezing is being done, give a moderate force which will not cause evident pain, and carry out slow pinch—squeezing until the local skin becomes reddish and congested.

Application

As one of the most commonly used and the most effective manipulations in infant *Tuina*, it can play its part in regulating *Yin* and *yang*, strengthening the spleen to benefit the stomach, dredging the channels and collaterals, promoting the circulation of *Qi* and blood, expelling heat, and relieving pain. Applicable to the spine and back and prone to *Bu*, *Nie Ji* (pinch on the spine) is used to treat infantile food retention, diarrhea and vomiting. Pinch—squeezing is prone to *Xie* and applicable to smaller manipulated parts such as the points Dazhui (DU 14) and Tiantu (RN 22). Performed, it will produce the effect of expelling heat and relieving vomiting.

9.8   *Fen* (laterally—divided push / pushing)

Explanation: Conducting separate pushing respectively on the two sides of a point or an operated part with the surfaces of the fingers of the two hands is called *Fen*.

Essentials

Put the whorled surface of the thumb of either hand on the operated part and conduct such lateral pushing as " ← o → " or " ↙ o ↘ " with the two thumbs (Fig. 137). The strength should not be too strong, the movements should be gentle and harmonious, and the frequency should be within 100—120 times per minute.

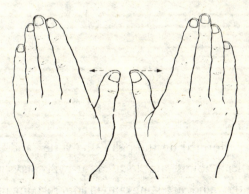

Fig. 137

Application

Performed on the face, the wrist, the chest, the abdomen and the back, this manipulation may play its part in regulating *Yin* and *Yang*, regulating *Qi* and blood, and promoting digestion to remove retended food.

9.9 *Dao* (pound / pounding)

Explanation: Tap gently the point with the tip of the middle finger or the dorsal protruded part of the proximal interphalangeal joint of the flexed middle finger. This is called *Dao*.

Essentials

Operate with one hand, exert force with the wrist, do *Dao* with the finger tip or the protruded part of the interphalangeal joint, and get the tapping light, skilled and elastic (Fig. 138). The frequency is usually slow, 100 times or so per minute.

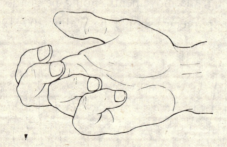

Fig. 138

Application

Usually performed on the palm, the vertex and the portion where superficial joints are located, it will play its part in tranquilizing the mind, arresting convulsion, relaxing muscles and tendons, and promoting the circulation of *Qi* in the channels.

10   Commonly Used Points in Infant *Tuina*

10.1   Points on the Head and Neck

Tianmen

Location: on anywhere of the straight line from the midpoint of the line between the two eyebrows up to the anterior hair line.

Operation: push straight from the below to the above alternately with the two thumbs. This is called *Kai* Tianmen (opening Tianmen) (Fig. 139).

Times: 30—50.

Function: inducing diaphoresis to relieve external syndrome, alleviating convulsion, tranquilizing the mind, causing resuscitation, restoring consciousness, and stopping headache.

Indications: common cold due to wind—cold, headache, fever, absence of sweat, symptoms due to fear, and listlessness.

Kangong

Location: on anywhere of the transverse line from the medial end of either eyebrow to the lateral end.

Operation: sit at the bed on which the infant is got to lie on the back, give a nipping—press to the midpoint of either supercillary arch with the two thumbs, and, then, conduct *Fen* from the ophryon to the lateral end of either eyebrow with the radial aspect of either thumb. This is called *Tui* Kangong (push-

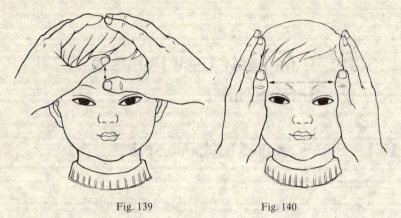

Fig. 139   Fig. 140

ing Kangong) (Fig. 140).

Times: 30–50.

Function: inducing diaphoresis to relieve external syndrome, restoring consciousness, impromving eyesight, and alleviating headache.

Indications: headache due to common cold, dizziness, conjunctival congestion with pain, infantile convulsion, myopia and strabismus.

Taiyang (EX–HN5)

Location: in the depression about 1 *Cun* posterior to the midpoint of the line from the lateral end of the eyebrow to the outer canthus.

Operation: sit upright by the end of a bed on which the infant is got to lie on the back, conduct straight *Tui* from the outer canthus to the ear with the radial border of the thumb, and do the above on the both sides with the two thumbs and this is called *Tui* Taiyang (pushing Tiayang); carry out *Rou* on the point with the tip of the middle finger and this is called *Rou* and *Yun* Taiyang (kneading and arc–pushing Taiyang) (Fig. 141). Kneading towards the eye is *Bu* (reinforcement), while kneading toward the ear is *Xie* (reduction).

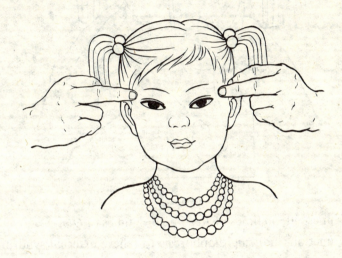

Fig. 141

Times: 30–50.

Function: expelling wind, relieving external syndrome, clearing away heat, improving eyesight, and alleviating headache.

Indications: headache, fever, chills without sweat, and myopia and strabismus as well.

Erhougaogu

Location: in the place posterior to the ear where the mastoid process of temporal bone is located.

Operation: stand behind the infant who is in the prone position or sitting upright, conduct *Rou* or *Qia* with the tips of the two thumbs or the two middle fingers. This is called *Rou* or *Qia*

Erhougaogu (kneading or nipping Erhougaogu) (Fig. 142).

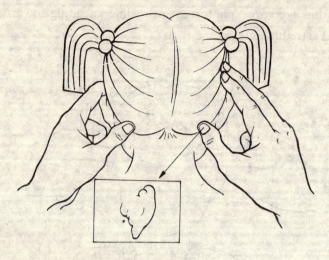

Fig. 142

Times: 30—50 times of *Rou* and 3—5 times of *Qia*.

Function: inducing diaphoresis to relieve external syndrome and alleviating pain in the head and neck.

Indications: headache, infantile convulsion, dysphoria, and pain in the neck with motor impairment.

Baihui (DU 20)

Location: at the point of intersection of the line connecting the apexes of the two auricles and the line connecting the tip of the nose and the midpoint of the posterior hairline.

Operation: sit to the end of a bed on which the infant is got to lie on the back or stand behind the infant who is got to sit upright, prop one side of its head or its forehead with the left hand, and conduct *An* or *Rou* with the thumb of the other hand. This is called *An* or *Rou* Baihui (pressing or kneading Baihui) (Fig. 143).

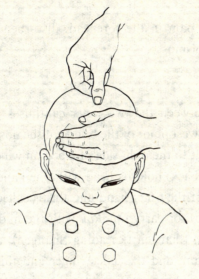

Fig. 143

Times: 30—50 times of *An* and 100—200 times of *Rou*.

Function: tranquilizing the mind, relieving convulsion, elevating *Yang* to astring prolapse.

Indications: headache, vertigo, infantile convulsion, epilepsy, prolapse of rectum and enuresis.

Yintang (EX—HN3)

Location: at the midpoint of the line connecting the medial ends of the two eyebrows.

Operation: sit to the right side of the infant in the supine position and conduct *An* or *Rou* on the point with the tip of a finger. This is called *An* or *Rou* Yintang(pressing or kneading Yintang) (Fig. 144).

Times: 50—100.

Function: tranquilizing the mind, inducing resuscitation and relieving pain.

Indications: pain in the forehead, disturbed sleep, rhinitis, myopia and strabismus.

Shangen

Location: between the two inner canthuses and in the depression of the lowest point of the bridge of the nose.

Operation: sit to the right side of a bed on which the infant is got to lie on the back, hold its head with one hand, conduct *Qia* with the thumb of the other hand and this is called *Qia* Shangen (nipping Shangen), or carry out *Rou* with the middle finger and this is called *Rou* Shangen (kneading Shangen), and undertake *Nie* with the thumb and the index finger and this is called *Nie* Shangen (pinching Shangen) (Fig. 145).

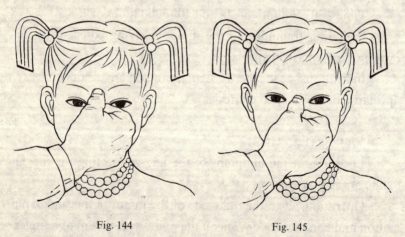

Fig. 144   Fig. 145

Times: 3—5 times of *Qia*, 30—50 times of *Rou* and 20—30 times of *Nie*.

Function: inducing resuscitation, improving vision and calming the mind.

Indications: infantile convulsion.

Shuigou (DU 26)

Location: below the nose, above the upper lip, at the junction of the superior 1 / 3 and the inferior 2 / 3 of the philtrum.

Operation: sit or stand at the side of the infant who is in the supine position or sitting upright, conduct first *Qia* with the thumb nail and then *Rou* with the thumb belly and this is called *Qia-rou* Shuigou (nipping—kneading Shuigou) (Fig. 146).

Times: 3—5 times or do it until the patient comes to.

Function: inducing resuscitation and restoring consciousness.

Indications: infantile convulsion, syncope, facial paralysis, tic, and spasm of the lips.

Chengjiang (RN 24).

Location: in the centre of the mentolabial groove.

Operation: stand to the right side of the infant who is got to lie on the back or sit upright, conduct *Qia* with the nail of the thumb and this is called *Qia* Chengjiang (nipping Chengjiang), carry out *Rou* with the belly of the thumb and this is called *Rou* Chengjiang (kneading Chengjiang) (Fig. 147).

Times: conduct *Qia* 3—5 times or until the patient comes to, and carry out *Rou* 30—50 times.

Function: restoring consciousness, inducing resuscitation, relieving convulsion, and alleviating pain.

Indications: facial paralysis, toothache, syncope due to summer—heat evil, and epilepsy.

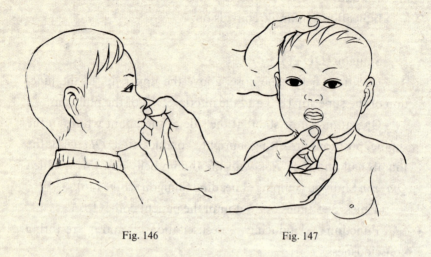

Fig. 146   Fig. 147

Fengchi (GB20)

Location: between m. sternocleidomastoideus and m. trapezius, 0.5 *Cun* superior to the posterior hairline, and on the same level with Fengfu (DU 16).

Operation: stand behind the infant who is got to sit upright, conduct *Na* on the point with the two thumbs, this is called *Na* Fengchi (grasping Fengchi) (Fig. 148).

Times: 5—10.

Function: inducing diaphoresis to relieve external syndrome, expelling wind and dispersing cold.

Indications: common cold, headache, vertigo, stiff and painful neck with motor impairment, myopia, strabismus, and infantile myogenic torticollis.

Yaguan

Location: 1 *Cun* inferior to the ear, in the depression of the mandible.

Operation: stand laterally and anteriorly to the infant who is got to sit upright, conduct *An* with the thumb or *Rou* with the middle finger on the point, and this is called *An* Yaguan (pressing Yaguan) or *Rou* Yaguan (kneading Yaguan) (Fig. 149).

Times: 5—10 times of *An* and 30—50 times of *Rou*.

Function: relieving lockjaw and stopping toothache.

Indications: lockjaw, facial paralysis, toothache, and swelling and pain of parotid gland.

Tianzhugu

Location: on anywhere of the straight line from the midpoint of the posterior hairline to Dazhui (DU 14).

Operation: stand behind the lateral side of the infant who is got to sit upright, conduct straight *Tui* from the above to the below with the thumb or the index and middle fingers and this is called *Tui* Tianzhugu (pushing Tianzhugu) (Fig. 150).

Times: 100—300.

Function: lowering the adverse flow of *Qi*, arresting vomiting, expelling wind and dispersing cold.

Indications: nausea, vomiting, commoncold due to wind—cold, headache, stiff neck, myopia and strabismus.

Xinmen

Location: 2 *Cun* straight above the midpoint of the anterior hairline, in the bone depression anterior to Baihui (DU 20).

Operation: stand to the left or right side of the infant who is got to sit upright, support its head with the index, middle, ring and small fingers of the two hands, conduct *Tui* from the anterior hairline toward the point alternately with the two thumbs (with the *Tui* stopped at the bone border before the closure of fontanel) and this is called *Tui* Xinmen (pushing Xinmen), carry out gentle *Rou* on this point and this is called *Rou* Xinmen (kneading Xinmen) (Fig. 151).

Times: 50—100 times of either *Tui* or *Rou*.

Function: relieving convulsion, calming the mind and inducing resuscitation.

Indications: headache, stuffy nose, infantile convulsion, epistaxis and dysphoria.

10.2 Points on the Chest and Abdomen

Tiantu (RN 22)

Location: in the centre of the suprasternal fossa.

Operation: stand at the right side of the infant who is got to lie on the back, conduct *An* or *Rou* on the point with the tip of the middle finger and this is called *An* or *Rou* Tiantu (pressing or kneading Tiantu) (Fig. 152). Pinch the local skin with the thumbs and the index fingers of the two hands and conduct centrewise squeezing, which is called *Ji—nie* Tiantu (squeezing—pinching Tiantu).

Times: 10—15.

Function: promoting the flow of *Qi* to resolve sputum, lowering the adverse flow of *Qi* to relieve asthma, and arresting vomiting.

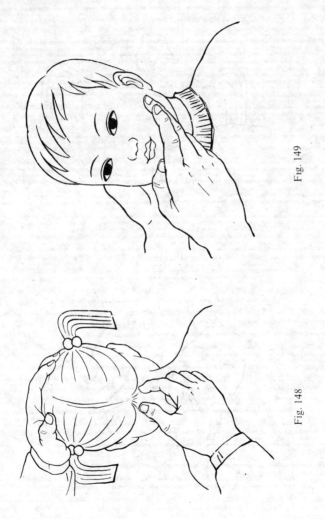

Fig. 149

Fig. 148

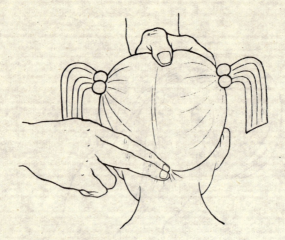

Fig. 150

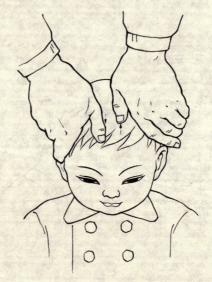

Fig. 151

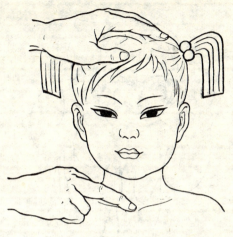

Fig. 152

Indications: asthma due to accumulation of phlegm, dyspnea, cough, choking sensation in the chest, difficulty in coughing out sputum, retention of food, nausea and vomiting.

Danzhong (RN 17)

Location: on the anterior midline, midway between the nipples, at the level of the fourth intercostal space.

Operation: stand to the right side of the infant who is got to lie on the back or to sit upright, conduct *Fen* from Danzhong towards the both sides with the radial aspects of the two thumbs and this is called *Fen* Danzhong (laterally–divided pushing Danzhong) (Fig. 153). Carry out *Tui* from the sternal end down to Danzhong with the bellies of the index and middle fingers, which is called *Xiatui* Danzhong (downward–pushing Danzhong). Undertake *Rou* on the point with the whorled surface of the middle finger, which is called *Rou* Danzhong (kneading Danzhong) (Fig. 154).

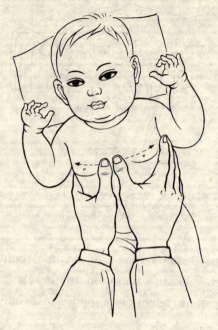

Fig. 153

Times: 100—200 times of either *Tui* or *Rou* and 50—100 times of *Fen*.

Function: soothing the chest to regulate the flow of *Qi*, ventilating the lung to arrest cough and resolve phlegm.

Indications: chest oppression, chest pain, cough, asthma, rale in the throat, nausea and vomiting.

Rugen (ST 18)

Location: 0.2 *Cun* inferior to the nipple.

Operation: conduct *Rou* on the point with the tip of the middle finger and this is called *Rou* Rugen (kneading Rugen).

Times: 20—50.

Function: soothing the chest to regulate *Qi*, arresting cough and resolving phlegm.

Indications: chest oppression, chest pain, cough, asthma, and rale in the throat.

Rupang

Location: 0.2 *Cun* lateral to the nipple.

Operation: get the infant to lie on the back or to sit upright, conduct *Rou* on the point with the tip of the middle finger, and this is called *Rou* Rupang (kneading Rupang) (Fig. 155).

Times: 20—50.

Function: soothing the chest to regulate *Qi*, arresting cough and resolving phlegm.

Indications: chest oppression, chest pain, cough, asthma, and rale in the throat.

Zhongwan (RN 12)

Location: 4 *Cun* superior to the navel.

Operation: get the infant to lie on the back, conduct *An* or *Rou* on the point with the finger tip or the palm root and this is called *An* or *Rou* Zhongwan (pressing or kneading Zhongwan), carry out *Mó* with the palm or the closed four fingers and this is called *Mó* Zhongwan (rubbing Zhongwan) (Fig. 156).

Times: conduct *Rou* 100—300 times and *Mó* for 5 minutes.

Function: strengthening the spleen, regulating the stomach, promoting digestion, and activating the middle—*Jiao*.

Indications: food retention, abdominal distension, abdominal pain, vomiting, diarrhea, poor appetite and eructation.

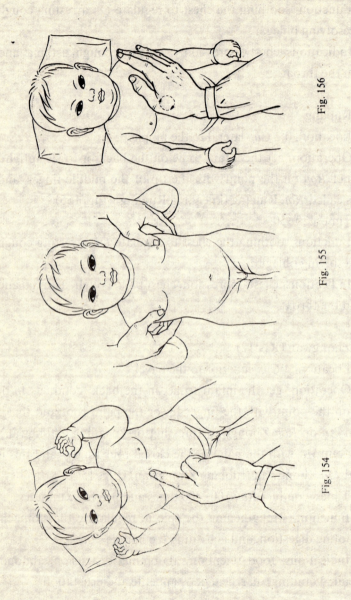

Fig. 156

Fig. 155

Fig. 154

Xielei

Location: the hypochondriac region below the armpit and above Tianshu (ST 25).

Operation: stand before or behind the infant who is got to sit upright with its head in its hands, conduct *Cuo—mó* with the two palms from under the armpits to the points Tianshu, and this is called *Cuo—mó* Xielei (doing foulage and rubbing on Xielei) (Fig. 157).

Times: 50—100.

Function: soothing the liver to promote the flow of *Qi*, resolving phlegm, and removing accumulation.

Indications: retention of food, accumulation of phlegm, stagnation of *Qi*, chest oppression, pain in the hypochondriac region, asthma due to accumulation of profuse sputum, rapid breathing, infantile malnutrition and hepatosplenomegaly.

Shenque (RN 8)

Location: in the centre of the umbilicus.

Operation: get the infant to lie on the back, conduct *Rou* on the point with the tip of the middle finger or the palm root and this is called *Rou* Shenque (kneading Shenque); carry out *Mó* on it with the index, middle and ring fingers or the palm and this is called *Mó* Shenque (rubbing Shenque) (Fig. 158).

Times: undertake *Rou* 100—300 times and *Mó* for 3—5 minutes.

Function: warming up *Yang*, dispersing cold, and invigorating *Qi* and blood.

Indications: diarrhea, vomiting, abdominal distension, abdominal pain, retention of food, constipation, borborygmus and prolapse of rectum.

Tianshu (ST 25)

Location: 2 *Cun* lateral to the umbilicus.

Operation: sit to the right or left side of the infant who is got to lie on the back, conduct *Rou* on the point with the index or middle finger and this is called *Rou* Tianshu (kneading Tianshu); carry out *Na* on it with the thumb and the index finger and this is called *Na* Tianshu (grasping Tianshu) (Fig. 159).

Times: 50—100 times of *Rou* and 3—5 times of *Na*.

Function: activating the function of the large intestine, regulating the flow of *Qi* and removing retended food.

Indications: diarrhea, constipation, abdominal distension and pain, dysentery and indigestion.

Fu

Location: the abdomen.

Operation: sit to the right side of the infant who is got to lie on the back, conduct *Mó* with the palm or the surface of the four fingers on the abdomen clockwise or counterclockwise, and this is called *Mó* Fu (rubbing Fu) (Fig. 160).

Times: carry out the *Mó* for 3—5 minutes.

Function: strengthening the spleen to activate the function of the stomach, regulating the flow of *Qi* and promoting digestion.

Indications: abdominal distension and pain, food retention, constipation, diarrhea, poor appetite, indigestion and ascaris intestinal obstruction.

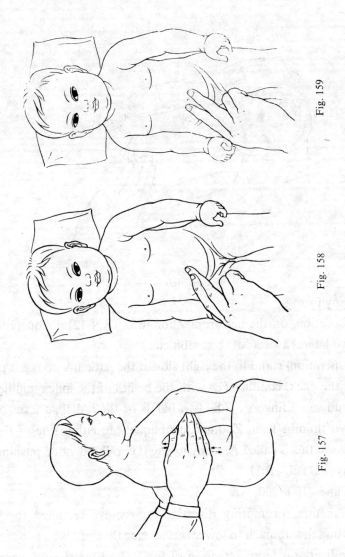

Fig. 157

Fig. 158

Fig. 159

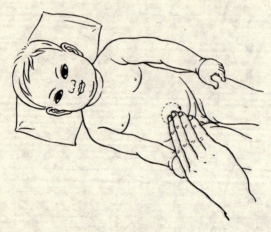

Fig. 160

Fuyinyang

Location: on the line from Zhongwan (RN 12) obliquely to the two lateral aspects of the umbilicus.

Operation: stand to the right side of the patient who is got to lie on the back, conduct *Fen* with the bellies of the index middle, ring and small fingers of the two hands or the radial surfaces of the two thumbs from Zhongwan obliquely to either side of the umbilicus, this is called *Fen* Fuyinyang (laterally-divided pushing Fuyinyang) (Fig. 161).

Times: 100—200.

Function: promoting digestion to remove retended food, regulating the stomach to lower the adverse flow of *Qi*.

Indications: fever, retention of food, chest oppression, vomiting of sour and foul things, abdominal distension and pain and indigestion.

Dujiao

Location: 2 *Cun* lateral to the umbilicus and 2 *Cun* inferior to the umbilicus.

Operation: get the infant to lie on the back, put either thumb on the point Dujiao and the index, middle fingers of either hand on either conjunction of the waist and the back, get the thumb and the index, middle fingers to work together to conduct *Na* on the abdominal tendons in depth, this is called *Na* Dujiao (grasping Dujiao) (Fig. 162).

Times: 2—3.

Function: relieving spasm and pain, promoting the flow of *Qi* to alleviate distension.

Indications: abdominal pain due to cold—heat, abdominal distension and diarrhea.

Dantian

Location: in the lower abdomen, 2.5 *Cun* inferior to the umbilicus.

Operation: sit at the right side of the infant who is got to lie on the back, conduct *Rou* or *Mó* on Dantian with the former carried out with the middle finger or the hand and the latter performed with the palm or the hand, and this is called *Rou* or *Mó* Dantian (kneading or rubbing Dantian) (Fig. 163).

Times: 50—100 times of *Rou* and 3—5 minutes of *Mó*.

Function: reinforcing the kidney to consolidate the fundamental, warming and tonifying the kidney—*Yang*, and separating the useful from the waste.

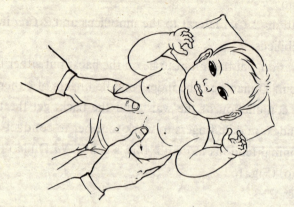

Fig. 161

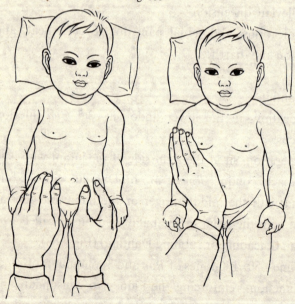

Fig. 162   Fig. 163

Indications: enuresis, prolapse of rectum, anuresis, scanty

and dark urine, distension and pain in the lower abdomen, and hernia.

10.3 Points on the Back

Dazhui (DU 14)

Location: below the spinous process of the 7th cervical vertebra.

Operation: stand at the right side of the infant who is got to sit upright, conduct *An—rou* on the point with the thumb or the middle finger of the right hand, and this is called *Rou* Dazhui (kneading Dazhui) (Fig. 164).

Times: 100—300.

Function: clearing away heat to relieve superficial syndrome.

Indications: common cold, fever, headache, stiff neck, hectic fever, night sweat, cough and asthma.

Feishu (BL 13)

Location: 1.5 *Cun* lateral to the inferior of the spinous process of the 3rd thoracic vertebra.

Operation: stand to the right side of the infant who is got to lie on the abdomen, conduct *An—rou* on the point with the thumbs or the index and middle fingers of the two hands, and this is called *Rou* Feishu. (kneading Feishu). Outward—kneading is *Xie* (reduction), while kneading toward the vertebrae, *Bu* (reinforcement) (Fig. 165).

Times: 100—300.

Function: regulating the lung—*Qi*, reinforcing the weakened body and arresting cough.

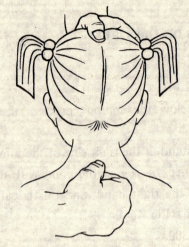

Fig. 164

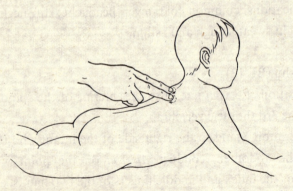

Fig. 165

Indications: cough, asthma, choking sensation in the chest, chest pain and fever.

Fengmen (BL 12)

Location: 1.5 *Cun* lateral to the inferior of the spinous process of 2nd thoracic vertebra.

Operation: get the infant to sit upright or to lie on the abdomen, conduct *An* or *Rou* on Fengmen with the tips of the index and middle fingers of the right hand, and this is called *An* or *Rou* Fengmen (pressing or kneading Fengmen).

Times: 30—50.

Function: expelling wind, dispersing cold, facilitating the flow of the lung—*Qi* to relieve asthma.

Indications: common cold due to wind—cold, cough, asthma, fever, headache, stiffness and pain of the nape and back, and disturbed sleep.

Yaoshu (DU 2)

Location: in the depression 3.5 *Cun* lateral to the 3rd lumbar vertebra.

Operation: get the infant to be in the prone position, conduct *An* and then *Rou* on the point with the thumbs, and this is called *An* and *Rou* Yaoshu (pressing and kneading Yaoshu).

Times: 30—50.

Function: clearing and activating the channels and collaterals, tonifying the kidney to strengthen the loins.

Indications: aching in the loins, five kinds of flaccidity in infants, five kinds of retardation, and paralysis of the lower limbs.

Notes: Five kinds of flaccidity in infants refers to flaccidity of neck, debility of nape, flaccidity of extremities, flaccidity of muscle and flaccidity in mastication. Five kinds of retardation means retardation in standing, walking, hair—growing, tooth eruption and the faculty of speech.

Pishu (BL 20)

Location: 1.5 *Cun* lateral to the inferior of the spinous process of the 11th thoracic vertebra.

Operation: stand to the right side of the infant in the prone position, conduct *An—rou* on the point with the surfaces of the thumbs or the index and middle fingers of the two hands sand this is called *Rou* Pishu (kneading Pishu)

Times: 100—200.

Function: strengthening the spleen, regulating the stomach, activating the function of the spleen to resolve dampness.

Indications: vomiting, diarrhea, infantile malnutrition, jaundice, edema, distending pain in the epigastrium, indigestion, chronic infantile convulsion, and listlessness.

Shenshu (BL 23)

Location: 1.5 *Cun* lateral to the inferior of the spinous process of 2nd lumbar vertebra.

Operation: stand to the right side of the infant in the prone position, conduct *An—rou* on the point with the two thumbs or the tips of the index and middle fingers of the right hand, and this is called *Rou* Shenshu (kneading Shenshu).

Times: 50—100.

Function: nourishing *Yin*, reinforcing *Yang*, invigorating the kidney.

Indications: lumbago due to weakness of the kidney, diarrhea, constipation, pain in the lower abdomen, and flaccidity of the lower limbs.

Qijiegu

Location: on anywhere of the straight line from Mingmen (DU 4) to the end of the caudal vertebra.

Operation: get the infant in the prone position, conduct straight *Tui* along the point with the radial aspect of the right thumb or the surface of the closed index and middle fingers. Pushing from the below to the above is called *Tui* Shangqijiegu (pushing upwards Qijiegu), while from the above to the below, *Tui* Xiaqijiegu (pushing downwards Qijiegu) (Fig. 166).

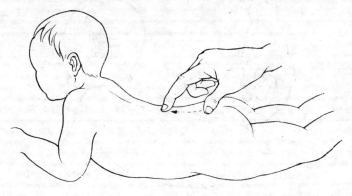

Fig. 166

Times: 100—300.

Function: *Tui* Shangqijiegu has the effect of warming up *Yang* and arresting diarrhea, while *Tui* Xiaqijiegu, purging heat to relax the bowels. The former is *Bu* (reinforcement), while the latter, *Xie* (reduction).

Indications: *Tui* Shangqijiegu is effective in treating diarrhea and protracted dysentery due to cold of deficiency type, and enuria and prolapse of rectum due to sinking of the weakened *Qi* of the middle—*Jiao*, while *Tui* Xiaqijiegu, abdominal distension and constipation due to heat in the intestines, diarrhea due to damp—heat, diarrhea due to overeating and acute dysentery.

Guiwei

Location: at the end of caudal vertebra.

Operation: stand at the right side of the infant in the prone position, conduct *Rou* on the point with the tip of the thumb or the middle finger of the right hand, and this is called *Rou* Guiwei (kneading Guiwei) (Fig. 167).

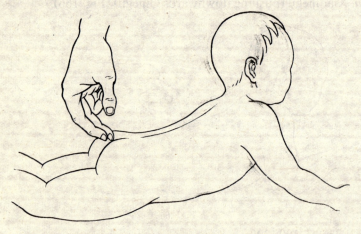

Fig. 167

Times: 100—300.

Function: promoting the flow of *Qi* in the *Du* Channel, regulating the function of the large intestine, arresting diarrhea and relaxing the bowels.

Indications: diarrhea, constipation, prolapse of rectum and enuresis.

Jizhu

Location: on anywhere of the straight line from Dazhui (DU 14) to Guiwei.

Operation: stand at the right or left side of the infant in the prone position, conduct *Tui* in a straight line from the above to the below with the surface of the index and middle fingers and this is called *Tui Ji* (pushing Jizhu) (Fig. 168–1), carry out *Nie* from the below to the above with the thumbs, the index and middle fingers of the two hands and this is called *Nie Ji* (pinching Jizhu) (Fig. 168–2). Usually, 3 times of pinching is followed by 1 time of lifting of the skin, and this is called "pinching 3 times and lifting 1 time", which comprises 1 section. Before *Nie Ji* is undertaken, perform gentle pressing and rubbing on the back so as to relax the muscles.

Times: 100–300 times of *Tui* and 3–5 sections of *Nie*.

Function: *Tui Ji* has the effect of clearing away heat, while *Nie Ji*, regulating *Yin* and *Yang*, supplementing *Qi* and blood, clearing and activating the channels and collaterals, coordinating *Zang* and *Fu*, reinforcing the primordial *Qi* and strengthening the body.

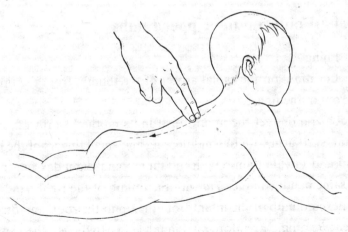

Fig.168–1

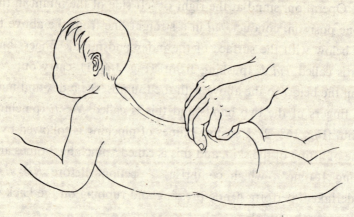

Fig. 168—2

Indications: *Tui Ji* is effective in treating fever, infantile convulsion and morbid night crying, while *Nie Ji*, such chronic diseases due to congenital defect or due to lack of proper care after birth as infantile malnutrition, diarrhea, abdominal pain, vomiting and constipation.

10.4 Points on the Upper Limbs

Pijing

Location: on the radial aspect of the thumb, from the tip to the root of the finger.

Operation: get the infant to sit in its mother's arms, fix the infant's left arm with the middle, ring and small fingers of the left hand and flex its thumb with the thumb and the index finger of the same hand, conduct *Tui* with the thumb of the right hand on the flexed thumb of the infant from the tip to the root, and this is called *Bu* Pijing (reinforcing Pijing) (Fig. 169); get the flexed thumb of the infant stretched straight, carry out *Tui* from the root to the tip, and this is called *Xie* Pijing (reducing Pijing); undertaking forceful *Tui* to and fro is called *Bu* and *Xie* Pijing (reinforcing and reducing Pijing).

Times: 100—500.

Function: *Bu* Pijing has the effect of strengthening the spleen, regulating the stomach and invigorating *Qi* and blood, while *Xie* Pijing, clearing away heat, promoting diuresis, removing stagnation of *Qi*, dispelling stagnated food and resolving phlegm.

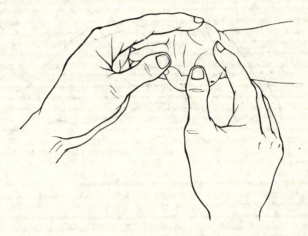

Fig. 169

Indications: weak constitution, poor appetite, emaciation with sallow complexion, vomiting, diarrhea, constipation, dysentery, jaundice, cough with phlegm due to dampness, and urticaria.

Weijing

Location: on the red—white border of the radial aspect of the major thenar of the palm.

Operation: get the infant to sit in its mother's arms with its left side of the body toward you, fix its arm with your left hand to expose Weijing, conduct *Tui* from the palm root to the root of the thumb with your right thumb or your right index and middle fingers, this is reinforcement and called *Bu* Weijing (reinforcing Weijing), carrying out *Tui* from the root of the thumb to the root of the palm is reduction and called *Xie* Weijing (reducing Weijing) (Fig. 170).

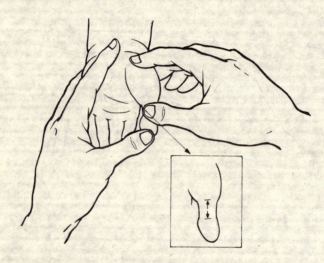

Fig. 170

Times: 100–500.

Function: *Bu* Weijing has the effect of strengthening the spleen and stomach to promot digestion, while *Xie* Weijing, purging stomach–fire, lowering the adverse flow of *Qi*, arresting vomiting, relieving restlessness and quenching thirst.

Indications: weakness of the spleen and stomach, indigestion, loss of appetite, abdominal distension, and such disorders due to excess of the stomach–fire as high fever, dysphoria, thirst, constipation, epistaxis, abdominal pain, vomiting and poor appetite.

Ganjing

Location: on the whorled surface of the tip of the index finger.

Operation: get the infant to sit in its mother's arms with its left side toward you, hold the hand of the infant with your left hand with the fingers of its hand upwards and the dorsum of its hand outwards, conduct *Tui* from the transverse striation of the ending knuckle of the index finger via the fingerprint region to the tip with the thumb of your right hand, this is reduction and called *Xie* Ganjing (reducing Ganjing) (Fig. 171); carrying out the same *Tui* but in the opposite direction is reinforcement and called *Bu* Ganjing (reinforcing Ganjing).

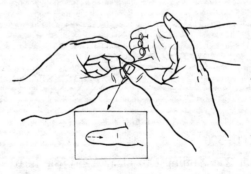

Fig. 171

Times: 100–500.

Function: *Xie* Ganjing can calm the liver to purge fire, relieve convulsion, alleviate mental depression and restlessness, while *Bu* Ganjing, nourish the liver and replenish the kidney.

Indications: dysphoria, conjunctival congestion, infantile

convulsion, bitter taste, dry throat, and restlessness and feverish sensation in the chest, palms and soles.

Xinjing

Location: on the whorled surface of the ending knuckle of the middle finger.

Operation: get the infant to sit in its mother's arms with its left side toward you, fix its hand with your left hand, conduct straight *Tui* toward the tip of its finger with the belly of the thumb of your right hand, this is reduction and called *Xie* Xinjing (reducing Xinjing) (Fig. 172);carrying out the same *Tui* but in the opposite direction is reinforcement and called *Bu* Xinjing (reinforcing Xinjing).

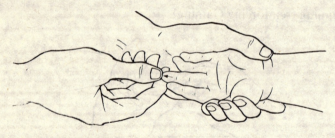

Fig. 172

Times: 100—500.

Function: *Xie* Xinjing can clear away the heart—fire, while *Bu* Xinjing, enrich the heart—blood and calm the mind.

Indications: such disorders due to excess of heart—fire as high fever, coma, flushed face, aphthae, scanty and dark urine, restlessness and feverish sensation in the chest, palms and soles and convulsion, and dysphoria and half—closed eyes in sleep due to deficiency of the heart—blood.

Feijing

Location: on the whorled surface of the ending knuckle of the ring finger.

Operation: get the infant to sit in one's arms, fix the left hand of the infant with your left hand to expose its ring finger, conduct straight *Tui* toward the finger tip with the thumb of your right hand, this is reduction and called *Xie* Feijing (reducing Feijing); carrying out the same *Tui* but in the opposite direction is reinforcement and called *Bu* Feijing (reinforcing Feijing) (Fig. 173).

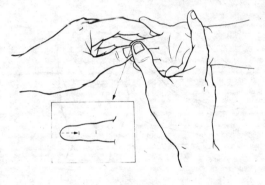

Fig. 173

Times: 100-300.

Function: *Xie* Feijing can clear away heat from the lung, relieve cough and resolve phlegm, while *Bu* Feijing, warm up the lung to arrest cough and invigorate the lung−*Qi*.

Indications: fever due to common cold, cough, asthma, rale in the throat, pale complexion, spontaneous sweating, night sweating, convulsion, dry nasal cavity, prolapse of rectum, enuresis, constipation and measles without adequate eruption.

Shenjing

Location: on the palm surface of the small finger, slightly inclining towards the ulnar aspect, from the finger tip up to the palm root.

Operation: get the infant to sit in one's arms with its left side towards you, hold its hand with the palm upwards with your left hand, conduct *Tui* from the palm root to the tip of the small finger with the thumb of your right hand, this is reinforcement and called *Bu* Shenjing (reinforcing Shenjing); carrying out the same *Tui* but in the opposite direction is reduction and called *Xie* Shenjing (reducing Shenjing) (Fig. 174).

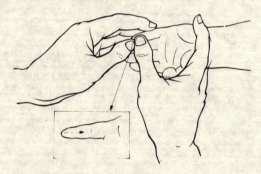

Fig. 174

Times: 100—500.

Function: *Bu* Shenjing can nourish the kidney to enhance *Yang* and strengthen the muscles and bones, while *Xie* Shenjing, remove damp—heat in the lower—*Jiao*.

Indications: congenital weakness, debility due to prolonged disease, diarrhea before dawn, enuresis, asthma due to deficiency, conjunctival congestion, stabbing pain and dribbing in micturition due to accumulation of heat in the urinary bladder, flaccidity of bone and general weakness, all of which should be treated through *Bu* Shenjing; and pain in the small intestine due to stagnancy of *Qi* which is treated through *Xie* Shenjing.

Sihengwen

Location: on the palm surface, along the transverse striations of the 1 st interphalangeal joint of each of the index, middle, ring and small fingers.

Operation: get the infant in the sitting or supine position, hold the hand of the infant with your left hand and get its palm upward and the fingers slightly flexed, conduct *Qia* on the transverse striation of the index finger and get the *Qia* followed by *Rou* performed with the nail of your right thumb, and, then, do the above successively on the middle, ring and small fingers, and this is called *Qia* Sihengwen (nipping Sihengwen). Or, get the four fingers of the infant closed and carry out *Tui* from the transverse striation of the index finger up to that of the small finger with the thumb surface of your right hand, which is called *Tui* Sihengwen (pushing Sihengwen).

Times: conduct *Qia* on each of the four fingers 5 times and carry out *Tui* 100—300 times.

Function: abating fever, removing restlessness, dissipating blood stasis, regulating *Qi* and blood and relieving flatulence.

Indications: infantile malnutrition, abdominal distension and fullness, incoordination of *Qi* and blood, indigestion, infantile convulsion, asthma and cracked lips.

Xiaohengwen

Location: on the palm surface, along the transverse striations of the metacarpophalangeal articulations of the index, middle, ring and small fingers.

Operation: get the infant to sit in one's arms, fix its left hand and make the palm upward with your left hand, conduct *Qia* successively on the transverse striations of the metacarpophalangeal articulations of the index, middle, ring and small fingers with the thumb nail of your right hand, carry out *Rou* following *Qia*, and this is called *Qia* Xiaohengwen (nipping Xiaohengwen); performing *Tui* on the transverse striations of the metacarpophalangeal articulations of the four fingers with the radial aspect of the thumb is called *Tui* Xiaohengwen).

Times: conduct *Qia* on each of the four fingers 5 times and perform *Tui* 100—300 times.

Function: abating fever, relieving distension and dissolving lumps.

Indications: cracked lips, fever, restlessness, aphthae and abdominal distension.

Dachang

Location: on the radial border of the index finger, on anywhere of the straight line from the tip of the index finger to the part between the index finger and the thumb.

Operation: get the infant to sit in one's arms, prop with your left hand the infant's left hand with the part between its index finger and its thumb upward and its thumb in between your index and middle fingers and perform *Tui* from the tip to the root of its index finger with the radial border of your right thumb, and this is reinforcement and called *Bu* Dachang (reinforcing Dachang) or *Cetui* Dachang (pushing laterally Dachang) (Fig. 175); conducting the same *Tui* but in the opposite direction is reduction and called *Xie* Dachang (reducing Dachang).

Times: 100—500.

Function: *Bu* Dachang can gain the effect of astringing intestine to correct diarrhea and warming the middle—*Jiao* to treat prolapse, while *Xie* Dachang, clearing the intestines to remove damp—heat and stagnancy.

Indications: diarrhea, dysentery, constipation, abdominal distension and pain, prolapse of rectum and swelling of anus.

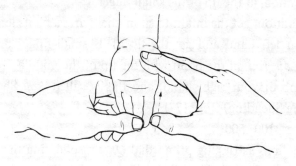

Fig. 175

Xiaochang

Location: on the ulnar border of the small finger and on anywhere of the straight line from the finger tip to the finger root.

Operation: get the infant to sit in one's arms, hold its left hand with your left hand and get the ulnar aspect of its small finger downward, conduct straight *Tui* on the finger from tip to root with the surface of the index and middle fingers of your right hand, this is reinforcement and called *Bu* Xiaochang (reinforcing Xiaochang); carrying out the same *Tui* but in the opposite direction is reduction and called *Xie* Xiaochang (reducing Xiaochang) (Fig. 176).

Times: 100—300.

Function: *Xie* Xiaochang can remove the damp—heat in the lower—*Jiao* and separate the useful from the waste, while *Bu* Xiaochang, warm up the lower—*Jiao*, disperse cold and induce diuresis.

Indications: scanty and dark urine, watery stools, enuresis, anuresis and aphthae

Shending
Location: at the tip of the small finger.

Operation: get the infant to sit in one's arms, fix its left hand with your left hand and get the tip of its small finger upward, conduct *An—rou* on the point with the tip of the middle finger or the thumb of your right hand, and this is called *Rou* Shending (kneading Shending) (Fig. 177).

Times: 100—500.

Function: astringing primordial *Qi*, consolidating the superficial to arrest sweating.

Indications: spontaneous sweating, night, sweating, or profuse sweating and infantile metopism.

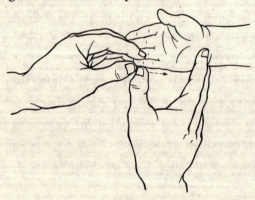

Fig. 176

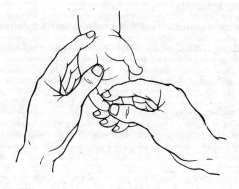

Fig. 177

Shenwen

Location: on the transverse striation of the 2nd interphalangeal joint of the palmar surface of the small finger.

Operation: get the infant to sit in one's arms, conduct *An−rou* on the point with the tip of the middle finger or the thumb, and this is called *Rou* Shenwen (kneading Shenwen) (Fig. 178).

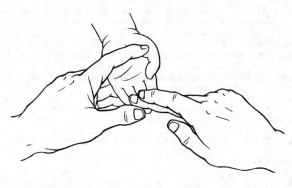

Fig. 178

Times: 100−500.

Function: expelling wind, improving eyesight and dissipating blood stasis and masses.

Indications: conjunctival congestion with swelling and pain, thrush, and disorders due to sanking of noxious heat into the interior.

Zhangxiaohengwen

Location: on the palmar surface, below the root of the small finger, and at the end of the palmar crease of the ulnar aspect of the hand.

Operation: get the infant to sit in one's arms or to lie on the back, hold the index, middle, ring and small fingers of the left hand of the infant with your left hand, conduct *An—rou* on the point with the tip of the middle finger or the thumb of your right hand, and this is called *Rou* Zhangxiaohengwen (kneading Zhangxiaohengwen).

Times: 100—500.

Function: clearing away heat, dissipating masses, soothing the chest, ventilating the lung, dissolving phlegm and arresting cough.

Indications: asthma and cough due to phlegm—heat, fever, pneumonia, aphthae, pertussis and slobbering.

Zongjin

Location: at the midpoint of the transverse striation of the palmar aspect of the wrist.

Operation: get the infant to sit in one's arms or to lie on the back, hold the four fingers (except for the thumb) of its right hand with your left hand, conduct *Qia* on Zongjin with the thumb nail of your right hand, and this is called *Qia* Zongjin (nipping Zongjin); carry out *An—rou* on it with the tip of the thumb or the middle finger, and this is called *Rou* Zongjin (kneading Zongjin) (Fig. 179).

Times: 100—300 times of *Rou* and 3—5 times of *Qia*.

Function: clearing away heat in the Heart Channel, dissipating masses, relieving spasm and regulating the flow of *Qi* throughout the body.

Indications: aphthae, morbid night crying, tidal fever, toothache and convulsion.

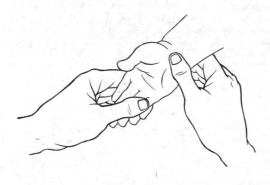

Fig. 179

Banmen

Location: on the flat surface of the major thenar of the palm.

Operation: get the infant to sit in one's arms or to lie on the back, hold the four fingers (except for the thumb) of its left hand with your left hand and get the major thenar of its palm upward, conduct *Rou* on the thenar with the tip of the thumb or the middle finger of your right hand, and this is called *Rou* Banmen (kneading Banmen) (Fig. 180); carrying out *Tui* from the root of the thumb to the carpal transverse striation is called "pushing from Banmen to carpal transverse striation" (Fig. 181), undertaking the same *Tui* but in the opposite direction is called "pushing from carpal transverse striation to Banmen".

Times: 100—300.

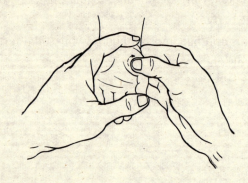

Fig. 180

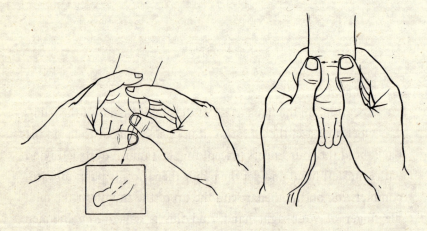

Fig. 181   Fig. 182

Function: "*Rou* Banmen" can strengthen the spleen, regulate the stomach, promote digestion and remove stagnancy; "pushing from Banmen to carpal transverse striation", arrest diarrhea; "pushing from carpal transverse striation to Banmen", relieve vomiting.

Indications: retention of food, abdominal distension, poor appetite, belching, diarrhea and vomiting.

Dahengwen

Location: at the transverse striation of the palmar aspect of the wrist with *Yangchi* near the thumb root and *Yinchi* near the root of the small finger.

Operation: get the infant in the sitting position, support its wrist joint with the index, middle, ring and small fingers of your two hands, conduct *Fen* from the midpoint of the carpal transverse striation (where Zongjin is located) to the left and right with your two thumbs and this is called *Fen* Dahengwen or *Fen Yinyang* (laterally—divided pushing Dahengwen or *Yinyang*) (Fig. 182); pushing from the left and right (Yangchi and Yinchi) to Zongjin is called *He Yinyang* (balancing *Yin* and *Yang*).

Times: 30—50.

Function: *Fen Yinyang* can balance *Yin* and *Yang*, regulate *Qi* and blood, eliminate stagnancy and promote digestion, while *He Yinyang* resolve phlegm and dissipate masses.

Indications: alternate cold and fever, dysphoria, indigestion of milk, abdominal distension, diarrhea, vomiting, asthma and cough due to accumulation of phlegm, choking sensation in the chest, dysentery and infantile convulsion due to fright.

Yunshuirutu and Yunturushui

Location: on anywhere of the arc—line from the root of the thumb to the root of the small finger and along the border of the palm.

Operation: get the infant to sit or lie on the back, hold its left hand and get the five fingers closed with your left hand, conduct *Tui* with the thumb of your right hand from the root of its thumb along the border of the palm via Xiaotianxin to the root of its small finger, and this is called "Yunturushui"; carry out the same *Tui* but in the opposite direction and this is called "Yunshuirutu".

Times: 100—300.

Function: Effect of Yunturushui is clearing away damp—heat in the spleen and stomach, inducing diuresis and arresting diarrhea, while effect of Yunshuirutu, strengthening the spleen to activate its function in transporting, moistening dryness to free the movement of the bowels.

Indications: dark urine, difficulty in urination, abdominal distension, dysentery, vomiting, diarrhea, constipation, infantile malnutrition and poor appetite.

Neilaogong

Location: in the centre of the palm, at the midpoint appearing between the middle finger and the ring finger when the fingers are bent.

Operation: get the infant to sit or lie on the back, use your left hand to hold the four fingers (except for the thumb) of the infant's one hand with the palm upward, conduct *Rou* on the point with the tip of the middle finger of your right hand, and this is called *Rou* Neilaogong (kneading Neilaogong); carry out *Yun* from the root of the small finger via Xiaohengwen of the palm and Xiaotianxin to Neilaogong, and this is called *Yun* Neilaogong or Shuidilaoyue (arc−pushing Neilaogong or salvaging moon in the river).

Times: 100−300 times of *Rou* and 10−30 times of *Yun*.

Function: The effect of clearing away heat in the heart and eliminating restlessness can be gained through *Rou* Neilaogong, while the effect of removing heat of deficiency type in the Heart and Kidney Channels, through *Yun* Neilaogong.

Indications: fever, dysphoria, aphthae, erosion of gum and other symptoms due to internal heat.

Neibagua

Location: on anywhere of a circle on the palm surface. The centre of the circle is where Neilaogong is located and the radius of the circle is the 2 / 3 length from Neilaogong to the transverse striation at the root of the middle finger.

Operation: conduct *Yun* clockwise with the radial aspect of the thumb of the right hand and this is called *Yun* Neibagua or Bagua (arc−pushing Neibagua or Bagua).

Times: 100−300.

Function: relieving stuffiness of the chest to benefit the diaphragm, regulating the flow of *Qi* to dissolve phlegm, removing stagnated food and promoting digestion.

Indications: cough, dyspnea due to phlegm, chest oppression, poor appetite, abdominal distension vomiting and diarrhea.

Xiaotianxin

Location: in the depression where the hypothenar and the

major thenar meet.

Operation: get the infant to sit in one's arms or to lie on the back, hold its left hand with your left hand, conduct *Rou* on the point with the tip of the middle finger of your right hand, and this is called *Rou* Xiaotianxin (kneading Xiaotianxin) (Fig. 183) carrying out, *Qia* with the nail of the thumb is called *Qia* Xiaotianxin (nipping Xiaotianxin), performing *Dao* with the tip of the middle finger or the interphalangeal joint of the bent middle finger is called *Dao* Xiaotianxin (pounding Xiaotianxin).

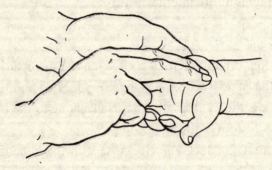

Fig. 183

Times: 100–300 times of *Rou*, 10–40 times of *Qia* and 10–40 times of *Dao*.

Function: clearing away heat, relieving convulsion, inducing diuresis and improving vision.

Indications: infantile convulsion, dysphoria, morbid night crying, conjunctival congestion with swelling and pain, aphthae, scanty and dark urine and smallpox without adequate eruption.

Shixuan (EX–UE 11)

Location: on the tips of the ten fingers, about 0.1 *Cun* distal to each of the nails.

Operation: get the infant to sit in one's arms or to lie on the back, fix the thumb, the index, middle, ring and small fingers of one hand of the infant with the thumb and the index finger of your left hand, conduct *Qia* with the nail of the thumb of your right hand on the five fingers one by one and do the same on the five fingers of the other hand of the infant, and this is called *Qia* Shixuan (nipping Shixuan)

Times: conduct *Qia* on each of the ten fingers 5 times or until the infant comes to.

Function: clearing away heat, inducing resuscitation and restoring consciousness.

Indications: high fever, infantile convulsion, spasm and syncope.

Laolong

Location: 0.1 *Cun* away from the proximal nail root of the middle finger.

Operation: get the infant in the supine position, fix the middle finger of one hand of the infant and expose the nail of it with the thumb, the index and middle fingers of your left hand, conduct *Qia* on the point with the thumb nail of your right hand, and this is called *Qia* Laolong (nipping Laolong) (Fig. 184).

Times: conduct *Qia* 5 times or until the infant comes to.

Function: restoring consciousness and inducing resuscitation.

Indications: acute convulsion, sudden loss of consciousness, high fever and spasm.

Ershanmen

Location: on the dorsum of the hand, in the depressions at the both sides of the capitulum of the 3rd metacarpal bone.

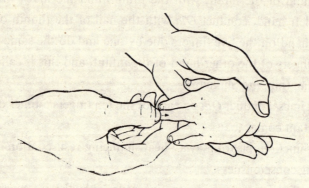

Fig. 184

Operation: get the infant in the sitting position, hold either of its hands with your left hand and have the palm downward, the wrist fixed by your index and middle fingers and the hand propped by your ring finger, conduct *Qia* on the point with the thumb nail of your right hand, and this is called *Qia* Ershanmen (nipping Ershanmen); carrying out *An—rou* with the radial border of the tip of the thumb or the index and middle fingers is called *Rou* Ershanmen (kneading Ershanmen) (Fig. 185).

Times: 5 times of *Qia* and 100—500 times of *Rou*.

Function: inducing diaphoresis to relieve superficial syndrome, abating fever and arresting asthma.

Indications: common cold due to wind—cold, fever without sweat, cough, asthma, acute convulsion, spasm and facial hemiparalysis.

Zuoduanzheng

Location: on the radial aspect of the middle finger, about 0.1

Cun lateral to the root of the nail.

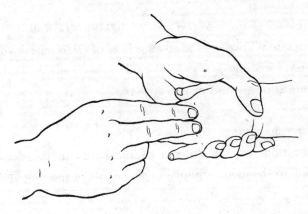

Fig. 185

Operation: get the infant in the sitting position, fix the middle finger of either of its hands with the thumb, the index and middle fingers of your left hand, conduct *Qia* on the point with the thumb nail of your right hand and, then, carry out *Rou*. This is called *Qia* and *Rou* Zuoduanzheng (nipping and kneading zuoduanzheng).

Times: 3—5 times of *Qia* and 50—100 times of *Rou*.

Function: treating diarrhea and dysentery.

Indications: diarrhea and dysentery.

Youduanzheng

Location: on the ulnar aspect of the middle finger about 0.1 *Cun* lateral to the nail root.

Operation: get the infant in the sitting position, fix the middle finger of one of its hands with the thumb, the index and middle fingers of your left hand, conduct first *Qia* and then *Rou* on the point with the thumb nail of your right hand, and this is called *Qia* and *Rou* Youduanzheng (nipping and kneading Youduanzheng).

Times: 3—5 times of *Qia* and 50—100 times of *Rou*.

Function: lowering the adverse flow of *Qi* to relieve vomiting and arrest bleeding.

Indications: vomiting and epistaxis.

Errenshangma

Location: on the dorsum of the hand, in the depression proximal to the metacarpophalangeal joints of the ring and small fingers.

Operation: get the infant in the sitting position, hold either of its hands and have the palm downward with your left hand, and conduct *Rou* on the point with the tip of the thumb of your right hand, which is called *Rou* Erma (kneading Erma).

Times: 100—500.

Function: nourishing *Yin*, reinforcing the kidney, regulating the flow of *Qi*, dissipating masses, inducing diuresis to treat stranguria.

Indications: cough and asthma due to heat of deficiency type, scanty and dark urine, coma, toothache, abdominal pain, teethgrinding in sleep, enuresis and diarrhea due to deficiency of the spleen and kidney.

Yiwofeng

Location: in the depression at the midpoint of the transverse striation of the dorsum of the wrist.

Operation: get the infant in the sitting position, hold its left hand whose palm is downward with your left hand, conduct *Rou* on the point with the tip of the thumb or the middle finger of your right hand, and this is called *Rou* Yiwofeng (kneading Yiwofeng) (Fig. 186).

Times: 100—300.

Function: warming the middle—*Jiao*, promoting the flow of *Qi*, arresting pain due to arthralgia—syndrome and relieving rigidity of the joints.

Indications: abdominal pain, borborygmus, arthralgia and common cold.

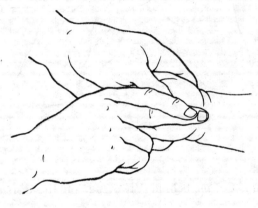

Fig. 186

Wailaogong

Location: on the dorsum of the hand, opposite to Neilaogong.

Operation: get the infant in the sitting position, conduct *Rou* with a finger tip, which is called *Rou* Wailaogong (kneading Wailaogong) (Fig. 187); carry out *Qia* with the nail of a thumb and this is called *Qia* Wailaogong (nipping Wailaogong).

Times: 100—300 times of *Rou* and 5 times of *Qia*.

Function: warming up *Yang*, dispelling cold, elevating the spleen *Yang* and inducing diaphoresis to relieve superficial syndrome.

Indications: common cold due to wind—cold, abdominal pain and distension, borborygmus, diarrhea, dysentery, prolapse of rectum, enuresis and hernia.

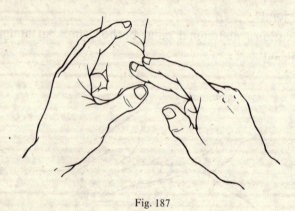

Fig. 187

Boyangchi

Location: 3 *Cun* behind Yiwofeng, on the dorsum of the hand.

Operation: get the infant in the sitting position, use your left hand to prop one of its wrists with the palm surface of the hand downward, conduct *Qia* on the point with the thumb nail of your right hand, and this is called *Qia* Boyangchi (nipping Boyangchi). Following that, carry our *Rou* with the tip of the thumb and this is called *Rou* Boyangchi (kneading Boyangchi).

Times: 100—300.

Function: relaxing the bowels and arresting headache.

Indications: constipation, common cold, headache, and

scanty and dark urine.

Sanguan

Location: on the radial aspect of the forearm, on anywhere of the straight line from Yangchi (SJ 4) to Quchi (LI 11).

Operation: conduct *Tui* from the wrist to the elbow with the radial aspect of the thumb or the surface of the middle finger of your right hand and this is called *Tui* Sanguan (pushing Sanguan) (Fig. 188). Get the thumb of the infant flexed and carry out *Tui* from the lateral aspect of the flexed thumb to the elbow, which is called *Datui* Sanguan (pushing Sanguan in a great extent).

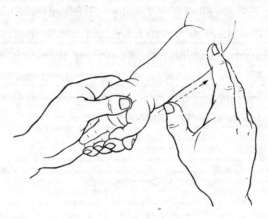

Fig. 188

Times: 100—300.

Function: invigorating *Qi*, promoting the circulation of *Qi*, warming up *Yang*, expelling cold, inducing diaphoresis to relieve superficial syndrome.

Indications: deficiency of *Qi* and blood, debility after illness, cold limbs due to deficiency of *Yang*, abdominal pain, diarrhea, skin eruption, miliaria alba, measles without adequate eruption, common cold due to wind—cold, and all the others due to deficiency and cold.

Tianheshui

Location: along the midline of the forearm, on anywhere of the straight line connecting Zongjin and Hongchi.

Operation: get the infant in the sitting position, hold its left hand with your left hand and have the palm upward, the forearm propped by your straightened index finger and the palm root pinched by your thumb, conduct *Tui* from its wrist to the elbow with the surface of the index and middle fingers of your right hand, and this is called *Xie* Tianheshui (reducing Tianheshui) (Fig. 189). Use alternately your index and middle fingers wet with water to carry out beating just like striking the strings along the way from Zongjin to Hongchi, and, at the same time, puff across the tail of beating, and this is called *Damaguotianhe* (crossing the milk way while beating your horse).

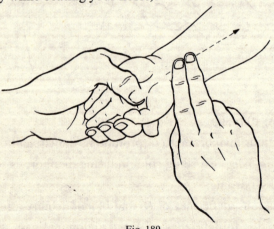

Fig. 189

Times: 100—300 times for either of *Xie* Tianheshui and

Damaguotianhe.

Function: clearing away heat, relieving superficial syndrome, purging fire and removing restlessness.

Indications: all the symptoms due to heat such as fever caused by exogenous pathogenic factors, tidal fever, internal heat, dysphoria, thirst, playing with the tongue, inflammation of the sublingual soft tissue, aphthae, dry mouth and throat, morbid night crying and convulsion.

Liufu

Location: on the ulnar aspect of the forearm and along the straight line from Yinchi to the elbow.

Operation: conduct *Tui* from the elbow to the wrist with the surface of the thumb or the index and middle fingers and this is called *Tui* Liufu (pushing Liufu) (Fig. 190).

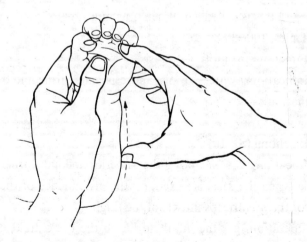

Fig. 190

Times: 100—300.

Function: clearing away heat, cooling blood and removing toxins.

Indications: all the symptoms due to heat of excess type such as high fever, restlessness, thirst, eruptions, infantile convulsion, thrush, swollen and rigid tongue, inflammation of the sublingual soft tissue, sore throat, mumps and constipation.

10.5   Points on the Lower Limbs

Jimen

Location: on the medial aspect of the thigh and along the straight line from the superior border of the knee to the groin.

Operation: get the infant to lie on the back with its thigh slightly abducted, put one hand on the lateral aspect of its knee joint, conduct *Tui* from the medial border of the knee up to the groin with the surface of the index and middle fingers of the other hand, and this is called *Tui* Jimen (pushing Jimen).

Times: 100−300.

Function: promoting diuresis.

Indications: watery stools, anuresis, dark urine and difficulty in urination.

Baichong (SP 10)

Location: 2 *Cun* above the superior medial corner of the patella when the knee is flexed, on the prominence of the medial head of the quadriceps muscle of the thigh.

Operation: get the infant to lie on the back, hold its ankle with the left hand and have its leg slightly abducted, conduct *An* or *Na* on the point with the thumb or the thumb and the index finger, and this is called *An* or *Na* Baichong (pressing or grasping Baichong) (Fig. 191).

Times: 5 times of *An* or *Na*.

Function: clearing and activating the channels and collaterals and relieving convulsion.

Indications: paralysis of the lower limbs and convulsion of the extremities.

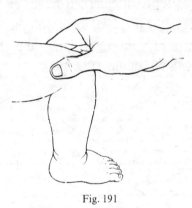

Fig. 191

Zusanli (ST 36)

Location: 3 *Cun* below Dubi (ST 35), one finger breadth from the anterior crest of the tibia.

Operation: get the infant to lie on the back, fix its ankle with the left hand, conduct *An—rou* on the point with the thumb tip of the right hand, and this is called *An—rou* Zusanli (press—kneading Zusanli).

Times: 50—100.

Function: strengthening the spleen, regulate the stomach, promoting the flow of *Qi* through the middle—*Jiao*, and removing stagnancy and obstruction in the channels and collaterals.

Indications: abdominal distension and pain, diarrhea, vomiting and paralysis of the lower limbs.

Weizhong (BL 40)

Location: in the centre of the popliteal fossa, between the two tendons.

Operation: get the infant to lie on the back with the knee 90 ° flexed, fix its foot with the left hand, and lift, grasp and pluck the tendons in the popliteal fossa with the thumb, the index and middle fingers of your right hand, and this is called *Na* Weizhong (grasping Weizhong) (Fig. 192).

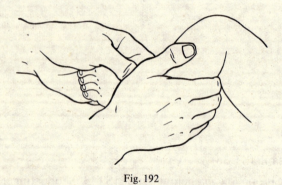

Fig. 192

Times: 5.

Function: relieving convulsion, clearing and activating the channels and collaterals, and strengthening the back and loins.

Indications: infantile convulsion, paralysis of the lower limbs, and soreness of the loins and back.

Houchengshan

Location: in the depression below the belly of the gastrocnemius muscle.

Operation: get the infant in the prone position, pluck the point with the middle finger of the right hand or grasp the point with the thumb and the index finger of the same hand, and this is called *Na* Houchengshan (grasping Houchengshan).

Times: 5.

Function: clearing and activating the channels and collaterals, and relieving convulsion.

Indications: pain and spasm in the leg, flaccidity of the lower limbs and infantile convulsion.

Qianchengshan

Location: beside the tibia of the shank, opposite to Houchengshan.

Operation: get the infant in the supine position, conduct *Qia* or *Rou* on the point with the thumb nail or surface of the right hand, and this is called *Qia* or *Rou* Qianchengshan (nipping or kneading Qianchengshan).

Times: 5 times of *Qia* and 30 times of *Rou*.

Function: relieving convulsion.

Indications: infantile convulsion and spasm of the lower limbs.

Sanyinjiao (SP 6)

Location: 3 *Cun* above the medial malleolus.

Operation: get the infant to lie on the back, fix its left or right foot with the left hand, conduct *An—rou* on the point with the tip of the thumb or the middle finger of the right hand, and this is called *An—rou* Sanyinjiao (press—kneading Sanyinjiao) (Fig. 193).

Times: 100–200.

Function: promoting blood circulation, clearing and activating the channels and collaterals, removing damp–heat in the lower–*Jiao*, and clearing and regulating water passage.

Indications: arthralgia of the lower limbs, enuresis, frequent urination, difficulty and pain in micturition, uroschesis and infantile convulsion.

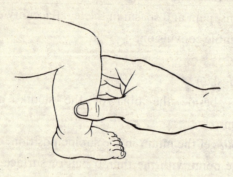

Fig. 193

Jiexi (ST 41)

Location: at the midpoint of the dorsal crease of the ankle joint, between the tendons of the long extensor muscle of the great toe and the long extensor muscle of the toes.

Operation: conduct *An–rou* on the point with the tip of the thumb and this is called *An–rou* Jiexi (press–kneading Jiexi) (Fig. 194).

Times: 50–100.

Function: relieving convulsion, arresting vomiting and diarrhea and treating rigidity of the joints.

Indications: infantile conculsion, vomiting, diarrhea and rigidity of the ankle joint.

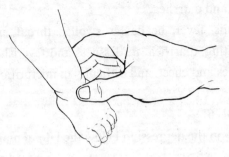

Fig. 194

Yongquan (KI 1)

Location: in the depression at the centre of the sole when the foot and toes are flexed.

Operation: get the infant to lie on the back, hold its heel with the left hand, conduct *Tui* towards the toes with the tip of the thumb, and this is called *Tui* Yongquan (pushing Yongquan); carry out *Rou* on the point with the tip of a finger and this is called *Rou* Yongquan (kneading Yongquan) (Fig. 195).

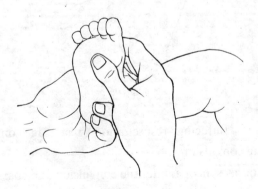

Fig. 195

Times: 50—100 times for either *Tui* or *Rou*.

Function: *Tui* Yongquan can conduct the fire back to its origin and abate fever of deficiency type, while *Rou* Yongquan, arrest vomiting and diarrhea.

Indications: fever, headache, swollen throat, infantile convulsion, vomiting, diarrhea, restlessness and feverish sensation in the palms, soles and chest, and difficulty in micturition.

Pucan (BL 61)

Location: in the depression below the lateral malleolus of the heel.

Operation: sit at the end of a bed on which the infant is got to be in the prone position, conduct *Na* on the point and this is called *Na* Pucan (grasping Pucan), carry out *Qia* on this point and this is called *Qia* Pucan (nipping Pucan) (Fig. 196).

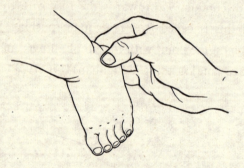

Fig. 196

Times: 5.

Function: inducing resuscitation, restoring consciousness and relieving convulsion.

Indications: syncope, infantile convulsion and spasm.

Translator's Notes:

In this chapter, there have appeared quite a lot of terms expressed in Chinese phonetic words, such as "*Bu* Pijing", "*Xie* Xinjing", "Yunshuirutu", "Shuidilaoyue", etc. In the following chapter, they will be used again and again to introduce the way of treating common infantile diseases. English—speaking overseas readers have to understand them. fully and keep in mind what is included in each of them. Why we don' t use English terms instead is that no English terms can express their exact meanings. If we did so, those English—speaking overseas readers would be misled.

11   Treatment of Common Infantile Diseases

11.1   Fever

Abnormal high body temperature is called fever. Infantile fever may be treated with *Tuina* unless it is due to infectious diseases and their like. Moreover, sure curative effects can be achieved sooner.

Etiology and Pathogenesis

It is caused by affection of exogenous pathogenic factors, accumulation of milk and food or impairment of *Yin*—fluid due to congenital defect and malnutrition after birth.

Clinical Manifestations

Fever due to exopathogens: chills, fever, stuffy nose, nasal discharge, cough, thin tongue coating and superficial venule of index finger. That mainly due to wind—cold is marked by serious chills, slight fever, watery nasal discharge, anhidrosis, and superficial reddish venule of index finger. That mainly due to wind—heat is manifested as severe fever, mild chills, turbid nasal discharge, sweating, and superficial purplish venule of index finger.

Fever due to *Yin*—deficiency: fever occurring after noon, flushed cheeks, feverish sensation in the palms, soles and chest, emaciation, dysphoria, night sweating, poor appetite, reddened tongue with little coating, and purplish dark superficial venule of index finger.

Fever due to heat of excess type in the lung and stomach:

high fever, dysphoria, hotness in the palms and chest, flushed face, shortness of breath, fullness in the epigastrium and abdomen, constipation, loss of appetite, thirst with desire for drink, reddened tongue with yellowish coating, and purplish uneven superficial venule of index finger.

Treatment

1. Fever due to exopathogens

(1) Therapeutic method: clearing away heat to relieve superficial syndrome.

(2) Prescription: *Tui* Tianmen 300 times, *Tui* Kangong 300 times, *Yun* Taiyang (EX–HE 5) 300 times, and *Yun* Erhougaogu 100 times.

(3) Modification: If the fever is due to wind–cold, 100 times of *An–rou* Fengchi (GB 20) and 2 times of *Na* Jianjing (GB 21) are added. If the fever is due to wind–heat, 50 times of *Nie–ji* (pinch–squeezing) Dazhui (Du 14) and 100 times of *Rou* Hegu (LI 4) are added.

(4) Treatment Course: Treatment is given once daily and 3 times of treatment make 1 course.

(5) Operation:

A. Peppermint water and juice of onion and ginger are used as medium with the former for fever due to wind–heat, the latter for fever due to wind–cold.

B. Get the infant held in its mother's arms or in the sitting position with its face towards you and carry out the manipulations according to the requirement. Fever due to wind–heat, for example, is treated like this: first, *Rou* Hegu at the both sides, second, *Tui* Tianmen from the below to the above alternately with the radial aspects of the two thumbs, third, *Fen* Kangong from Yintang (EX—HN 3) to the both sides, and, finally, *Yun* Taiyang towards behind the ears.

C. Get the infant's back towards you, *Yun* Erhougaogu at the both sides, *An—rou* Fengchi for fever due to wind—cold, *Nie—ji* Dazhui for fever due to wind—heat, and, finally, *Na* Jianjing (GB 21).

2. Fever due to *Yin*—deficiency

(1) Therapeutic method: nourishing *Yin* and clearing away heat.

(2) Prescription: *Bu* Pijing 300 times, *Bu* Feijing 300 times, *Bu* Shenjing 300 times, *Rou* Erma 500 times, *Xie* Tianheshui 300 times, *Fen* Yinyang 50 times, *Yun* Bagua 50 times, and *Rou* Yongquan (KI 1) 300 times.

(3) Treatment course: Treatment is given once daily, and 3 times of treatment make 1 course of treatment.

(4) Operation:

A. Warm water is used as medium.

B. Get the infant held in its mother's arms and conduct the manipulations on one arm of the infant like this: *Tui* Pijing and Feijing from the tip to the root of the finger, *Tui* Shenjing from the root to the tip of the finger, *Yun* Bagua clockwise, *Rou* Erma, *Fen* Yinyang on the wrist, and, finally, *Tui* Tianheshui from the wrist to the elbow.

C. *Rou* Yongquan at the both sides.

3. Fever due to heat of excess type in the lung and stomach

(1) Therapeutic method: clearing away internal heat.

(2) Prescription: *Xie* Feijing 300 times, *Xie* Weijing 500 times *Xie* Dachang 500 times, *Xie* Tianheshui 200 times, *Tui* Liufu 300 times, *Yun* Bagua 50 times, *Mó* Zhongwan (RN 12) for 3

minutes, and *Tui* Xiaqijiegu 100 times.

(3) Treatment course: Treatment is given once daily, 3 times make 1 course of treatment.

(4) Operation:

A. Egg white is used as medium.

B. Get the infant held in its mother's arms and perform the manipulations on either of its arms like this: *Tui* Feijing, Weijing and Dachang from the root to the tip of the finger successively, *Yun* Bagua, *Tui* Tianheshui from the wrist to the elbow, and, finally, *Tui* Liufu from the elbow to the wrist.

C. Get the infant to lie on its back with its abdomen exposed and *Mó* Zhongwan on the abdomen clockwise with one hand which has been dipped in egg white.

D. Get the infant in the prone position with its lumbosacral portion exposed and *Tui* Xiaqijiegu from the 4th lumbar vertebra to the coccyx.

Points for Attention

1. Find out the causes of fever and treat that due to infection with corresponding antibiotics.

2. Physical methods for lowering body temperature may be added if the fever is very high.

3. Treatment may be given twice daily if the lowered fever re−rises after 1 time of Tuina therapy is carried out.

11.2 Cold

Cold, a syndrome, is common in the four seasons, especially in fall and winter. In infants, it is rapid in onset and easy to complicate. This is due to the physiological and pathological features of infants.

Etiology and Pathogenesis

Infants tend to be attacked by wind pathogen and get cold whenever sudden change of weather or improper exposure to cold or heat occurs.

Clinical Manifestations

Type of wind—cold: aversion to cold, mild fever, anhidrosis, stuffy nose, watery nasal discharge, sneezing, cough, thin sputum, light—red tongue with thin white coating, and slightly reddish superficial venule of index finger.

Type of wind—heat: severe fever, slight chills, sweating, stuffy nose, turbid nasal discharge, flushed face, congested throat, yellowish sputum, reddened tongue with thin yellowish coating, and red—purplish superficial venule of index finger.

Treatment

1. Type of wind—cold

(1) Therapeutic method: expelling wind, dispersing cold and relieving superficial syndrome.

(2) Prescription: *Tui* Tianmen 300 times, *Tui* Kangong 300 times, *Yun* Taiyang (EX—HN 5) 40 times, *Yun* Erhougaogu 40 times, *Na* Fengchi (GB 20) 10 times, *Rou* Yingxiang (LI 20) 20 times, *Rou* Yiwofeng for 3 minutes, *Tui* Sanguan 100 times, and *Rou* Feishu (BL 13) 50 times.

(3) Treatment course: Treatment is given once daily and 3 times make 1 course of treatment.

(4) Operation:

A. Water in which ginger or onion has been steeped is used as medium.

B. Get the infant held in its mother's arms and carry out the manipulations on one of its arms like this: first, *Rou* Yiwofeng on the palm and, then, *Tui* Sanguan from the wrist towards the elbow.

C. Get the infant in the sitting position with its face towards you and conduct the manipulations on its face like this: *Rou* Yingxiang with the two thumbs or the index and middle fingers apart of one hand, *Tui* Tianmen from the below to the above, *Fen* Kangong from Yintang (EX—HN 3) towards the both sides, *Yun* Taiyang towards behind the ears, and *Yun* Erhougaogu at the both sides and, then, *Na* gently Fengchi (GB 20). after the infant is got to turn round.

D. Get the infant in the prone position with its back exposed and *Rou* Feishu 50 times with a finger.

2. Type of wind—heat

(1) Therapeutic method: expelling wind, clearing away heat and relieving superficial syndrome.

(2) Prescription: *Tui* Tianmen 300 times, *Tui* Kangong 300 times, *Yun* Taiyang (EX—HN 5) 40 times, *Yun* Erhougaogu 40 times, *Rou* Yingxiang (LI 20) 20 times, *Rou* Dazhui (DU 14) 200 times, *Tui* Tianzhugu 200 times, *Xie* Feijing 300 times, *Tui* Liufu 200 times, and *Rou* Xiaotianxin 200 times.

(3) Treatmen course: Treatment is given once daily, 6 times make 1 course of treatment.

(4) Operation:

A. Water in which peppermint has been steeped is used as medium.

B. Get the infant held in its mother's arms and do the manipulations on one of its arms according to the following requirements: first, *Tui* Feijing from the root to the tip of the finger, second, *Rou* Xiaotianxin, finally, *Tui* Liufu from the elbow to the wrist.

C. Get the infant to be in the sitting position with its face towards you and carry out the manipulations on its face in the following order: *Rou* Yingxiang with the two thumbs or the index and middle fingers apart of one hand, *Tui* Tianmen from the below to the above, *Fen* Kangong from Yintang (EX−HN 3) towards the both sides, *Yun* Taiyang towards behind the ears, and, then, get the infant to turn round, *Yun* Erhougaogu at the bothe sides, *Tui* Tianzhugu from the above to the below, and *Rou* Dazhui.

(5) Modification:

A. If it is complicated by sputum, what is added is: *Rou−an* (knead−pressing) Tiantu (RN 22) 30 times, *Fen* Danzhong (RN 17) 100 times, and *Rou* Rugen (ST 18) 30 times.

B. If it is accompanied by food retention, what is added is: *Xie* Pijing 100 times, *Xie* Weijing 100 times, *Yun* Banmen 100 times, and *Mó* the abdomen for 5 minutes.

C. If terror is also a factor responsible for the fever, what is added is: *Xie* Ganjing 300 times, *Xie* Xinjing 300 times, and *Rou* Xiaotianxin 20 times.

11.3   Cough

With its onset usually in spring, cough is one of the common symptoms of diseases of the lung system. Clinically, it falls into two kinds: that due to exopathogens and that due to inner injury. In infants, the former is more, and responds to *Tuina* therapy better, than the latter.

Etiology and Pathogenesis

1. Attack of wind−cold or wind−heat on the lung and linger-

ing of pathogens in the superficies of the body lead to the impairment of the purifying and descending function of the lung. In this case, the *Qi* will go up adversely and this is responsible for cough.

2. Dysfunction of the lung—*Qi* in ventilating due to weakness of the lung or deficiency of the lung—*Yin* results in accumulation and retention of body fluid. The retended body fluid will turn into sputum. Failure of foodstuff to be transported and transformed due to frequent deficiency of the spleen causes production of cold—dampness in the interior. This cold—dampness will turn into sputum, too. Stagnated sputum will bring about adverse flow of *Qi* and induce cough.

Clinical Manifestations

Cough due to exopathogens: cough with sputum, stuffy nose, nasal discharge, aversion to cold, fever, headache, general aching, thin tongue coating and floating pulse. Cough due to wind—cold is marked by thin sputum, watery nasal discharge, severe chills, thin whitish tongue coating and pale—red superficial venule of index finger, while cough due to wind—heat, by yellowish thick sputum, yellowish nasal discharge, severe fever, thin yellowish tongue coating and bright—red superficial venule of index finger.

Cough due to inner injury: protracted cough, mild fever, cough with little or much sputum, poor appetite, lassitude and emaciation.

Treatment

1. Cough due to exopathogens

(1) Therapeutic method: expelling wind, relieving superficial syndrome, ventilating the lung and arresting cough.

(2) Prescription: *Tui* Tianmen 100 times, *Tui* Kangong 100 times, *Yun* Taiyang (EX–HN 5) 100 times, *Xie* Feijing 100 times, *Yun* Bagua 100 times, *Tui* Danzhong (RN 17) 100 times, *Rou* Danzhong 100 times, *Rou* Rupang 20 times, *Rou* Rugen (ST 18) 20 times, *Xie* Tiantu (RN 22) 20 times, and *Fen* Jianjiagu (scapula) 100 times.

(3) Modification *Tui* Sanguan 300 times and *Rou* Ershanmen 100 times for cough due to wind–cold; *Tui* Liufu 300 times, *Xie* Tianheshui 300 times and *Tui* Tianzhugu 100 times for cough due to wind–heat.

(4) Treatment course: Treatment is given once daily and 6 times make 1 course of treatment.

(5) Operation:

A. Ginger juice or water in which peppermint has been steeped is used as medium.

B. Get the infant held in its mother's arms and conduct the manipulations on one of its arms according to the requirements. It is done like this: first, *Tui* Feijing from the root to the tip of the finger, *Yun* Bagua, and *Rou* Ershanmen if the cough is due to wind–cold, second, *Tui* Tianheshui from the wrist to the elbow or *Tui* Sanguan or *Tui* Liufu from the elbow to the wrist according to the different pathogenic factors of cough, finally, *Tui* Tianmen from the below to the above, *Fen* Kangong from Yintang (EX–HN 3) towards the both sides and *Yun* Taiyang towards behind the ears.

C. Get the infant to lie on the back with its chest exposed, *Fen* Danzhong with the thumbs and, then, *Rou* Danzhong, *Rou* Tiantu, *Rou* Rupang and *Rou* Rugen.

D. Get the infant in the prone position, *Tui* Tianzhugu on

the neck from the above to the below to treat cough due to wind—heat, then, expose its back and *Fen* Jianjiangu with the two thumbs.

2. Cough due to inner injury

(1) Therapeutic method: strengthening the spleen, resolving sputum, ventilating the lung and relieving cough.

(2) Prescription: *Bu* Feijing 300 times, *Bu* Pijing 300 times, *Yun* Bagua 300 times, *Tui* Danzhong (RN 17) 100 times, *Rou* Rupang 100 times, *Rou* Rugen (ST 18) 100 times. *Rou* Zhongwan (RN 12) 100 times, *Rou* Feishu (BL 13) 100 times, *Rou* Pishu (BL 20)100 times,and *Nie Ji* 3 times.

(3) Treatment course: Treatment is given once daily and 6 times make 1 course of treatment.

(4) Operation:

A. Talcum powder is used as medium.

B. Get the infant held in its mother's arms and conduct the manipulations on one of its arms according to the requirements. First, *Tui* Feijing and Pijing one after the other from the tip to the root of the finger and, then, *Yun* Neibagua clockwise.

C. Get the infant to lie on the back with its chest exposed, carry out *Fen* first and then downward—*Tui* and *An—rou* as well on Danzhong, conduct *Rou* on Rupang and Rugen, and, finally, expose the abdomen of the infant and undertake *Rou* on Zhongwan.

D. Get the infant to be in the prone position with its back exposed, conduct *Rou* on Feishu and Pushu, carry out *Tui* and *Rou* on the spine from the above to the below with the root of your palm and do this 2 times, undertake *Nie* (pinching) on the spine 3 times from the below to the above, and, finally, perform gentle *Rou* up and down with your palm root.

Points for Attention

1. During the treatment, pay attention to keep the infant warm lest it be attacked by cold.

2. Cough due to inner injury may be seen in many kinds of diseases. To treat it, medicines should be administered if necessary.

11.4　Asthma

Asthma refers to paroxysmal dyspnea. It is characterized by prolonged exhalation and rales in the throat. Severe asthma makes the patient breathe with the mouth opened and the shoulders lifted and even unable to lie flat. This disease is common in spring and fall and responds well to *Tuina* therapy.

Etiology and Pathogenesis

1. General weakness of the body, insufficiency of the lung, spleen and kidney and failure of food stuff and water to be transported and transformed normally lead to the production of phlegm. The accumulated phlegm blocks the respiratory passage and disturbs breathing, causing asthma.

2. When the weather changes suddenly or the temperature is irregulated, the lung will be attacked by pathogens. The attacked lung dysfunctions in ventilating and descending. In this case, the flow of *Qi* will be obstructed, causing asthma.

Clinical Manifestations

Asthma of heat type: cough, shortness of breath, rales in the throat, yellow thick sputum, dysphoria, deep—colored urine, fever, flushed face, reddened tongue with yellowish thick coating, and deep—red superficial venule of index finger.

Asthma of cold type: cough, shortness of breath, rales in the throat, whitish and foamy watery sputum, cold limbs, pale complexion, clear and abundant urine, thin and whitish tongue coating, and purplish red superficial venule of index finger.

Asthma of deficiency type: shortness of breath, faint coughing, languor in speaking, pale complexion, emaciation, profuse sweat, aversion to wind, poor appetite, pale tongue with thin whitish coating, and pale superficial venule of index finger.

Treatment

1. Asthma of cold type

(1) Therapeutic method: warming the lung, resolving phlegm, relieving asthma and arresting cough.

(2) Prescription: *Bu* Feijing 100 times, *Tui* Danzhong (RN 17) 100 times, *Rou* Danzhong 100 times, *Rou* Tiantu (RN 22) 30 times, *Cuo−mó* the hypocondriac regions for 2 minutes, *An−rou* Feishu (BL 13) 100 times, *Yun* Bagua counterclockwise 100 times, *Tui* Sanguan 100 times, *Rou* Fengchi (GB 20) 50 times, and *Rou* Yiwofeng 50 times.

(3) Treatment course: Treatment is given once daily and 6 times make 1 course of treatment.

(4) Operation:

A. Talcum powder is used as medium.

B. Get the infant held in its mother's arms and conduct the manipulations on one of its arms according to the requirements. It is done in the following order: *Tui* Feijing from the tip to the root of the finger, *Yun* Bagua counterclockwise, *Rou* Yiwofeng, and *Tui* Sanguan from the wrist to the elbow.

C. Get the infant to lie on the back with its chest exposed, *Fen* Danzhong, downward−*Tui* Danzhong, *Rou* Danzhong, *Rou*

·Tiantu, and *Cuo—mó* the hypochondriac regions with the two palms.

D. Get the infant to take the prone position with its neck and back exposed, *Rou* Fengchi and *An—rou* Feishu.

2. Asthma of heat type

(1) Therapeutic method: clearing away heat, resolving sputum, regulating the flow of *Qi* and relieving asthma.

(2) Prescription: *Xie* Feijing 200 times, *Nie—ji* (pinching—squeezing) Tiantu (RN 22) 100 times, *Fen* Danzhong (RN 17) 30 times, *Xie* Dachang 200 times, *Fen* Jianjiagu (scapula) 30 times, *An* Feishu (BL 13) 30 times, *Xie* Tianheshui 200 times, *Tui* Tianzhugu 50 times, and *Tui Ji* 20 times.

(3) Treatment course: Treatment is given once daily and 6 times of treatment make 1 course.

(4) Operation:

A. Talcum powder is used as medium.

B. Get the infant held in its mother's arms and carry out the manipulations on one of its arms according to the requirements in the following order: *Tui* Feijing from the root to the tip of the finger, *Tui* Dachang, and *Tui* Tianheshui from the wrist to the elbow.

C. Get the infant to lie on the back with its chest exposed, conduct *Ji—nie* (squeeze—pinching) towards the centre of Tiantu from the both sides or from the above and below, and, then, *Fen* Danzhong.

D. Get the infant to take the prone position with its neck and back exposed, *Tui* Tianzhugu from the above to the below, *An—rou* Feishu, *Fen* Jianjiagu (scapula) with the two thumbs, and *Tui Ji* from the above to the below (up to the coccyx).

3. Asthma of deficiency type

(1) Therapeutic method: improving inspiration by invigorating the kidney—*Qi* and astringing the lung—*Qi* to relieve asthma.

(2) Prescription: *Bu* Feijing 300 times, *Bu* Shenjing 300 times, *Tui* Sanguan 100 times, *Rou* Dantian 100 times, *An* Mingmen (DU 4) 100 times, *Rou* Feishu (BL 13) 200 times, *Rou* Shenshu (BL 23) 200 times, *Bu* Pijing 500 times, *Rou* Pishu (BL 20) 100 times, *Fen* Danzhong (RN 17) 100 times, and *Rou* Tiantu (RN 22) 100 times.

(3) Treatment course: Treatment is given once daily and 10 times of treatment make 1 course.

(4) Operation:

A. Talcum powder is used as medium.

B. Get the infant held in its mother's arms and conduct the manipulations on one of its arms according to the requirements. The manipulations are carried out in the following order: *Tui* Feijing and Pijing one after the other from the tip to the root of the finger, *Tui* Shenjing from the root to the tip of the finger, and *Tui* Sanguan from the wrist to the elbow.

C. Get the infant to lie on the back with its chest and abdomen exposed, *Fen* Danzhong, *Rou* Tiantu, and then, *Rou* Dantian.

D. Get the infant to take the prone position with its back exposed, *Rou* Feishu, Pishu and Shenshu successively, and, finally, *An* Mingmen.

Points for Attention

This disease tends to recur and the course of treatment may be properly prolonged.

11.5 Anorexia

Anorexia is a common syndrome in infants which is marked by long-time poor appetite, and even food refusal.

Etiology and Pathogenesis

Improper diet or feeding and long-time food preference impair the function of the spleen and stomach in transportation and transformation, causing this disease.

Clinical Manifestations

1. Type of failure of the spleen to transport and transform nutrients: pale complexion, loss of appetite or taste, food refusal, emaciation usually with normal mental state and basically normal stool and urine, thin and whitish tongue coating, and forceful pulse.

2. Type of deficiency of the *Qi* of the spleen and stomach: listlessness, sallow complexion, anorexia, food refusal, undigested food in feces or formless feces occurring after a little intake of food, tending to sweat, thin and clean tongue coating, and weak pulse.

Treatment

1. Type of failure of the spleen to transport and transform nutrients.

(1) Therapeutic method: strengthening the spleen to improve its function in transporting and transforming nutrients.

(2) Prescription: *Xie* Pijing 500 times, *Bu* Pijing 500 times, *Rou* Banmen 300 times, *Tui* Sihengwen 50 times, *Fen* Fuyinyang 300 times, *Rou* Zusanli (ST 36) 300 times, and *Nie Ji* 5 times.

(3) Operation:

A. Talcum powder is used as medium.

B. Get the infant to sit upright, fix its left hand with your left hand, *Xie* and *Bu* Pijing, *Rou* Banmen, and, then, *Tui* Sihengwen.

C. Stand at the righ side of the infant who is got to take the supine position, conduct *Fen* from Zhongwan (RN 12) to the both sides with the surfaces of the two thumbs, and, then, carry out *Rou* on Zusanli.

D. Stand at the right side of the infant who is got to take the prone position, conduct *Nie* from the coccyx to Dazhui (DU 14) 5 times with the thumbs and the index fingers and give a forceful lift whenever *Nie* is being carried out on Feishu, Pishu and Ganshu during the last two times, and, finally, perform *An−rou* on each of Ganshu, Pishu and Weishu 3−5 times.

2. Type of deficiency of the *Qi* of the spleen and stomach

(1) Therapeutic method: warming the stomach, strengthening the spleen and invigorating *Qi* and blood.

(2) Prescription: Bu Pijing 500 times, *Tui* Sanguan 300 times, *Rou* Wailaogong 100 times, *Yun* Neibagua 100 times, *Rou* Zhongwan (RN 12) 300 times, *Nie Ji* 5 times, *Bu* Dachang 500 times in case of indigestion, and *Xie* Dachang 300 times in case of enteritis.

(3) Operation:

A. Talcum powder is used as medium.

B. Get the infant to take the sitting position, fix its left hand, *Bu* Pijing, *Yun* Neibagua, and, finally, *Rou* Wailaogong.

C. Get the infant to lie on the back and *Rou* Zhongwan with one of your hands.

D. Get the infant to take the prone position, conduct *Nie* and *Na* on the skin from the coccyx to Dazhui (DU 14) 5 times with the thumb and the index and middle fingers, 1 time of lifting is done after 3 times of pinching during the last two times of *Nie* and *Na*, and, finally, carry out forceful *An* on Pishu on the both sides 3—5 times and do the same on Shenshu.

Treatment is given once daily and 6—10 times of treatment make 1 course. If cure has not come after 6 times of continual treatment, another 4 times are given after one day of interval.

11.6　Morbid Night Crying

Morbid night crying is common in infants within 1 year old. It is marked by calmness as usual in the day, and crying starting as soon as the night comes and even lasting through the night. The duration of this morbid condition may be several days or several months.

Etiology and Pathogenesis

1. Cold pathogen invades *Zang* and *Fu* and condenses in the channels and collaterals. The channels and collaterals obstructed by the cold pathogen cause pain. The pain makes the infant cry, especially in the night.

2. Up—stirring of fire pathogen disturbs the heart and has abundant heart—fire produced, causing dysphoria and insomnia of the infant.

3. Sudden terror attacks the heart and has the flow of its *Qi* disordered, causing mental derangement and convulsion of the infant.

4. Undigested milk over—taken leads to distension of the epigastrium and abdomen, causing calmless sleep of the infant.

Clinical Manifestations

1. Type of spleen—cold: crying in the night, timidness, lassitude, low and timid voice, blue—pale complexion, cold limbs,

clear urine, abdominal pain relieved by warmth and pressure, and light—red superficial venule of index finger.

2. Type of heart—heat: loud crying in the night, dysphoria, flushed face, reddish lips, hot air exhaled from the mouth, constipation, dark urine, warm hands and feet, and blue—purple superficial venule of index finger.

3. Type of terror: complexion sometimes blue and sometimes pale, sad and nervous night crying, calmlessness, sleep occurring only in its mother's arms, and attack of terror happening now and then.

4. Type of food retention: night crying, distension and fullness in the abdomen, sharper crying occurring when the abdomen is pressed, anorexia, milk regurgitation, stools with tart and foul flavor, and purple uneven superficial venule of index finger.

Treatment

1. Type of spleen—cold

(1) Therapeutic method: warming the middle—*Jiao*, strengthening the spleen and calming the mind.

(2) Prescription: *Qia—rou* Xiaotianxin 20 times, *Rou* Jingning 100 times, *Rou* Wailaogong 30 times, *Bu* Pijing 300 times, *Tui* Sanguan 300 times, and *Mó* the abdomen for 5 minutes.

(3) Treatment course: Treatment is given once daily and 6 times of treatment make 1 course.

(4) Operation:

A. Talcum powder is used as medium.

B. Get the infant held in its mother's arms and conduct the manipulations on one of its arms according to the requirements like this: *Tui* Pijing from the tip to the root of the finger, *Rou*

Jingning, *Rou* Wailaogong, and, then, *Tui* Sanguan from the wrist to the elbow.

C. Get the infant to lie on the back with its abdomen exposed and carry out slow *Mó* on the abdomen with one palm clockwise and counterclockwise alternately for 5 minutes.

D. Perform gentle and rapid *Qia—rou* on Xiaotianxin 20 times.

2. Type of heart—heat

(1) Therapeutic method: clearing away heat and calming the mind.

(2) Prescription: *Rou* Jingning 100 times, *Dao* Xiaotianxin 20 times, *Xie* Ganjing 200 times, *Xie* Xinjing 200 times, *Xie* Tianheshui 300 times, and *Tui* Liufu 200 times.

(3) Treatment course: Treatment is given once daily and 6 times of treatment make 1 course.

(4) Operation:

A. Talcum powder or warm water is used as medium.

B. Get the infant held in its mother's arms and undertake the manipulations on one of its arms according to the requirements in the following order: *Tui* Ganjing and Xinjing one after the other from the root to the tip of the finger, *Tui* Tianheshui from the wrist to the elbow, *Tui* Liufu from the elbow to the wrist, *Rou* Jingning, and *Dao* Xiaotianxin.

3. Type of terror

(1) Therapeutic method: relieving muscular spasm and tranquilizing the mind.

(2) Prescription: *Rou* Baihui (DU 20) 10 times, *Xie* Ganjing 100 times, *Xie* Xinjing 300 times, *Xie* Feijing 200 times, *Bu* Pijing 300 times, *Rou* Jingning 20 times, and *Qia—rou* each of the

phalangeal joints of the five fingers 3 times.

(3) Treatment course: Treatment is given once daily and 3 times of treatment make 1 course.

(4) Operation:

A. Talcum powder is used as medium.

B. Get the infant held in its mother's arms and perform the manipulations on one of its hands according to the requirements in the following order: *Tui* Ganjing, Xinjing and Feijing successively from the root to the tip of the finger, *Tui* Pijing from the tip to the root of the finger, *Rou* Jingning, and *Qia—rou* the phalangeal joints of the five fingers.

4. Type of food retention

(1) Therapeutic method: promoting digestion to remove retended food and regulating the function of the stomach.

(2) Prescription: *Xie* Weijing 200 times, *Xie* Dachang 200 times, *Yun* Banmen 100 times, *Yun* Bagua clockwise 100 times, *Rou* Zhongwan (RN 12) for 3 minutes, *An—rou* Tianshu (ST 25) 10 times, and *Rou* Xiaotianxin 30 times.

(3) Treatment course: Treatment is given once daily and 6 times of treatment make 1 course.

(4) Operation:

A. Talcum powder is used as medium.

B. Get the infant held in its mother's arms and conduct the manipulations on either of its hands according to the requirements in the following order: *Tui* Weijing and Dachang from the root to the tip of the finger, *Yun* Banmen, *Yun* Bagua clockwise, and *Rou* Xiaotianxin.

C. Get the infant to lie on the back with its abdomen exposed, *Rou* Zhongwan, and *An—rou* Tianshu.

Points for Attention

1. Night crying here does not include that due to parasitic infestation or fever or other factors.

2. Keep the infant warm lest it be attacked by cold while the manipulations are being done.

11.7 Constipation

Constipation refers to retention of feces, prolonged duration of defecation or dyschesia due to hard feces occurring when the infant has a desire for defecation. It is common in infants and preschool young children.

Etiology and Pathogenesis

1. Insufficiency of Qi and blood: Inability of the large intestine to transport feces due to Qi deficiency and failure of the large intestine to be moistened by body fluid due to blood deficiency are responsible for constipation. Insufficiency of Qi and blood is resulted from general debility or prolonged diseases.

2. Improper diet: Over—intake of fatty food pungent in flavor and heat in nature leads to accumulation of heat pathogen in the intestines and stomach and stagnation of Qi, and febrile disease exhausts and impairs body fluid. If so, $Fu-Qi$ will be stagnated and feces fails to be transported.

Clinical Manifestations:

1. Constipation of deficiency type: dyschesia, dry hard or soft feces, pale complexion and lips and nails, emaciation, lassitude, clear and profuse urine, cold pain in the abdomen relieved by warmth but worsened by cold, and cold limbs.

2. Constipation of excess type: dry feces, flushed face, fever, saburra, red lips, dark and scanty urine, poor appetite,

eructation, acid regurgitation, or distension and fullness in the abdomen, yellowish dry tongue coating, and purple superficial venule of index finger.

Treatment

1. Type of excess type

(1) Therapeutic method: clearing away heat, promoting bowel movement and activating the flow of *Qi* to reduce stagnation.

(2) Presciption: *Xie* Dachang 300 times, *Tui* Liufu 200 times, *Yun* Neibagua 50 times, *An−rou* Boyangchi 50 times, *Mó* the ab-domen clockwise 100 times, *Tui* Xiaqijiegu 200 times, and *Cuo−mó* the hypochondriac regions 50 times.

(3) Treatment Course: Treatment is given once daily and 3 times of treatment make 1 course.

(4) Operation:

A. Talcum powder is used as medium.

B. Get the infant to take the sitting position, hold its left hand with your left hand, *Xie* Dachang, *Tui* Liufu, *Yun* Neibagua, *An−rou* Boyangchi, and *Cuo−mó* its hypochondriac regions from the axillary fossa to the point Tianshu (ST 25) with your both palms.

C. Stand to the right side of the infant who is got to lie on the back, and conduct *Mó* on its abdomen clockwise with the fin-gers or palm of your right hand.

D. Stand to the right side of the infant who is got to take the prone position, and carry out *Tui* on Xiaqijiegu from the 4th lumbar vertebra to the end of the coccyx with the surface of the thumb or the index and middle fingers of your right hand.

2. Type of deficiency

(1) Therapeutic method: nourishing *Yin*, moistening dryness, invigorating *Qi* and enriching blood.

(2) Prescription: *Bu* Pijing 300 times, *Xie* Dachang 100 times, *Tui* Sanguan 200 times, *Rou* Erma 50 times, *Rou* Shenshu (BL 23) 50 times, *An–rou* Zusanli (ST 36) 50 times, and *Nie Ji* 5 times.

(3) Treatment Course: Treatment is given once daily and 6 times of treatment make 1 course.

(4) Operation:

A. Talcum powder is used as medium.

B. Get the infant to take the sitting position. fix its left hand with your left hand, *Bu* Pijing, *Xie* Dachang, and *Tui* Sanguan.

C. Get the infant to lie on the back and conduct *An–rou* on Zusanli.

D. Get the infant to take the prone position, carry out *Nie Ji* from the coccyx to Dazhui (DU 14) with your two thumbs and perform *An–rou* on Shenshu 3–5 times.

11.8　Vomiting

Vomiting is common in infants. It may be seen in many kinds of diseases.

Etiology and Pathogenesis

In children, the stomack–*Qi* is weak due to congenital defect. Once there is affection of exopathogens, over–intake of food or drink, traumatic injury, frightening, or accumulation of heat pathogen or cold of deficiency type in the spleen and stomach, the descending stomach–*Qi* will go upwards adversely, causing vomiting.

Clinical Manifestations

1. Vomiting of cold type: intermittent vomiting aggravated

by cold, clear vomit without foul odor, lassitude, pale face and lips, cold body and limbs, abdominal pain relieved by warmth, loose stools, pale tongue with thin whitish coating, and reddish superficial venule of index finger.

2. Vomiting of heat type: vomiting occurring just after food intake and vomit with tart and foul odour, which may be accompanied by fever, thirst, drinking a lot, dysphoria, reddened lips, foul stools or constipation, dark urine, yellow greasy tongue coating, and purplish superficial venule of index finger.

3. Vomiting of improper-diet type: frequent vomiting of things with sour and foul odour, nausea, eructation with foul odour of the retended food, comfort after vomiting, foul breathing, fullness and distension in the epigastrium and abdomen, stools with sour and foul odour or constipation, thich greasy tongue coating, slippery forceful pulse, and dark-purple superficial venule of index finger.

Treatment

1. Vomiting of cold type

(1) Therapeutic method: warming the stomach, expelling cold, regulating the function of the stomach and checking the adverse flow of *Qi*.

(2) Prescription: *Bu* Pijing 500 times, *Tui* Sanguan 500 times, *Rou* Wailaogong 500 times, conduct *Tui* from Hengwen to Banmen 200 times, *Rou* Zhongwan (RN 12) 300 times, *Na-an* Jianjing (GB 21) 3-5 times, and *Rou* Zusanli (ST 36) 100 times.

(3) Treatment Course: Treatment is given once daily 3 times of treatment make 1 course.

(4) Operation:

A. Ginger juice is used as medium.

B. Get the infant to sit upright, hold its left hand with your left hand, and conduct the following manipulations with your right hand: *Tui* Sanguan, *Bu* Pijing, *Tui* from Hengwen to Banmen, and *Rou* Wailaogong.

C. Get the infant to take the supine position and carry out *Rou* on Zhongwan and Zusanli with the middle finger or the palm root of your right hand, and, then, get the infant to take the sitting position and conduct *An—na* on Jianjing.

2. Vomiting of heat type

(1) Therapeutic method: clearing away heat to regulate the stomach and checking the adverse flow of *Qi* to arrest vomiting.

(2) Prescription: *Xie* Pijing 300 times, *Xie* Weijing 100 times, *Xie* Feijing 300 times, *Shuidilaoyue* 50 times, *Tui* Liufu 300 times, *Rou* Yongquan (LI 1) 100 times, and *Tui* Tianzhugu 300 times.

(3) Treatment Course: Treatment is given once daily and 3 times of treatment make 1 course.

(4) Operation:

A. Talcum powder or cold water is used as medium.

B. Get the infant to take the sitting position, fix its left hand and do the following manipulations: *Xie* Pijing, Weijing and Feijing one after the other, perform *Shuidilaoyue*, *Tui* Liufu and *Tui* Tianzhugu.

C. Get the infant to lie on the back, fix its foot with your left hand, and *Rou* Yongquan leftward with your right thumb.

3. Vomiting of improper—diet type

(1) Therapeutic method: promoting digestion to eliminate undigested food and regulating the stomach to check the adverse flow of *Qi*.

(2) Prescription: *Xie* Banmen 500 times, *Xie* Dachang 500

times, *Tui* Liufu 300 times, *Yun* Neibagua 100 times, *Rou* Zhongwan (RN 12) 300 times, *Fen* Fuyinyang 200 times, *Mó* the abdomen 100 times, *Tui* Xiaqijiegu 200 times, *An—rou* Zusanli (ST 36) 20 times, and *Nie—ji* (pinch—squeezing) Tiantu (RN 22) up to the appearance of local blood—stasis.

(3) Treatment Course: Treatment is given once daily and 3 times of treatment make 1 course.

(4) Operation:

A. Talcum powder is used as medium.

B. Get the infant to lie on the back, conduct *Tui* from Zhongwan to the both sides with the two thumbs until the distension and fullness of the abdomen are relieved, carry out *Mó* on Zhongwan with the palm, and perform *An—rou* on Zusanli.

C. Get the infant to take the sitting position in its mother's arms and do the following manipulations with your left hand: *Xie* Banmen, *Xie* Dachang, *Yun* Neibagua, and *Tui* Liufu.

D. Get the infant to take the prone position and *Tui* Xiaqijiegu with the surface of the index and middle fingers.

E. Get the infant to take the sitting position in its mother's arms again, conduct *Ji—nie* (squeeze—pinching) on the skin around Tiantu (RN 22) with the thumbs and the index fingers until 5 "◇"—shaped marks appear on the skin with every two marks 2 cm apart, and let the mother pat the back of the infant gently if it is crying while the manipulation is being done.

11.9 Diarrhea

Diarrhea in infants is also called indigestion. It is characterized by frequent defecation and loose or watery stools.

Etiology and Pathogenesis

1. Affection of exopathogen: Exogenous dampness pathogen disturbs the spleen—*Yang*. And the spleen dysfunctions in transporting and transforming nutrients with diarrhea resulting.

2. Interior impairment due to improper diet: Improper feeding marked by giving too much milk, or food fatty, greasy, raw, cold or dirty to an infant leads to the impairment of its spleen and stomach and causes diarrhea.

3. Weakness of the spleen and stomach: Insufficiency of the spleen due to congenital defect or prolonged disease or dysfunction of the spleen and stomach due to exogenous pathogenic factors will also cause diarrhea.

Clinical Manifestations

1. Diarrhea due to cold—dampness: watery and foamy stools without deep color and foul odour, borborygmus, abdominal pain, pale complexion, no thirst, clear and profuse urine, white and greasy tongue coating, soft pulse and reddish superficial venule of index finger.

2. Diarrhea due to damp—heat: fever or no fever, yellowish—brown watery stools with foul odour, feverish sensation in the reddened anus, thirst, reddened tongue with yellowish greasy coating, and purplish superficial venule of index finger.

3. Diarrhea due to improper diet: pain and distension and fullness in the abdomen, crying or giving vent before diarrhea, pain relieved after diarrhea, profuse stools usually with tart and foul odour, foul breathing, anorexia sometimes accompanied by vomiting of things with sour and foul odour, thick and greasy tongue coating, and slippery pulse.

4. Diarrhea due to weakness of the spleen: intermittent diarrhea or protracted and unhealing diarrhea, thin stools with

whitish lumps of milk or undigested food, defecation occurring whenever food is taken, poor appetite, pale complexion, pale tongue with thin whitish coating, and deep weak pulse.

Treatment

1. Diarrhea due to cold—dampness

(1) Therapeutic method: warming up the middle—*Jiao* to expel cold and resolving dampness to relieve diarrhea.

(2) Prescription: *Bu* Pijing 200 times, *Bu* Dachang 150 times, *Tui* Sanguan 300 times, *Rou* Wailaogong 200 times, *Mó* the abdomen 100 times, and *Tui* Shangqijiegu 200 times.

(3) Treatment Course: Treatment is given once daily and 3 times of treatment make 1 course.

(4) Operation:

A. Ginger juice or talcum powder is used as medium.

B. Get the infant to take the sitting position, fix its left hand and do the following manipulations with your right hand: *Bu* Pijing, *Tui* Sanguan, *Bu* Dachang, and *Rou* Wailaogong.

C. Get the infant to lie on the back and conduct *Mó* on its abdomen counterclockwise and then clockwise with the surface of the fingers or the palm of your right hand.

D. Get the infant to take the prone position and perform *Tui* on Shangqijiegu from the end of the coccyx to the 4th lumbar vertebra with the surface of the thumb or the index and middle fingers.

2. Diarrhea due to damp—heat

(1) Therapeutic method: clearing away heat, removing dampness, regulating the middle—*Jiao* and relieving diarrhea.

(2) Prescription: *Xie* Pijing 200 times, *Xie* Dachang 200 times, *Xie* Xiaochang 100 times, *Tui* Liufu 300 times, *Rou*

Tianshu (ST 25) 50 times, and *Rou* Guiwei 50 times.

(3) Treatment Course: Treatment is given once daily and 3 times of treatment make 1 course.

(4) Operation:

A. Cold water or talcum powder is used as medium.

B. Get the infant to take the sitting position, fix its left hand and do the following manipulations: *Tui* Liufu, *Xie* Pijing, *Xie* Dachang and *Xie* Xiaochang.

C. Get the infant to lie on the back and conduct *Rou* on Tianshu with the tips of the two thumbs or the tips of the index and middle fingers of one hand.

D. Get the infant to take the prone position and carry out *Rou* on Guiwei with the tip of the middle finger.

3. Diarrhea due to improper diet

(1) Therapeutic method: promoting digestion, removing undigested food, regulating the middle—*Jiao* and aiding in the transportation and transformation of nutrients.

(2) Prescription: *Xie* Pijing 300 times, *Xie* Banmen 200 times, *Yun* Neibagua 100 times, *Xie* Dachang 100 times, *Mó* the abdomen 200 times, and *Rou* Zhongwan (RN 12) 50 times.

(3) Treatment Course: Treatment is given once daily and 3 times of treatment make 1 course.

(4) Operation:

A. Talcum powder is used as medium.

B. Get the infant to take the sitting position, fix its left hand and undertake the following manipulations:*Xie* Pijing, *Xie* Banmen, *Yun* Neibagua and *Xie* Dachang.

C. Get the infant to take the supine position and conduc the following manipulations with the tip of the middle finger or the surface of the four fingers and the palm of your righ hand: *Rou* Zhongwan and *Mó* the abdomen clockwise and then counterclockwise.

4. Diarrhea due to weakness of the spleen

(1) Therapeutic method: strengthening the spleen, invigorating *Qi*, warming up *Yang* and relieving diarrhea.

(2) Prescription: *Bu* Pijing 300 times, *Bu* Dachang 200 times, *Tui* Sanguan 300 times, *Mó* the abdomen 100 times, *Tui* Shangqijiegu 200 times, and *Nie Ji* 3—5 times.

(3) Treatment Course: Treatment is given once daily and 6 times of treatment make 1 course.

(4) Operation:

A. Talcum powder is used as medium.

B. Get the infant to take the sitting position, fix its left hand with your left hand and perform the following manipulations: *Bu* Pijing, *Tui* Sanguan and *Bu* Dachang.

C. Get the infant to lie on the back and conduct *Mó* on its abdomen counterclockwise with the surface of the four fingers or the palm of your right hand.

D. Get the infant to take the prone position, *Tui* Shangqijiegu with the surface of the index and middle fingers, and, then, *Nie Ji* from the coccyx to Dazhui (DU 14) 5 times with the thumb working together with the index and middle fingers and 1 time of lifting of the skin is done after every 3 times of *Nie* while the last two times of *Nie Ji* are carried out.

11.10　Proctoptosis

Proctoptosis refers to prolapse of the anus and rectum. It is common in young children.

Etiology and Pathogenesis

It is caused by:

1. congenital defect and debility in the convalescence.

2. injury of the vital—Qi due to protracted diarrhea, which leads to deficiency and sinking of Qi of the middle—$Jiao$.

3. dry feces due to accumulation of heat in the large intestine and sinking of damp—heat.

Clinical Manifestations

1. Type of Qi deficiency: prolapse of the anus and rectum with severe swelling and pain, which is accompanied by pale or sallow complexion, emaciation, listlessness, pale tongue with thin coating, and light—colored superficial venule of index finger.

2. Type of excess heat: prolapse of the anus and rectum with swelling, stabbing pain and itching, which is accompanied by dry mouth, yellow tongue coating, defecation with dry feces, urination with scanty and dark urine, and purple superficial venule of index finger.

Treatment

1. Type of Qi deficiency

(1) Therapeutic method: Bu the middle—$Jiao$, invigorating Qi, elevating the spleen—Qi and correcting prolapse.

(2) Prescription: Bu Pijing 300 times, Bu Feijing 200 times, Bu Dachang 100 times, Tui Sanguan 300 times, $An–rou$ Baihui (DU 20) 200 times, Rou Guiwei 50 times, Tui Shangqijiegu 100 times, and $Nie\ Ji$ 3—5 times.

(3) Treatment Course: Treatment is given once daily and 15 times of treatment make 1 course.

(4) Operation:

A. Talcum powder is used as medium.

B. Get the infant to be in the sitting position, fix its left hand and do the following manipulations: *Bu* Pijing, *Tui* Sanguan, *Bu* Feijing and *An—rou* Baihui.

C. Get the infant to take the prone position, *Rou* Guiwei, *Tui* Shangqijiegu, and *Nie Ji*.

2. Type of excess heat

(1) Therapeutic method: clearing away heat, removing dampness and iducing bowel movement.

(2) Prescription: *Xie* Pijing 300 times, *Xie* Dachang 200 times, *Xie* Xiaochang 200 times, *Tui* Liufu 100 times, *An—rou* Boyangchi 50 times, *Rou* Tianshu (ST 25) 100 times, *Tui* Xiaqijiegu 50 times, and *Rou* Guiwei 50 times.

(3) Treatment Course: Treatment is given once daily and 6 times of treatment make 1 course.

(4) Operation:

A. Talcum powder is used as medium.

B. Get the infant to take the sitting position, fix its left hand with your left hand, conduct *Tui* Liufu, *Xie* Pijing, *Xie* Dachang, *Xie* Xiaochang and *An—rou* Boyangchi.

C. Get the infant to lie on the back and carry out *Rou* Tianshu with the tips of the index and middle fingers.

D. Get the infant to take the prone position, perform *Rou* Guiwei and *Tui* Xiaqijiegu.

11.11　Malnutrition

Malnutrition in infants is due to insufficient intake or absorption of nutrients.

Etiology and Pathogenesis

1. Malnutrition due to insufficient intake of food:

Inadequate breast milk, weaning before the scheduled time or improper feeding provide nutrients not enough to meet the needs of the infant's body.

2. Injury of the spleen and stomach due to improper diet:

Over or irregular feeding of milk or food fatty, sweet, raw or cold impairs the spleen and stomach. The impaired spleen and stomach dysfunction in transporting and transforming foodstuff, leading to food retention and failure of nutrients to be absorbed.

Clinical Manifestations

1. Malnutrition due to insufficient intake of food: pale complexion, withered yellowish sparse hair, disturbed sleep, low crying, cold limbs, maldevelopment, loose stools, pale tongue with thin coating, and light—colored superficial venule of index finger.

2. Injury of the spleen and stomach due to improper diet: emaciation, light body weight, fullness in the abdomen, poor appetite, listlessness, disturbed sleep, abnormal feces usually with disagreeable odor, and thick greasy tongue coating.

Treatment

1. Type of malnutrition due to insufficient intake of food

(1) Therapeutic method: warming up the middle—Jiao, strengthening the spleen and invigorating Qi and blood.

(2) Prescription: Bu Pijing 300 times, Bu Feijing 300 times, Rou Wailaogong 200 times, Tui Sanguan 300 times, Rou Zhongwan (RN 12) 200 times, An—rou Zusanli (ST 36) 200 times, and Nie Ji 5 times.

(3) Treatment course: Treatment is given once daily and 12 times of treatment make 1 course.

(4) Operation:

A. Talcum powder or Chineses holly leaf ointment is used as

medium.

B. Get the infant to take the sitting position and conduct the following manipulations on the left hand of the infant: *Bu* Pijing, *Bu* Feijing, *Rou* Wailaogong clockwise, and *Tui* Sanguan.

C. Get the infant to lie on the back with its abdomen exposed, *Rou* Zhongwan clockwise with the four fingers (except for the thumb)of your right hand, and, then, fix the lower limbs of the infant with your left hand and *An-rou* Zusanli with the thumb of your right hand.

D. Get the infant to take the prone position, conduct *Nie Ji* from Changqiang (DU 1) To Dazhui (DU 14) 5 times and give 1 time of lifting of the skin after every 3 times of *Nie* while the last two times of *Nie Ji* are carried out, and, finally, perform *An* with the two thumbs on each of Xinshu (BL 15), Ganshu (BL 18), Pishu (BL 20) and Weishu (BL 21) 3 times.

2. Type of injury of the spleen and stomach due to improper diet

(1) Therapeutic method: promoting digestion, removing undigested food and regulating the function of the spleen and stomach.

(2) Prescription: *Bu* Pijing 300 times, *Rou* Banmen 300 times, *Yun* Neibagua 200 times, *Rou* Zhongwan (RN 12) 200 times, *Fen* Fuyinyang 200 times, *Tui* Sihengwen 200 times, *Rou* Tianshu (ST 25) 200 times, and *An-rou* Zusanli (ST 36) 200 times.

(3) Treatment course: Treatment is given once daily and 12 times of treatment make 1 course.

(4) Operation:

A. Talcum powder is used as medium.

B. Get the infant to take the sitting position, conduct *Bu* Pijing, *Rou* Banmen, *Yun* Neibagua clockwise, and *Tui* Sihengwen.

C. Get the infant to lie on the back, carry out *Rou* Zhongwan clockwise with the four fingers (except for the thumb) of your right hand, and, then, *Rou* Tianshu clockwise with the bellies of the index and middle fingers.

D. Get the infant to lie on the back, fix its lower limbs with your left hand and undertake *An—rou* on Zusanli.

11.12　Abdominal Pain

Abdominal pain is a clinical symptom common in infants. It may be caused by many kinds of diseases. But what we are going to deal with is that mainly due to attack of cold pathogen on the abdomen, food retention, cold of deficiency type of the spleen and stomach or enterositosis.

Etiology and Pathogenesis

1. Affection of cold: If an infant is improperly taken care of when the weather changes suddenly, its abdomen will be attacked by wind—cold. If it is feeded in wind or over—feeded on cold fruit, cold pathogen will be accumulated in its body, leading to stasis of *Qi* and restriction of middle—*Jiao Yang*. In this case, *Qi* can not flow freely and pain results.

2. Food retention: If an infant is feeded improperly or feeded on too much food and drink or on raw and cold food, the food will stay in the middle—*Jiao*, undigested. If so, *Qi* will flow adversely and the food will fail to be transported and transformed, causing pain due to abdominal distension.

3. Cold of deficiency type of the spleen and stomach: If there is *Yang* deficiency or debility in the convalescence, the middle—*Jiao Yang* will be weakened together with the

spleen—*Yang*. If so, the food taken fails to be transported and transformed, cold—dampness stays in the interior, and the flow of *Qi* is blocked, with pain caused.

4. Enterositosis: Round worms move in the intestines or the biliary tract, or many of them gather into lumps. If so, the function of *Qi* will be disturbed, resulting in pain due to *Qi* stasis.

Clinical Manifestations

1. Pain due to cold pathogen: sudden pain usually occurring after affection of cold or intake of raw and cold food which is aggravated by cold but relieved by warmth, the pain moving up and down and usually in the form of colicky one which makes the infant cry and calmless, pale complexion, watery stools, pale tongue with white slippery coating, and reddish superficial venule of index finger.

2. Pain due to food retention: distension and tenderness in the abdomen, anorexia, foul breathing, eructation, acid regurgitation, breaking wind with disagreeable odor, tart and foul stools with undigested food, or abdominal pain with desire for diarrhea, pain relieved after diarrhea, sleep in the night which is now and then disturbed by crying, thick and greasy tongue coating, slippery pulse, and purplish uneven superficial venule of index finger.

3. Pain due to cold of deficiency type: dull and protracted abdominal pain relieved by warmth and pressure, sallow complexion, emaciation, poor appetite, diarrhea easy to induce, pale tongue with thin coating, light—colored superficial venule of index finger, and thready soft pulse.

4. Pain due to enterositosis: abdominal pain taking place and disappearing suddenly especially around the umbilicus, occasion-

ally palpable peristalic lumps, round worms having been found in feces, emaciation, anorexia, or paroxia, paroxysmal drilling pain occurring when worms are moving in the biliary tract, and vomiting.

Treatment

1. Pain due to cold pathogen

(1) Therapeutic method: warming up the middle—*Jiao*, expelling cold, regulating the flow of *Qi* and relieving pain.

(2) Prescription: *Bu* Pijing 200 times, *Rou* Wailaogong 300 times, *Tui* Sanguan 300 times, *Rou* Yiwofeng 300 times, *Mó* the abdomen 200 times, and *Na* Dujiao 3—6 times.

(3) Treatment course: Treatment is given once daily and 6 times of treatment make 1 course.

(4) Operation:

A. Talcum powder is used as medium.

B. Get the infant to take the sitting position and conduct the following manipulations successively on its left hand: *Bu* Pijing, *Rou* Wailaogong, *Rou* Yiwofeng, and *Tui* Sanguan.

C. Get the infant to lie on the back, carry out *Mó* on the abdomen clockwise with your palm, and, then, perform *Na* on Dujiao.

2. Pain due to food retention

(1) Therapeutic method: promoting digestion, removing undigested food, regulating the middle—*Jiao* and relieving pain.

(2) Prescription: *Bu* Pijing 200 times, *Xie* Dachang 300 times, *Rou* Banmen 300 times, *Yun* Neibagua 150 times, *Rou* Zhongwan (RN 12) 200 times, *Rou* Tianshu (ST 25) 200 times, and *Fen* Fuyinyang 200 times.

(3) Treatment course: Treatment is given once daily and 6

times of treatment make 1 course.

(4) Operation:

A. Talcum powder is used as medium.

B. Get the infant to take the sitting position and undertake the following manipulations one after the other on its left hand: *Bu* Pijing, *Xie* Dachang, *Rou* Banmen, and *Yun* Neibagua clockwise.

C. Get the infant to lie on the back with its abdomen exposed, *Rou* Zhongwan clockwise, *Rou* Tianshu, and *Fen* Fuyinyang.

3. Pain due to cold of deficiency type

(1) Therapeutic method: warming and reinforcing the spleen and kidney, invigorating *Qi* and relieving pain.

(2) Prescription: *Bu* Pijing 300 times, *Bu* Shenjing 300 times, *Tui* Sanguan 300 times, *Rou* Wailaogong 200 times, *Rou* Zhongwan (RN 12) 200 times, *Rou* the umbilicus 200 times, and *An–rou* Zusanli (ST 36) 200 times.

(3) Treatment course: Treatment is given once daily and 12 times of treatment make 1 course.

(4) Operation:

A. Chinese holly leaf ointment is used as medium.

B. Get the infant to take the sitting position and carry out the following manipulations one after the other on its left hand: *Bu* Pijing, *Bu* Shenjing, *Tui* Sanguan, and *Rou* Wailaogong clockwise.

C. Get the infant to lie on the back with its abdomen exposed, *Rou* Zhongwan with the tip of the middle finger, *Mó* the umbilicus with the palm, and, finally, *An–rou* Zusanli.

4. Pain due to enterositosis

(1) Therapeutic method: warming up the middle-*Jiao*, promoting the flow of *Qi*, calming worms and relieving pain.

(2) Prescription: *Rou* Yiwofeng 300 times, *Rou* Wailaogong 300 times, *Tui* Sanguan 300 times, *Mó* the abdomen 200 times, and *Rou* the umbilicus 200 times.

(3) Treatment course: Treatment is given once daily and 6 times of treatment make 1 course.

(4) Operation:

A. Liquid paraffin is used as medium.

B. Get the infant to take the sitting position and conduct the following manipulations one after the other on its left hand: *Rou* Yiwofeng, *Rou* Wailaogong, and *Tui* Sanguan.

C. Get the infant to lie on the back with its abdomen exposed, carry out *Mó* on its abdomen with your palm, and conduct *Rou* on its umbilicus with your palm root.

D. Get the infant to take the prone position and perform *An* and Rou on Ganshu (BL 18) and Danshu (BL 19) with your thumbs until the pain is relieved.

11.13 Uroschesis

Uroschesis is a symptom manifested as retention of lots of urine in the urinary bladder but dysuria.

Etiology and Pathogenesis

1. Accumulation of damp-heat: When damp-heat retends in the urinary bladder or the kidney-heat transfers to it, the dampness and heat will be combined each other and disturb the function of the urinary bladder, causing uroschesis.

2. Insufficiency of the kidney-*Qi*: When the kidney-*Yang* is insufficient, the fire from the gate of life will be declined. If so, *Qi*

fails to be transmitted, retended water fails to be removed, the urinary bladder fails to perform its function, and uroschesis results.

Clinical Manifestations

1. Accumulation of damp–heat: anuresis or oliguria, dark urine, burning sensation in urination, distension and fullness in the lower abdomen, bitter and sticky taste in the mouth, or thirst without desire for drink, or constipation, reddened tongue with yellowish greasy coating, and purplish superficial venule of index finger.

2. Insufficiency of the kidney −*Qi*: anuresis, or difficult urination with dribbling urine, weakness of the loins and knees, aversion to cold, pale complexion, listlessness, pale tongue, deep thready pulse, and light–colored superficial venule of index finger.

Treatment

1. Accumulation of damp–heat

(1) Therapeutic method: clearing away damp–heat in the lower–*Jiao* and inducing diuresis.

(2) Prescription: *Xie* Xiaochang 300 times, *Rou* Xiaotianxin 200 times, *An−rou* Dantian 300 times, *Tui* Jimen (SP 11) 500 times, and *An−rou* Sanyinjiao (SP 6) 200 times.

(3) Treatment course: Treatment is given once daily and 3 times of treatment make 1 course.

(4) Operation:

A. Talcum powder is used as medium.

B. Get the infant to sit upright and perform the following manipulations on its left hand: *Xie* Xiaochang and, then, *Rou* Xiaotianxin.

C. Get the infant to take the supine position, *An–rou* Dantian clockwise with the tip of the middle finger, the palm root or the surface of the four fingers (except for the thumb), *Tui* Jimen with the closed index and middle fingers of your right hand, and, finally, *An–rou* Sanyinjiao.

2. Insufficiency of the kidney–*Qi*

(1) Therapeutic method: warming up *Yang*, invigorating *Qi*, strengthening the kidney and inducing diuresis.

(2) Prescription: *Bu* Shenjing 300 times, *Bu* Pijing 300 times, *Rou* Erma 300 times, *Tui* Sanguan 200 times, *Tui* Jimen (SP 11) 500 times, and *Mó* the umbilicus for 1–2 minutes

(3) Treatment course: Treatment is given once daily and 3 times of treatment make 1 course.

(4) Operation:

A. Ginger juice or talcum powder is used as medium.

B. Get the infant to sit upright, hold its left hand with your left hand and carry out the following manipulations one after the other: *Bu* Shenjing, *Bu* Pijing, *Rou* Erma and *Tui* Sanguan.

C. Get the infant to lie on the back, conduct *Mó* on the umbilicus counterclockwise with the palm or the surface of the four fingers (except for the thumb), and, then, perform *Tui* on Jimen with the index and middle fingers.

11.14   Enuresis

Also called bed–wetting, enuresis refers to subconscious spontaneous urination in the course of sleep of the infants beyond 3 years old.

Etiology and Pathogenesis

1. Cold of deficiency type in the lower–*Jiao*: Congenital de-

fect of the kidney—*Qi* is responsible for cold of deficiency type in the lower—*Jiao*. If there has existed cold of deficiency type in the lower—*Jiao*, the urinary bladder will fail to perform its function and enuresis results.

2. *Qi* deficiency of the spleen and lung: *Qi* deficiency of the organs in the upper body will involve the ones in the lower body, which makes the water passages fail to be controlled and causes enuresis.

Clinical Manifestations

1. Cold of deficiency type in the lower —*Jiao*: 1—2 times or more of bed—wetting taking place during sleeping, which is accompanied by pale complexion, mental retardation, soreness and weakness of the loins and knees, clear and profuse urine, even cold limbs and chills, pale tongue, and deep slow weak pulse.

2. *Qi* deficiency of the spleen and lung: frequent subconscious urination with little urine occurring during sleeping usually in the convalescence, which is accompanied by pale complexion, listlessness, weak limbs, poor appetite, loose stools, pale tongue, and slow or deep thready pulse.

Treatment

1. Cold of deficiency type in the lower—*Jiao*

(1) Therapeutic method: warming up and replenishing the kidney—*Yang* to strengthen the lower—*Jiao*.

(2) Prescription: *Bu* Shenjing 300 times, *Tui* Sanguan 200 times, *Rou* Wailaogong 100 times, *An—rou* Baihui (DU 20)200 times, *Mó* Dantian 200 times, *An—rou* Shenshu (BL 23), and *An—rou* Sanyinjiao (SP 6) 100 times.

(3) Treatment course: Treatment is given once daily and 12 times of treatment make 1 course.

(4) Operation:

A. Talcum powder is used as medium.

B. Get the infant to take the sitting position and do the following manipulations one by one on the left hand of the infant: *Bu* Shenjing, *Tui* Sanguan, *Rou* Wailaogong clockwise, *An* Baihui and *Rou* Baihui clockwise.

C. Get the infant to lie on the back with its abdomen exposed, conduct *Mó* on Dantian with the palm and, then, perform *Rou* on Sanyinjiao.

D. Get the infant to take the prone position and carry out *An—rou* with the surface of the thumb on Shenshu on the both sides.

2. *Qi* deficiency of the spleen and lung

(1) Therapeutic method: tonifying the kidney to replenish *Qi* and control urination.

(2) Prescription: *Bu* Pijing 300 times, *Bu* Feijing 300 times, *Rou* Erma 200 times, *Bu* Shenjing 200 times, *An—rou* Baihui (DU 20) 50 times, *Mó* Guanyuan (RN 4) 300 times, *An—rou* each of Baliao (BL 31—34) 5—10 times, and *Rou* Guiwei 100 times.

(3) Treatment course: Treatment is given once daily and 12 times of treatment make 1 course.

(4) Operation:

A. Ginger juice or talcum powder is used as medium.

B. Get the infant to sit upright and carry out the following manipulations on its left hand one after the other: *Bu* Pijing, *Bu* Feijing, *Bu* Shenjing, *Rou* Erma, *An* Baihui, and *Rou* Baihui clockwise.

C. Get the infant to lie on the back and conduct *Mó* on Guanyuan clockwise with the palm.

D. Get the infant to take prone position, perform with the thumb *An* first and *Rou* second on each of the following points: Shangliao (BL 31), Ciliao (BL 32), Zhongliao (BL 33), Xialiao (BL 34) and, then, conduct *Rou* on Guiwei.

11.15 Thrush

Thrush is characterized by the walls of the mouth cavity and the surface of the tongue coated with white erosive points.

Etiology and Pathogenesis

Heat accumulated in the Heart, Spleen and Stomach Channels goes up to burn the mouth and tongue, causing thrush.

Deficiency of both *Qi* and *Yin* due to weakness of the spleen and stomach and impairment of the kidney—*Yin* renders water to fail to control fire, leading to flaring—up of fire of deficiency type which is also responsible for thrush.

Clinical Manifestations

1. Type of heat accumulated in the heart and spleen: congestive mucous membrane of mouth coated with patchy cream white things, flushed face, red lips, foul breathing, constipation, restlessness, crying of the infant when it is sucking, salivation, scanty and dark urine, reddened tongue with white greasy coating, and slippery or slippery rapid pulse.

2. Type of deficiency of both *Qi* and *Yin*: not obviously congested mucous membrane of mouth on which there are white points, flushed cheeks, debility, poor appetite, listlessness, dry mouth not accompanied by thirst, loose stools, clear urine, light—red tongue, and thready weak pulse.

Treatment

1. Type of heat accumulated in the heart and spleen

(1) Therapeutic method: clearing away heat, removing toxins and dispersing fire.

(2) Prescription: *Xie* Pijing 500 times, *Xie* Weijing 300 times, *Xie* Xinjing 500 times, *Rou* Shenwen 300 times, *Xie* Xiaochang 500 times, *Shuidilaoyue* 100 times, *Rou* Xiaotianxin 100 times, *Xie* Tianheshui 500 times, and *Tui* Liufu 300 times.

(3) Treatment Course: Treatment is given once daily and 6 times of treatment make 1 course.

(4) Operation:

A. Clear water is used as medium.

B. Get the infant to sit in its mother's arms and conduct the manipulations on its left hand in the following order: *Xie* Pijing, *Xie* Weijing, *Xie* Xinjing, *Rou* Shenwen' *Xie* Xiaochang and *Rou* Xiaotianxin.

C. Conduct *Shuidilaoyue*.

D. Clear Tianheshui and *Tui* Liufu.

2. Type of deficiency of both *Qi* and *Yin*

(1) Therapeutic method: strengthening the spleen, invigorating *Qi*, nourishing *Yin* and lowering fire.

(2) Prescription: *Bu* Shenjing 300 times, *Bu* Pijing 500 times, *Rou* Erma 300 times, *Yun* Neibagua 30 times, *Mó* Zhongwan (RN 12) 300 times, *Rou* Yongquan (KI 1) 200 times, *Nie Ji* 3—5 times.

(3) Treatment Course: Treatment is given once daily and 12 times of treatment make 1 course.

(4) Operation:

A. Talcum powder is used as medium.

B. Get the infant to sit in its mother's arms and carry out the manipulations on its left hand in the following order: *Bu*

Shenjing, *Bu* Pijing, *Yun* Neibagua clockwise, *Rou* Erma and *Rou* Yongquan.

C. Get the infant to take the supine position and conduct *Mó* on Zhongwan with the surface of the index, middle and ring fingers.

D. Get the infant to take the prone position and perform the manipulation of *Nie Ji*. A forceful lifting of the skin around Dazhui (DU 14) is given while the last two times of *Nie Ji* are undertaken. Finally, conduct *An—rou* on Dazhui 3 times.

Points for Attention

1. Care for the oral hygiene of infants. To prevent ulceration of oral mucosa, a piece of newly—produced black cloth having been dipped into sesame oil may be used to smear the walls of mouth cavity.

2. Antibiotic abuse is strictly prohibited especially for infants with weak constitution.

3. Breast—feeding mothers should eat light food with plenty of nutrients.

11.16 Myopia

Myopia is an eye disorder characterized by near vision. The congenital one is inherited from the parents with high myopia but it is less common. The acquired one is developed gradually due to over—use of the eyes in the dim light before one's youth or due to weaker constitution in one's young days caused by food prefer-ence. Clinically, myopia is subdivided into pseudomyopia (regulative) and true myopia (axial). Fatigue of the ciliary muscle due to over—use of the eyes makes the refractive power of the lens fail to be regulated, leading to pseudomyopia, which may be cured or relieved through rest. Optic axis is too long, which makes refractive regulation fail to be undertaken and leads to true myopia, which can be corrected only with the help of dispersing lens. Myopia in the beginning may be both pseudomyopia and true myopia.

Etiology and Pathogenesis

1. When the heart—*Yang* is deficient, enough blood and *Qi* fail to be sent up to the eyes, the eyes can not be nourished normally with enough essence and blood, and the normal vision becomes a near one.

2. When the *Yin* of the liver and kidney are deficient, enough essence and blood fail to be sent up to the eyes, the eyes can not be nourished normally, either, and the normal vision becomes a near one.

Clinical Manifestations

Clinical manifestations of myopia are different according to the seriousness of myopia itself and its complications. Common pure mild myopia is only marked by near vision without other symptoms accompanying. Some patients prefer indoor activities to outdoor ones because they can not see far things as clearly as the normal persons do.

Myopia complicated by astigmatism tends to cause fatigue and discomfort of the eyes. If the eyes are used continuously for a longer time, there will appear soreness of the eyes, headache, etc., all of which may be relieved after rest. Vitreous opacity is usually seen in patients with moderate myopia, who feel there are shifting stars before their eyes. Fatigue of the eyes occurs more often in patients with high myopia, who will suffer from monocular latent or manifest exotropia. Exotropia may lead to disuse myopia in the end.

Treatment

By treatment of myopia with *Tuina* is meant the treatment of the mild or moderate one usually seen in primary and middle—school pupils. Remarkable short—term curative effects can be achieved if myopia due to over—tenseness and contraction of the ocular muscles and prominence of the lens is treated with *Tuina*.

1. Therapeutic method: regulating *Qi* and blood and removing obstructions in the channels and collaterals.

2. Prescriptions: *Rou* Jingming (BL 1) 300 times, *Tui* Cuanzhu (BL 2) 300 times, *Tui* Tianying 300 times, *Tui* Taiyang (EX—HN 5) 300 times, *Tui* Sibai (ST 2) 200 times, *Tui* Yifeng (SJ 17) 300 times, *An* Fengchi (GB 20) 300 times, *An—rou* Tianzhugu 300 times, *Tui* Kangong 300 times, and *Mó* either of the upper and lower orbits 100 times.

3. Operation:

The patient is got to lie on the back first and then to take the sitting position. The manipulations are carried out one after the other according to the requirements and the prescription.

Modification

1. If there exists deficiency of the heart—*Yang*, 100 times of *Rou* the left and right Xinshu (BL 15) and 150 times of *Rou* Shenshu (BL 23) are added in addition to the manipulations in the prescription.

2. For patients with insufficiency of the *Yin* of the liver and kidney, the manipulations added are: *Rou* Ganshu (BL 18) 100 times, *Rou* Shenshu (BL 23) 200 times, *Rou* Zuguangming (GB 37) 100 times, and *Rou* Yongquan (KI 1) 100 times.

Points for Attention

1. Treatment is given once daily and 12 times of treatment make 1 course. If the vision is improved after 1 course of treatment, the treatment should be continued for another 2—3 courses. For young pupils, 1—2 courses of treatment are suggested during either of the spring and summer vocations.

2. The physician should do the manipulations gently with clean hands whose fingernails have been trimmed and each manipulation should be performed to the extent that the patient has had a sensation of soreness and distension.

11.17   Rickets

Rickets is a chronic deficiency disease. It is common in infants below 3 years old. But the higher incidence is seen in babies within 6—12 months.

Etiology and Pathogenesis

TCM believes that weakness of the spleen and stomach due to malnutrition before and after the birth of an infant is the cause of this disease.

Clinical Manifestations

In the early stage: dysphoria, disturbed sleep in the night, listlessness, profuse sweating in the head and neck, poor appetite, muscular relaxtion, yellowish sparse hair, baldness in the occiput, soft skull, delay of the close of the fontanel, sallow complexion, weakness of the limbs, tending to be frightened, loose stools, and thin whitish tongue coating.

In the advanced stage: skeleton deformity marked by square skull, delay of the close of the extremely large fontanel, emaciation, general debility, listless facial expression, retardation of ·

movement, delay of tooth eruption, chicken breast, thickness of the ends of the epiphyses in the tibial and malleolar portions, "O / X-shaped" legs, and deformation of the spinal column.

Treatment

1. Therapeutic method

(1) In the early stage: strengthening the spleen and tonifying the kidney.

(2) In the advanced stage: strengthening the spleen, tonifying the kidney and correcting the deformation.

2. Prescription

Bu Pijing 300 times, *Bu* Shenjing 300 times, *Rou* Xiaotianxin 100 times, *Tui* Sanguan 100 times, *Rou* Shending 100 times, *Nie Ji* 3−5 times, and *An* each of Shenshu (BL 23), Pishu (BL 20), Weishu (BL 21) and Feishu (BL 13) 3−5 times.

3. Treatment Course: Treatment is given once daily and 30 times of treatment make 1 course.

4. Operation

(1) Get the infant to sit in its mother's arms, hold its left hand with your left hand, *Bu* Pijing and Shenjing one after the other, and *Rou* Shending and Xiaotianxin.

(2) Get the infant in the same position as the above with its forearm exposed, and *Tui* Sanguan with the surface of the index and middle fingers of your right hand.

(3) Stand at one side of the infant who is got to take the prone position, conduct routine *Nie Ji* with your two hands 4 times and carry out *Ti* (lifting) and *Nie* (pinching) at the same time in the course of the 4th time with especially forceful lifting given on Shenshu, Pishu, Weishu and Feishu, finally, perform *An−rou* on the above 4 points.

(4) Get the infant with chicken breast to take the sitting position and undertake gentle and rhythmic *Ya* (pressing) on the protruded portion 30—50 times with your two hands either of which is opposite to the other.

11.18   Cerebral Palsy

Complete or partial loss of the ability of the higher nerves to control the spinal nerves renders the tone of the involved muscles to be increased and their voluntary motion to be disordered, causing cerebral palsy.

Etiology and Pathogenesis

In TCM, this disease is included in the syndromes of "five kinds of retardation in infants" and "five kinds of flaccidity in infants". It is caused in this way. Deficiency of the liver—*Yin* and the kidney—*Yin* and weakness of the spleen and stomach lead to flaccidity of the tendons and bones and stagnation of *Qi* and blood. In this case, the muscles and tendons of the extremities can not be warmed and nourished. And cerebral palsy results.

Clinical Manifestations

There are many kinds of cerebral palsy, among which the commonest one is spastic bilateral paralysis or cerebral hemiplegia or monoplegia, and cerebellar ataxia comes the second.

As the infant is developing, the following are seen in it: difficulty in lifting its head by itself and in keeping itself in the sitting posture, laziness of the extremities seen especially in the lower limbs, the limbs hard to move due to hypermyotonia occurring when passive action is given, lying or walking with its legs crossed, scissors gait, spasm or deformation of the legs appearing as soon as it steps its toes on the floor, and the spasm of muscles increased whenever it wants to move but completely relieved when it has fallen into a deep sleep.

Spastic paralysis seen in clinical practice is different in seriousness and scope. If it is severe, the muscular tone is highly increased, while when it is mild, there only appears slight disorder of muscular movement. What is involved may be one limb, two upper limbs, two lower limbs, unilateral upper limb or the four limbs and the trunk. The involved upper limb / limbs is marked by adduction of the shoulder / shoulders, flexion of the elbow / elbows and the wrist / wrists, pronation of the forearm / forearms, adduction of the thumb / thumbs, and flexion of the four fingers into a fist. The involved lower limb / limbs is marked by flexion, adduction and intorsion of the hip / hips, flexion of the knee / knees, and foot drop and inversion. The involved trunk is marked by bending of the trunk backward or forward, and forward-bent or laterally-protruded chest and waist. In addition, aphasis, visual disturbance, dysaudia, dysnoesia and physical dysplasia are seen in a part of the diseased infants.

Treatment

1. Therapeutic method: dredging the channels and collaterals, moving the joints, strengthening the spleen, enhancing the kidney, invigorating *Qi*, and nourishing blood.

2. Prescription: *Bu* Pijing 500 times, *Bu* Shenjing 500 times, *Rou* Erma 200 times, *Yun* Neibagua 100 times, and *Dao* Xiaotianxin 50 times.

Modification

1. In case of paralysis of the upper limbs, the manipulations to be added are as follows: *Qia* 5-10 times on each of the

fingernail roots and each of the phalangeal joints of hand, *Rou* along part of the route of each of The Pericardium Channel of Hand—Jueyin, The Heart Channel of Hand—Shaoyin, The Tri—*Jiao* Channel of Hand—Shaoyang and The Large Intestine Channel of Hand—Yangming, and *Na* on Shaohai (HT 3) and Neiguan (PC 6).

2. In case of paralysis of the lower limbs, the manipulations to be added are as follows: *Qia* 5—10 times on each of the toe roots and each of phalangeal joints of foot, *Rou* along part of the route of each of The Stomach Channel of Foot—Yangming, The Gallbladder Channel of Foot—Shaoyang, The Liver Channel of Foot—Jueyin and The Spleen Channel of Foot—Taiyin, *Na* on Weizhong (BL 40), Chengshan (BL 57), Kunlun (BL 60), points on the both sides of the loins, Huantiao (GB 30) and Yanglingquan (GB 34).

3. Operation

(1) Talcum powder is used as medium.

(2) Get the infant to take the sitting position, hold the thumb of its right hand with your left hand, conduct *Tui* on Pijing and Shenjing one after the other, perform *Yun* on Neibagua, and undertake *Dao* on Xiaotianxin. Turn its hand over with the dorsum upward, carry out *Qia* with the thumb nail of your right hand successively on the roots of its fingernails and its phalangeal joints of hand until it feels painful. Finally, do *Qia* on the lower limbs in the same way.

(3) Get the infant to take the prone position, conduct *Dian* after gentle *Rou* with your middle finger along part of the route of each of The Pericardium Channel of Hand—Jueyin, The Heart Channel of Hand—Shaoyin, The Tri—*Jiao* Channel of

Hand—Shaoyang and The Large Intestine Channel of Hand—Yangming, and, then, undertake *Na* on Shaohai (HT 3) and Neiguan (PC 6). Finally, do the same on the lower limbs in the same way.

(4) If the trunk is involved, the infant may be got to take the prone position, and more forceful stimulation should be given to The Urinary Bladder Channel of Foot—Taiyang on the back.

(5) Get the infant to take the sitting or lying position and have its joints involved flexed, extended, adducted, inward—rotated and abducted.

4. Treatment course

1 course of treatment consists of 3 months, during which the treatment is given once daily.

If *Tuina* therapy is used to treat an infant with normal intelligence and mild or moderate paralysis, more evident curative effects will be seen after 3 months of treatment. However, if it is used to treat an infant with mental deficiency and more or the most severe paralysis, the effects will come after a longer time of treatment.

11.19 Myogenic Torticollis

Also called as congenital torticollis or primary torticollis, myogenic torticollis is characterized by slanting of the head of a diseased infant to the affected side with the face turned to the healthy side. Clinically, besides bony torticollis due to deformity of the spine, compensatory and postural torticollis due to visual disturbance caused by strabismus and nervous torticollis due to cervical muscular paralysis usually refer to myogenic torticollis due to spasm of unilateral sternocleidomastoid muscle.

Etiology and Pathogenesis

1. It has something to do with some congenital factors because it is often complicated by certain kinds of congenital deformity such as talipes valgus, talipes varus, dislocation of the hip joint, etc.

2. Someone believes that the head of a fetus happens to be in a wrong position when it is being delivered. This cuts off the blood supply to the middle portion of the sternocleidomastoid muscle and causes spasm of the muscle, leading to this disease in the end.

3. Most scholars think that when a fetus is being delivered, its unilateral sternocleidomastoid muscle is squeezed and pressed by the birth canal or the obstetric forceps. This cuts off the blood—flowing along the vessels within the muscle, which is responsible for the later patchy vascular embolism. The clots force the muscle to be in the shape of fusiform swelling, with cordlike contracture gradually formed and the disease resulted in.

4. A fetus in the womb has had its head set in the wrong position for a long time. This has its unilateral sternocleidomastoid muscle unable to get enough blood supply for a long time, leading to ischemic change of the muscle and causing this disease.

TCM considers the above reasonable.

Clinical Manifestations

After the delivery of the diseased fetus or within 1—2 weeks after that, there appear the following symptoms and signs: slanting of the head to one side, elliptic or cordlike tougher and painless mass occurring on one side of the neck and becoming obvious when the fetus turns its neck to the healthy side, the mass gradually growing contracted, tense, hard and even tougher, slanting of the head to the affected side and the slanting which becomes more and more obvious day by day, turning of the face to the healthy side and the turning which is limited due to pain in the front of the neck, disturbed development of the face, drop of the cheek on the affected side, shallower nasolabial groove, shorter distance between the corner of the mouth and the eye on the affected side, unsymmetrical development of the skull, unsymmetrical development maybe happening on the face if timely treatment is not given, and compensatory lateral prominence of the thoracic vertebrae usually seen in the advanced stage of this disease.

Treatment

Sure curative effects can be attained when *Tuina* is used to treat infantile myogenic torticollis. It produces little sufferings but needs longer course of treatment. In general, the earlier the treatment, the better the effects.

1. Therapeutic method: promoting blood circulation to remove blood stasis, softening the mass to subduing swelling, and correcting deformity.

2. Prescription: The manipulations are undertaken manily to subdue the mass of the sternocleidomastoid muscle at the affected side. The corresponding manipulations are conducted on Fengchi (GB 20) 300 times, on Erhougaogu 300 times, on Tianyou (SJ 16) 300 times, on Tianzhu (BL 10) 500 times, on Futu (LI 18) 500 times, on Jianjing (GB 21) 100 times, on Fengmen (BL 12) 50 times, and on Dazhu (BL 11) 50 times.

3. Operation:

(1) Talcum powder is used as medium.

(2) Get the infant to take the sucking posture in its mother's

arms with the affected side of its neck upward, conduct *Rou* on Fengchi, Tianzhu, Fengmen, Erhougaogu, Tianyou and Futū one after the other, carry out *Na* on the sternocleidomastoid muscle of the affected side along the route from the mastoid process to the clavicle and sternum with your thumb and index finger and do this 3—5 times with the mass and the area around it as the mainly—manipulated parts, and perform *Rou* on the sternocleidomastoid muscle of the affected side with the surface of your thumb for 3—5 minutes. Then, get the infant to take the upright posture in its mother's arms with its back towards you, undertake *Rou* on the processes of the cervical vertebrae with the whorled surface of your thumb for 1 minute, and finally, do straight *Tui* downward from Fengchi over the muscles of the two sides for 2 minutes with either of the two sides manipulated for 1 minute.

(3) Get the scapulae on the two sides of the infant body to be fully exposed, and conduct *An—rou* downward from the interior borders of the two scapulae with your two thumbs for 1minutes.

(4) Support the infant's shoulder of the affected side with one hand and put the other hand on the crown of the infant's head, get the head to slant gradually to the shoulder of the healthy side so as to lengthen the sternocleidomastoid muscle and do this 5—10 times.

4. Treatment course: Treatment is given once daily or every two days and 1 course of treatment consists of 1 month.

Points for Attention

Find out whether or not the torticollis is accompanied by congenital semiluxation of hip joint. If there exists the semiluxation, timely correction is needed.

12 Infant *Tuina* for Health-care

Infant *Tuina* can be done for the purpose of improving the immunologic function of an infant's body, so that its health may be built up so much that it can keep itself off some diseases. The manipulations of infant *Tuina* for health-care are easy to understand, easy to operate and easy to master.

The mother or father who wants to try infant *Tuina* for health-care on her / his infant must be patient and continue her / his performance according to the course of treatment. Any course must be carried on through to the end. In general, 6 days make 1 course of treatment. If the infant has an chronic disease, the mother or father may conduct her / his performance continually for 3-4 courses of treatment. Here are several kinds of infant *Tuina* for health-care.

12.1 Infant *Tuina* for Calming the Mind

An infant tends to be frightened by things that it has never seen and by sounds that it has never heard. Therefore, it tends to get the illness with the following symptoms: fright, crying, movements of the hands and feet and calmlessness. For this reason, to regulate and control the mind of an infant is especially important. Infant *Tuina* for calming the mind can be used to nourish the heart for tranquilizing the mind, replenish *Yin* and enrich blood.

1. Prescription: *Rou* Xinshu (BL 15) 50 times, *Fu-tui* (propping and pushing) the cervical vertebrae 50-100 times, and *Yuanhou Zhai Guo* (doing the manipulation as a monkey is pick-

ing apples) 30 times.

2. Operation:

(1) Talcum powder is used as medium.

(2) Let the mother hold the infant with her left arm to get the back of the infant toward you, or make the infant take the prone position on a bed, conduct gentle and rhythmic patting on its left upper back where Jueyinshu (BL 14) and Xinshu (BL 15) are located with your right cupped fist, and carry out *An—rou* 50 times on Xinshu on the two sides with the surfaces of the thumb and the index finger of either of your hands.

(3) Get the infant to be in the same position as the above and conduct the manipulation with your left hand like this: put the middle finger on Fengfu (DU 16), the index and ring fingers respectively on the two Fengchi (GB 20) at the both sides of the cervical vertebra and carry out *Tui* downward, repeat the above 50—100 times.

(4) Stand face to face with the infant who is got to sit in its mother's arms, hold the two auricular apexes with the index and middle fingers of your hands and do lifting 3—10 times (Fig. 197), hold the two ear lobes with the thumb and the index finger of either of your hands and do down—pulling 3—5 times (Fig. 198), and, then, rotate the head of the infant clockwise and counterclockwise 10—20 times.

3. Points for Attention

The manipulations are carried out once daily and 2—3 times make 1 course of treatment. 1 course may be followed by the other without any interval in between. The better time for performing the manipulations is before the infant's going to sleep or in the afternoon.

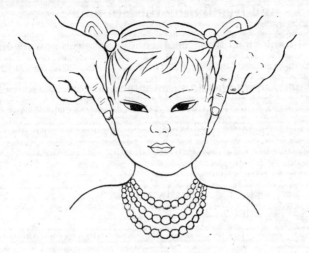

Fig. 197

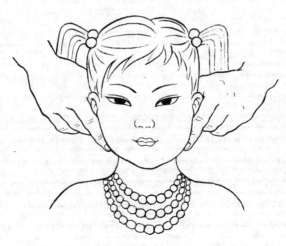

Fig. 198

12.2　Infant *Tuina* for Strengthening the Spleen and Regulating the Stomach

Infant *Tuina* for strengthening the spleen and regulating the stomach can be used to improve appetite, regulate *Qi* and blood and build up the health of an infant, so that its vital-*Qi* can be stored in the interior and the pathogens are kept off.

One or more points may be selected in infant *Tuina* for strengthening the spleen and regulating the stomach.

1. Prescription

(1) Prescription 1: *Mó* the abdomen.

(2) Prescription 2: *Nie Ji*.

(3) Prescription 3: *Bu* Pijing 500 times, *Rou* Zusanli (ST 36) 300 times, *Mó* the abdomen 300 times, and *Nie Ji* 3—5 times.

2. Operation:

(1) Talcum powder is used as medium.

(2) Get the infant to sit in its mother's arms, hold its left hand and conduct *Bu* on Pijing.

(3) Get the infant to lie on the back and carry out *Mó* on its abdomen with the palm of your right hand like this: move your palm from the right lower abdomen up to the right upper abdomen, transversely to the left upper abdomen, down to the left lower abdomen, and gently back to the right lower abdomen, i.e., in the direction of the ascending colon → the transverse colon → the descending colon → the ascending colon. Do the above 150 times and continue to perform *Mó* 150 times in the same way but in the opposite direction. Then, undertake *An—rou* on the two Zusanli with your two thumbs. It is better to conduct "*Mó* the abdomen followed by *An—rou* Zusanli" half an hour after

food—intake.

(4) Get the infant to take the prone position with its back exposed and conduct routine *Nie Ji* 5 times. But during the 4th and 5th times of operation, give a forceful lifting of the skin around the points of Shenshu (BL 23), Weishu (BL 21) and Pishu (BL 20) and, then, perform *An—rou* on the above points with your two thumbs.

3. Points for Attention

(1) The operation is given once daily within 7 days. After 3—day interval, the operation starts again and it is given in the same way as the above.

(2) The operation should not be given as an infant is suffering from an acute infectious disease. But it may be continued after the infant's recovery.

12.3 Infant *Tuina* for Strengthening the spleen to Reinforce the Lung

Infant *Tuina* for strengthening the spleen to reinforce the lung may function in improving the ability of the body to keep out the cold so that the onset of common cold can be prevented.

1. Prescription:

(1) Prescription 1: *Rou* Wailaogong (EX—UE 8) 300 times, *Huangfenrudong* (see it in "operation") 50 times.

(2) Prescription 2: *Bu* Pijing 300 times, *Mó* Xinmen 100 times, *Tui* Badao (see it in "operation") 50 times each, and *Rou* the palms 50 times and the soles 50 times, too.

2. Operation

The mixture of ginger juice and sesame oil is used as medium.

(1) Prescription 1 is suitable for those who are susceptible to common cold and cough. It is put into practice like this. Get the infant to sit in its mother's arms, hold its right hand with your left hand and conduct *Rou* on Wailaogong with the thumb of your right hand. Then, stand in front of the infant, fix its occiput with your left hand, put the index and middle fingers of your right hand respectively at the sides of the wings of its nose, carry out *Rou* up and down, and this is called *Huangfengrudong*. Finally, perform *An* on Jianjing (GB 21) 3—5 times.

(2) Prescription 2 is especially suitable for the infants who tend to be attacked by indigestion and common cold alternately or to have too good appetite before the onset of a disease. It is put into clinical practice in the following way.

A. Get the infant to sit in its mother's arms, fix its left hand with your left hand with its thumb exposed, and conduct the manipulation *Bu* Pijing. Then, carry out *Rou* on its palm and sole or soles with the middle finger of your right hand.

B. Spread the mixture of ginger juice and sesame oil over your palm and with it conduct gentle *Rou* on Xinmen (the fontanel of the infant). Be sure not to give forceful pressure to the fontanel.

C. Stand at one side of the infant who is got to lie on the back and undertake *Fen* with your two thumbs from the sternocostal joints of the infant between the 1st and 2nd ribs, between the 2nd and the 3rd ribs, between the 3rd and the 4th ribs and between the 4th and the 5th ribs, and this is called *Tui* Badao. Then, carry out *Rou* on Danzhong (RN 17) with your middle finger 50—100 times.

D. Get the infant to be held in its mother's arms with its

back towards you and conduct gentle patting on the portion where Feishu (BL 13) is located.

3. Points for Attention

The manipulations are carried out once daily, usually in the early morning. 7 times of performance make 1 course. Between every two courses, there are 3 days of interval.

12.4 Infant *Tuina* for Improving Intelligence and Building up Health

Infant *Tuina* for improving intelligence and building up health has the effect of developing the intelligence of an infant, building up its bodily and mental health and making it in the state of happiness.

1. Prescription

Tui Wujing (see it in "operation") 100 times, *Nie Shiwang* (see it in "operation") 20 times each, *Yao* (rotating) each of the joints of the limbs 20–30 times, *Nian* (twisting) each of the ten fingers and the ten toes 3–5 times and *Nie Ji* 3–5 times.

2. Operation

(1) Talcum powder is used as medium.

(2) Get the infant to sit or lie on the back, prop its left hand with the palm upwards with your left hand, conduct *Tui* again and again from the palm root of the infant's left hand towards the finger-tips with the closed five fingers of your right hand, and this is called *Tui Wujing*.

(3) Get the infant to be in the same position as the above, conduct *Nie* on the thumb, the index, middle, ring and small fingers of the right hand of the infant, and this is called *Nie Shiwang*. Then, carry out *Yao* (rotating) on each of the wrist joints, the el-

bow joints, the knees and the ankle joints. Finally, Twist the ten fingers and the ten toes with the surfaces of the thumb and the index finger of one of your hands.

(4) Get the infant to take prone position on its mother's thighs, perform *Nie Ji* with your thumbs and index fingers, give 3—5 times of forceful lifting of the skin around each of the points Shenshu (BL 21), Pishu (BL 20) and Xinshu (BL 15), and conduct *An—rou* on each of the above 3 points 3 times. Then, put the middle finger on The Du Channel with the index and ring fingers respectively on Fengmen (BL 12), carry out *Tui* from the above to the below and do this 10 times.

3. Points for Attention

Infant *Tuina* for improving intelligence and building up health is suitable for the infants below 3 years old. It may be conducted once daily. 1 course of treatment involves 7 times of operation. Between every two courses, there is an interval of 1 week.

7

推拿治疗学

序

《英汉实用中医药大全》即将问世，吾为之高兴。

歧黄之道，历经沧桑，永盛不衰。吾中华民族之强盛，由之。世界医学之丰富和发展，亦由之。然而，世界民族之差异，国别之不同，语言之障碍，使中医中药的传播和交流受到了严重束缚。当前，世界各国人民学习、研究、运用中医药的热潮方兴未艾。为使吾中华民族优秀文化遗产之一的歧黄之道走向世界，光大其业，为世界人民造福，徐象才君集省内外精英于一堂，主持编译了《英汉实用中医药大全》。是书之问世将使海内外同道欢呼雀跃。

世界医学发展之日，当是歧黄之道光大之时。

吾欣然序之。

中华人民共和国卫生部副部长
兼国家中医药管理局局长
世界针灸学会联合会主席
中国科学技术协会委员
中华全国中医学会副会长
中国针灸学会会长

胡熙明

1989 年 12 月

序

中华民族有同疾病长期作斗争的光辉历程，故而有自己的传统医学——中国医药学。中国医药学有一套完整的从理论到实践的独特科学体系。几千年来，它不但被完好地保存下来，而且得到了发扬光大。它具有疗效显著、副作用小等优点，是人们防病治病，强身健体的有效工具。

任何一个国家在医学进步中所取得的成就，都是人类共同的财富，是没有国界的。医学成果的交流比任何其他科学成果的交流都应进行得更及时，更准确。我从事中医工作 30 多年来，一直盼望着有朝一日中国医药学能全面走向世界，为全人类解除病痛疾苦做出其应有的贡献。但由于用外语表达中医难度较大，中国医药学对外传播的速度一直不能令人满意。

山东中医学院的徐象才老师发起并主持了大型系列丛书《英汉实用中医药大全》的编译工作。这个工作是一项巨大工程，是一种大型科研活动，是一个大胆的尝试，是一件新事物。对徐象才老师及与其合作的全体编译者夜以继日地长期工作所付出的艰苦劳动，克服重重困难所表现出的坚韧不拔的毅力，以及因此而取得的重大成绩，我甚为敬佩。作为一个中医界的领导者，对他们的工作给予全力支持是我应尽的责任。

我相信《英汉实用中医药大全》无疑会在中国医学史和世界科学技术史上找到它应有的位置。

中华全国中医学会常务理事
山东省卫生厅副厅长

张奇文

1990 年 3 月

出 版 前 言

中国医药学是我中华民族优秀文化遗产之一，建国以来由于党和国家对待中医药采取了正确的政策，使中医药理论宝库不断得到了发掘整理，取得了巨大的成绩。当前，世界各国人民对中国医药学的学习和研究热潮日益高涨，为促进这一热潮更加蓬勃的发展，为使中国医药学能更好地为全人类解除病痛服务，就必须促进中医中药在世界范围内的传播和交流，而要使这一传播和交流进行得更及时、更准确，就必须首先排除语言障碍。因此，编译一套英汉对照的中医药基本知识的书籍，供国内外学习、研究中医药时使用，已成为国内外医药学界和医药学教育界许多人士的迫切需要。

多年来，在卫生部门的号召下，在"中医英语表达研究"方面，已经作出了一些可喜的成绩。本书《英汉实用中医药大全》的编辑出版就是在调查上述研究工作的历史和现状的基础上，继续对中医药英语表达作较系统、较全面的研究，以适应中国医药学对外传播交流的需要。

这部"大全"的版本为英汉对照，共有 21 个分册，一个分册介绍论述中国医药学的一个分科。在编著上注意了中医药汉文稿的编写特色，在内容上注意了科学性、实用性、全面性和简明易读。汉文稿的执笔撰写者主要是有 20 年以上实践经验的教授、副教授、主任医师和副主任医师。各分册汉文稿撰写成后，均经各学科专家逐一审订。各分册英文主译、主审主要是国内既懂中医又懂英语的权威人士，还有许多中医院校的英语教师及医药卫生部门的专业翻译人员。英译稿脱稿后，经过了复审、终审，有些译稿还召开全国 22 所院校和单位人员参加的英译稿统稿定稿研讨会，对英译稿进行细致的研讨和推敲，对如何较全面、较系统、较准确地用英语表达中国医药学进行了探讨，从而推动整个译文达到较高水平，因此，这部"大全"可供中医院校高年级学生作为泛读教材使用。

这部"大全"的编纂得到了国家教育委员会、国家中医药管理局、山东省教育委员会、山东省卫生厅等各部门有关领导的支持。在国家教委高等教育司的指导下，成立了《英汉实用中医药大全》编译领导委员会。还得到了全国许多中医院校和中药生产厂家领导的支持。

希望这部"大全"的出版，对中医院校加强中医英语教学，对国内卫生界培养外向型中医药人才，以及在推动世界各国人民对中医药的学习和研究方面，都将产生良好的影响。

高等教育出版社

1990 年 3 月

前　言

　　《英汉实用中医药大全》是一部以中医基本理论为基础，以中医临床为重点，较为全面系统、简明扼要、易读实用的中级英汉学术性著作。它的主要读者是：中医药院校高年级学生和中青年教师，中医院的中青年医生和中医药科研单位的科研人员，从事中医对外函授工作的人员和出国讲学或行医的中医人员，西学中人员，来华学习中医的外国留学生和各类进修人员。

　　由于中国医药学为我中华民族之独有，因此，英译便成了本《大全》编译工作的重点。为确保译文能准确表达中医的确切含义，我们邀集熟悉中医的英语人员、医学专业翻译人员、懂英语的中医药人员乃至医古文人员于一堂，共同翻译、共同对译文进行研讨推敲的集体翻译法，这样，就把众人之长融进了译文质量之中。然而，即使这样，也难确保译文都能尽如人意。汉文稿虽反映了中国医药学的精髓和概貌，但也难能十全十美。我衷心地盼望读者能提出批评和建议，以便《大全》再版时修改。

　　参加本《大全》编、译、审工作的人员达 200 余名，他们来自全国 28 个单位，其中有山东、北京、上海、天津、南京、浙江、安徽、河南、湖北、广西、贵阳、甘肃、成都、山西、长春等 15 所中医学院，还有中国中医研究院，山东省中医药研究所等中医药科研单位。

　　山东省教育委员会把本《大全》的编译列入了科研计划并拨发了科研经费，山东省卫生厅和一些中药生产厂家也给了很大支持，济南中药厂的资助为编译工作的开端提供了条件。

　　本《大全》的编译成功是全体编译审者集体劳动的结晶，是各有关单位主管领导支持的结果。在《大全》各分册即将陆续出版之际，我诚挚地感谢全体编译审者的真诚合作，感谢许多专家、教授、各级领导和生产厂家的热情支持。

愿本《大全》的出版能在培养通晓英语的中医人才和使中医早日全面走向世界方面起到我所期望的作用。

主编　徐象才

于山东中医学院

1990 年 3 月

目　录

概　述

上篇　成　人　推　拿　·

下篇 小 儿 推 拿

说　　明

　　本书为《英汉实用中医药大全》的第 7 分册。

　　本分册主要由"成人推拿"和"小儿推拿"两部分组成。成人推拿部分包括"成人推拿简介"、"成人推拿常用手法"、"手法的练习方法与步骤"、"十四经及常用腧穴"、"练功"、"成人常见病症治疗"以及"成人保健推拿"等 7 章。小儿推拿部分包括"小儿推拿简介"、"小儿推拿手法"、"小儿推拿常用穴位"、"小儿常见病症治疗"以及"小儿保健推拿"第 5 章。其中，重点介绍的是 41 种成人常见病和 19 种小儿常见病的推拿疗法。全书共附插图 198 幅(283 个)，以方便读者阅读现解。

　　本分册的英文稿较为简明、准确、易读、易懂。其中，推拿手法、穴位及个别中医术语名称均用首字母大写的汉语拼音词表示；除穴位名称外，其他两种汉语拼音词均用斜体。

　　上海中医学院的郑凤胡教授审查了中文稿。山东中医学院的张赭、郭静、孔健、闫景波、张大勇、费丽萍、王欣、王磊、马君、孙世萍帮助做了部分翻译工作。

　　本书全部插图均由刘星池先生所绘。

主编

概　　述

　　中国的推拿是在中医理论的指导下，运用手法技巧刺激穴位或体表其他部位，以纠正人体的生理失衡而进行治疗的一种医学学科。是我国传统医学的重要组成部分。我国古代把治疗方法分为外治和内治两大类，推拿属於外治范围。

　　推拿的适应证极为广泛。它不仅能治疗各种软组织损伤，而且对内科、外科、妇科、神经科、五官科、儿科等多种疾病均有疗效，特别对小儿、老人尤为适宜。目前我国推拿医学已有成人推拿、小儿推拿、骨伤科推拿、美容推拿、保健推拿、康复推拿、运动医学推拿等分支。

　　具体来说，在成人推拿方面，颈椎病、腰肌劳损、腰椎间盘突出症、急性腰肌扭伤、类风湿性关节炎、胃脘痛、胃下垂、便秘、高血压、中风后遗症等都是传统适应症。其对糖尿病的治疗早已有报道。过敏性结肠炎和十二指肠球部溃汤经治疗可以很快痊愈。对慢性冠状动脉供血不足、心绞痛的推拿治疗也已取得明显的进展。著者从 1982 年以来开展对上述病症的研究和治疗，经治疗后的患者心电图、心功能、自觉症状等均有明显改善。小儿推拿对治疗婴幼儿腹泻、呕吐、腹痛、肠梗阻等消化系统疾病有十分满意的效果；对维生素 D 缺乏性佝偻病，营养不良、厌食、麻疹、百日咳、细菌性痢疾、上呼吸道感染、支气管哮喘、贫血和发烧等都有显效，对提高小儿的免疫能力方面有显著的作用，一些免疫功能低下而常患感冒的幼儿，经推拿治疗可长期不患感冒。

　　推拿能对人体的机能起双向调节的作用。如在肠蠕动亢进者的腹部和背部或上肢的相应穴位上进行推拿，可使亢进的机能受到抑制而恢复正常。而对肠蠕动功能减退者，推拿则可促使其肠蠕动恢复正常。人体得病常常由于细菌、病毒、原虫或物理、化学的因素导致生理机能的失常。用药物可抑制细菌、病毒的生长或杀灭之，但生理机能的失常有时并不因之而自然消失，因而有些疾病用药物常久治不愈。在这种情况下用推拿治疗，常常收到手到病除的功效。从中国传统医学的理论看，推拿治病，是通过对遍布全身的经络、穴位的作用，使内脏的功能得到调整。也就是说推拿可以疏通经络，活动血脉，调节阴阳，使人体功能正常。

近代的研究证实，推拿可以使血液和淋巴系统的微循环改善。这种改善不仅使各种软组织损伤、扭挫伤得以较快的恢复，而且由于控制内脏的微循环的神经系统开窍于皮肤，因而对体表一定穴位的推拿治疗又可以调节内脏的微循环。因此，推拿能够调节内脏的功能。推拿能调节中枢神经系统，因此可以治疗高血压和神经衰弱，可以调节体温使发烧的儿童退烧，可以进行推拿麻醉。

长期吞食大量的化学药品，在一些人身上会产生抗药性；有些药物的副作用还会给人们带来严重的后遗症。推拿疗法则是通过调节人体的机能来抵抗各种疾病的，不但没有副作用，而且能提高人体的免疫能力。此外它不给人们带来如同针刺那样的紧张心理，它基本上不消耗社会的物质财富，所以是一种廉价、高效，有益而无害的理想医疗方法。

当前在推拿领域需要做的工作很多；例如，首先要用现代医学理论对推拿治病的原理做更深入的研究；其次应该在临床上通过对更多的病症的治疗来扩大推拿的应用范围；第三应该把推拿向更多的国家作介绍，使这种非常理想的医疗方法为世界各国人民的健康事业作贡献。最后我们应该创造更多的推拿医疗和实验仪器，用于推拿的医疗科学研究和教育事业。

推拿不仅可以用于治病，而且可用于保健强身，消灭疾病于初起之时。汉代张仲景《金匮要略》中提出的："四肢才觉重滞，即导引、吐纳、针灸、膏摩，勿令九窍闭塞"。自我推拿作为一种防病保健手段在当时就被广泛应用。古人应用自我推拿使气血疏通，强筋健骨，除劳去烦而达到祛病延年的目的。祖国医学防治学中的精华之一就是不治已病治未病。现代老年医学和运动医学的研究结果表明，由于老年人的心理状态和病情的需要，保健推拿急待加强研究和发展，尽快总结出更符合老年人需要的保健推拿法。

1 中医推拿发展史略

推拿这种以"手"为治病工具的医疗方法，可以说是人类最早的医学形式之一，这在世界各古老民族的医学发展史中都可以得到佐证。因为，人们以手摩擦，按揉或捶打自己或同伴的肢体，以御寒取暖及解除疲劳，食胀与各种伤痛所造成的不适感等这类行为，是与人类生来就有的自卫防御本能有关，因此可以推想，生活在洪荒时期的人类祖先，在那个没有任何医疗工具，还未掌握应用药物治病方法的年代，所能采用只能是这种自摩自捏或相互捶打踩踏的自发的医疗方法了。这就是推拿的起源。而智慧的人类，把在实践中获得的经验，经过长期的积累、总结与创新，就逐渐形成了在现代被称之为"自然疗法"的推拿医学。

在中国，推拿的历史可以追溯到上古的黄帝时代，那时的推拿称案杌。到了两千多年前的春秋战国时期，当时被称为按摩的推拿疗法，已基本成为一种比较成熟的医疗手段而被广泛使用，如当时杰出的医学家扁鹊，在治疗虢太子的"尸厥症"时，就曾采用按摩等综合疗法，获得了起死回生的奇效。

至秦、汉、三国时期，由于在早期医疗实践中获得的经验与创造的方法逐步得到了充实、总结，因而诞生了我国——也是世界医学史上的第一部按摩专著《黄帝歧伯按摩经十卷》。可惜此书已佚失，今天我们已经无法从中了解按摩术在当时的发展全貌，但是，庆幸的是从与该书同时代成书的我国现存最早的医学巨著《黄帝内经》中，还是可以看到许多论述按摩的篇章。综观此书，所涉及的内容，在按摩医学的起源，手法，临床应用，适用范围，治病原理以及医学教学等各个方面，已无所不备。该书中提到的常用手法已有推、按、摩、跻、掣等十几种。适应症有惊恐，痿厥，寒热，脾风，经络不通，寒腹痛等，遍及各科的急、慢性病症。特别是在手法治病原理方面的见地已相当精辟，有的直至今日还在推拿临床与教学中起着指导作用。另外，在当时许多非医学的名著中，如《孟子》、《老子》、《荀子》、《墨子》，都可以看到有关按摩疗法在民间实用的记录。嗣后，医圣张仲景在《金匮要略》中，首先总结并提出了"膏摩"法，这是一种先将制成的中药膏剂涂沫在患者体表的经穴上，然后再用手法按摩治疗的方法。由于此法有手法与药物的协同作用，所以，不但提高了疗效，而且扩大了按摩疗法的适应范围。三国时期的名医华佗也用此法治疗伤寒与驱除肌肤的浮淫。从上述史料可以看出，此时的按摩术，不但已是一种常用的医疗手段而被普遍应用，而且受到许多当代著名医学家的重视与研究，以致专业技能与理论不断丰富与提高。这标志着此时的按摩术已从早期自发的医疗形式中脱胎而出，并奠定了它在中医临床医学体系中的学术地位。

至两晋南北朝，膏摩术有了进一步的发展。如王叔和在《脉经》里，提出用"风膏"治疗痹痛的方法；特别是葛洪在所著的《肘后备急方》中，首次系统总结了膏摩的方、药、证、法及摩膏的制作方法。书中介绍了8首膏摩方，适应症遍及内、外、妇、五官等各科常见病症。陶弘景也在《养性延命录》中著有占全书相当的篇幅、内容十分丰富的《导引按摩》专卷，介绍了许多成套的导引按摩动作，如啄齿，熨眼，按目，引耳，发举，摩面等等，为后世以养生，保健，疾病自疗为目的的自我推拿医疗体系开了先河。

隋唐时期推拿有很大的发展与提高。此时，在国家设立的"太医署"内，正式设置按摩科，按摩医生按等级分为按摩博士、按摩师、按摩工。博士在师与工的辅助下，负责日常的医疗工作和对按摩生进行有组织的按摩教学工作。此时，自我按摩与膏摩疗法得到了更加广泛的应用与提高，如在隋代巢元方的《诸病源候论》的每卷之末，都有按摩之法。唐代孙思邈的《千金方》更是发展了膏摩的方药并扩大了应用范围。本书特别对膏摩治疗小儿疾病有了系统的论述，如运用膏摩法治疗"中客忤，强项欲死"、"鼻塞不通有涕出"、"夜啼"、"腹胀满"、"不能乳食"等十多种小儿疾病。另外，在该书中还有"小儿虽无病，早起常以膏摩囟上及手足心，甚辟寒风。"的记载。此书是首次记载将膏摩法用于小儿保健的医学文献。由此可见，小儿推拿在唐朝时，就被广泛采用。孙氏还介绍了《老子按摩法》等按摩和导引的方法，其中，单是手法就有按、摩、擦、捻、抱、推、振、打、掖、捺等数十种之多。这个时期的医学名著《唐六典》说：按摩可治八疾：风、寒、暑、湿、饥、饱、劳、逸，足见按摩治病的适应范围已大大拓宽。《外合秘要》的主要贡献是：它不但大量介绍了按摩治病的经验，还辑录了大量的膏摩方剂，并一一注明了其出处。上述史料证明，在隋唐时期，按摩作为一个临床学科，在基础理论，诊断技术与治疗体系等方面，都已发展到了相当高的水平。

在这一时期，由于政治、经济、文化、交通等均有较大发展，对外文化交流出现了欣欣向荣的局面，推拿也随之传到了朝鲜、日本、印度等国家。

宋金元时期，政府的医疗机构虽不设按摩科，但北宋的"太医局"却设有"疡科"，元朝的"太医院"设"正骨兼金镞科"，有关按摩的医疗工作也都由该科承担，可以看出此时的按摩疗法主要应用在骨伤科疾病的治疗，这为后来逐渐形成正骨推拿医疗体系打下了基础。宋代医生还将按摩用于催产。此时的医学家不仅对按摩治病的效果、方法与适应范围有了更全面的认识；而且在如何辩证选用手法以及手法的作用原理等基础理论的研究方面也有了突破性的收获。如《圣济总录》说："可按可摩，时兼而用，通谓之按摩。按之弗摩，摩之弗按。按止以手，摩或兼以药。曰按曰摩，适所用也。……大抵按摩法，每以开达抑遏为义。开达则壅闭者以之发散，抑遏则剽悍者有所归宿。"这是对推拿理论发展的一大贡献。

明代是推拿发展的第二个兴旺发达的时期。在当时政府的医疗机构《太医院》中医十三科中，又有了"按摩科"。由于按摩在整体水平上的不断提高，尤其在治疗小儿疾病方面，已经积累了丰富的经验，至1601年，我国第一部小儿推拿专著《小儿按摩经》问世。不久《小儿推拿方脉活婴秘旨全书》、《小儿推拿秘诀》相继刊行。小儿推拿作为按摩的一个学术分支脱颖而出，在辩证、手法、穴位等方面形成了其独特的体系。另外，"推拿"这个我们在今天正式采用的学科名称，就是在这个时期首先提出来的。学科名称的沿革，标志着学科整体水平的提高，这在推拿发展史上具有深远的意义。

至清代，推拿虽未被官方重视，但在民间的应用与流传仍相当广泛。尤其在清朝的初、中叶，在小儿推拿方面还是有明显进展的，出现了一批著名的小儿推拿医生和对后世影响较大的专著如《小儿推拿广义》、《幼科推拿秘书》、《保赤推拿》、《厘正按摩要术》等。另外，在此时，推拿在治疗伤科疾病方面的成就也令人注目，如《医宗金鉴》一书，把摸、接、端、提、推、拿、按、摩列为伤科八法，可以说伤科推拿的医疗流派在此时已基本形成。

中华人民共和国成立之前的一个时期中，推拿没有得到足够的重视。但是由于推拿治病的独特疗效，故其应用仍非常普遍。许多民间的推拿医生对推拿潜心研究，努力继承，并在实践中不断有所创新，使得一指禅、擦法、内功推拿、点穴推拿、小儿推拿等各种学术流派保留了下来，对推拿医学的发展起到了承前启后的作用。

中华人民共和国成立以后，政府大力推行中医。因而，推拿学也受到了重视。1956年在上海开办了第一届推拿训练班，1958年成立了上海推拿门诊部与推拿专科学校。同时，全国很多医院陆续成立了推拿临床科室，吸收各地的民间推拿医生担任治疗工作。至 60 年代，在我国初步建立了一支推拿专业队伍。自 1974 年起，上海中医学院首先在针灸推拿骨伤系中设立了推拿专业。此后，北京、南京、福建、安徽等地的中医学院也相继成立了推拿专业，为培养高层次的推拿专业人才创造了条件。1987 年全国推拿学会成立。从此，国内外的学术交流活动得到了蓬勃的开展。近年来，推拿的专著与学术论文，无论在数量上还是质量上，都达到了历史的最高水平。推拿医学的基础与临床科研工作也得到了相应的开展。推拿治疗颈椎病、腰椎间盘突出症、小儿腹泻、冠心病、胆囊炎的成果已达到了世界先进水平。山东、上海等地也相继从运动生物力学的角度开展了推拿手法力学信息的研究，取得了一批有价值的研究成果。

目前，推拿医学在我国的发展正方兴未艾，在医疗、康复、预防、保健等各个医学领域中都有她的用武之地。随着国际科学文化交流的广泛开展，推拿疗法的安全、有效、对人体无害、无副作用等优越性，日益被世界人民所了解与接受。展望未来，我们相信古老而又年轻的中国推拿，将会以全新的面貌走向世界，为世界人民作出更大的贡献。

2　中医推拿流派概述

中医推拿，在其漫长的发展过程中，由于渊源，师承，主治对象以及政治、经济、社会、文化、地域、人情等复杂的原因与背景，形成了丰富多彩的流派与学术体系。如一指禅推拿、滚法推拿、内功推拿、整骨推拿、外伤按摩疗法、按摩疗法、小儿推拿、点穴推拿、脏腑经络推拿、保健推拿、养生按摩、胃病推拿、捏筋拍打疗法、指压推拿、指针疗法、指拨疗法、捏脊疗法、自我推拿、膏摩疗法、动功按摩、运动推拿、美容按摩、推拿麻醉、子午流注推拿、窍穴奇术推拿、经外奇穴推拿等等。综观各种推拿流派，大致有以下 3 个共同的特点：1. 有较长的发展历史，并在一定的地域范围内形成、流传、盛行；2. 有一定的理论指导，有丰富的医疗实践经验和擅长的主治范围，并有独特的练功与专业训练的方法；3. 各有一种主治手法或称流派手法。这些特点都往往带有明显的地域、人情色彩。

例如：一指禅指拿、自清代咸丰年间以来，一直流传于江南，特别在江苏、浙江、上海一带盛行。它以阴阳，五行，脏腑经络，营卫气血等中医基本理论为指导，以四诊八纲为诊察手段，强调审证求因、辩证论治；在手法方面，以一指禅推法为主治手法，以拿、按、摩、   、捻、抄、搓、缠、揉、摇、抖为辅助手法，手法运用要求柔和、深透、柔中寓刚，刚中带柔，刚柔相济，但特别强调手法要以柔和为贵。由于主治手法及几种主要辅助手法的技术难度较大，故其非常重视基本功的训练，并有一整套科学的专业技能训练方法，要求学员先练外壮功"易筋经"，并在米袋上进行手法基本动作的练习。一指禅推拿在治疗操作时，主要选用十四经络，十四经穴，经外奇穴及阿是穴，强调

"推穴道，走经络"。适应症比较广泛，无论是内因、外因所引起的经络、形体或内脏疾病，一般均可治疗，尤其擅长于治疗诸如头痛、失眠、劳倦内伤、胃脘痛、久泄、便秘、胸痹、痛经、月经不调等内、妇科杂病。

再如，在中国北方青岛、崂山、及胶东一带盛行的"点穴疗法"，是从我国传统武术中总穴、打穴、拿穴、踢穴等动作演化而来的推拿疗法。在武术中点穴既是一种击技的进攻手段，又是一种治疗损伤的方法。点穴疗法总结了它后一种功能的运用经验，将使人致伤，致命的超强度点击变化为人体生理所能接受的安全强度的点击，并在中医经络学说等理论的指导下，用于治疗疾病。其主治手法为点（击）法，主要辅助手法有：拍打法、叩打法、按压法、掐法、扣压法、抓拿法、捶打法、矫形法等。整个手法以各种点、打、推、捶等动作为基本形式。治疗风格峻猛刚健，速捷强劲。轻点在 10 公斤左右，重点可达 60~70 公斤。由于施术时，要求术者要有较强的指力，臂力与全身的支持力，故初学者要进行基本训练。首先进行是"点穴练功"，其主要功法有：蹲起功、运气拍打功、对拉功、仰卧功、撞背功、蜈蚣跳、鹰爪力、捶纸功、推山功及扎腰功等。临床治疗主要以各种瘫痪、麻痹、及风湿顽痹等为主。其治病理论为：当人体发生痿、痹等病证时，则邪正相搏，阴阳失调，经络之气亦随之逆乱，营卫气血的运行被阻，故在治疗时，要运用较强的点打各法"以其穴之前导之；或在对位之穴启之，使所闭之穴感受震激，渐渐开放，则所阻滞之气血，亦得缓缓通过其穴，以复其流行矣"，"经脉既舒，其病自除"。

从以上介绍的两种推拿流派的概况，可以看到，每种推拿流派，都以它们各自的历史渊源，医学理论，主治手法，训练方法以及医疗风格与适应范围而自成体系，构成了当代中医推拿的绚丽多姿与丰富内容。本书由于篇幅所限，不能将每种推拿流派的内容一一详解，只是综合了一指禅推拿，擦法推拿，内功推拿、点穴推拿、小儿推拿及保健推拿等部分流派的学术内容，分上、下 2 篇向读者作一概要介绍，希望能窥一斑而知全豹，引起大家学习中医推拿的兴趣，以使其为世界人民的健康事业作出更大贡献。

3 怎样学习中医推拿

中医推拿是一门理论性与实践性都比较强的中医临床学科。推拿专科医生不但要通晓中、西医学基础知识，掌握专业理论及临床诊病与辨证论治的本领，而且，还要具备推拿临床工作所需要的身体素质与熟练的手法操作技能。所以，在中国，中医院校推拿专业的学生，除学习一般中医本科学生必读的各门中、西医学基础与临床医学课程外，还需进行严格的身体素质锻炼与手法操作技能的基本训练。

在学习基础与临床医学课程时，除了学好中医的阴阳，五行，营卫，气血，经络，脏腑，病因，诊法，辨证论治等内容和西医的解剖，生理，病理，物理诊断等知识外，尤其要熟知十四经络的循行路线及与内脏的属络关系，常用十四经穴与经外奇穴的位置、取穴方法、性能与主治以及人体结构与运动生理学等。这都是指导推拿临床实践，实用价值较高的基本知识。

在专业技能训练方面，学员首先要根据本书"练功"一节所介绍的常用功法及其练功方法与步骤，认真练功，以全面提高自身的健康状况并获得推拿专业所要求具备的身体素质。同时，还要认真学习"常用手法"一节所介绍的各种手法的基本动作结构与技术要领，严格遵循所规定的训练方法与步骤，循序渐进，持之以恒地刻苦练习手法操作技能，保质保量地按步完成米袋练习，人体练习与常见病操作练习等 3 个基本阶段的训练任务。

总之，学习中医推拿，只要按照上述内容与方法，认真学习与刻苦训练，是一定能学会的。尤其是对具有一定医学基础知识的人来说，是不难在短期内入门的。但是，如果想要达到专科医师的水平，特别是要熟练掌握如一指禅推法、擦法等动作技术难度较高的手法，并能得心应手，运用自如，则不经过较长时间的专业训练，不积累一定的"功夫"，是不行的。

4　中医推拿作用原理简介

推拿为什么能治病?这是一个十分复杂的问题，有许多难题，诸如经络实质，手法运动生物力学特征，人体对手法刺激的接受，传递，转换，利用及产生效应的生物理化过程等等，还都处在研究阶段，要完全解开这些"谜"还需待时日。但是，从传统中医学的观点来看，推拿的作用原理主要是手法作用于人体经穴系统而起的效应。所以，推拿治病不外乎手法作用与经络作用两个方面。

经络遍布于全身，内属脏腑，外络于肢节，沟通和联结人体内外所有脏腑器官、孔窍、皮毛、筋肉与骨骼等组织；再通过气血在经络中运行，供应营养，传递信息与内外联络，形成了一个立体的整体性调节与控制系统。推拿时，术者精神集中，气息调匀，将一身之"气、力"调运到术手。术手紧贴在施术部位的着力点，并以一定的规范化动作结构在人体体表的经穴上进行操作。于是，由此而产生的具有特定"动力型式"（包括手法作用力的大小、频率、变化周期、节律与方向）的刺激信息就激发了经络与相应穴位的特异功能。这种功能以波动的形式沿着穴位→经络外行线→内行线→内脏的方向逐级地传递到人体内不同的组织层次，使人体整个经络、内脏系统进入了能发挥最大的自身调节与控制功能的激发状态，从而起到平衡阴阳，补虚泻实，调和营卫，通经活络，行气活血，调治脏腑，消炎止痛，滑利关节等治疗作用。

另外，推拿对人体局部软组织有理筋整复的作用。例如，当外伤所致肌腱滑脱，移位，关节半脱位，腰椎间盘髓核脱出、间隙变窄及腰椎后关节紊乱或滑膜嵌顿时，则可根据不同情况，运用旨在扶正理顺或弹筋拨络的摇，扳或拔伸牵引等手法，使上述各种因外伤所致的解剖学结构异常的情况得以纠正，从而使软组织与关节功能康复。

5 推拿手法现代研究简介

　　为了弄清手法动态力信息的真实面貌，手法动作结构与其所产生的动力型式之间内在的因果关系，和揭示推拿手法的动作原理与作用机制。我们于 1981 年研制了"TDL-1 型推拿手法动态测定器"（图 1），并用它与相应二次仪表组成"推拿手法力学信息测录系统"（图 2）。1984 年，又研制成"推拿力学信息计算机处理系统"（图 3）。几年来，我们应用上述仪器，先后对一指禅推拿、㨰法推拿、内功推拿、点穴推拿等中国当代部分著名推拿流派学术带头人的手法，进行了系统的运动生物力学研究，记录了大量的手法三维力学波形曲线图（图 4、5、6、7、8），并结合手法动作结构对图形进行了运动学与动力学分析及必要的数据处理，从而使这些以往只能"心授"不可"言传"的手法经验与技术诀窍，有了客观的定量指标与用科学语言表达的可能。并使我们能透过宏观的手法动作外观，窥探到微观的手法技能的奥秘。因为，手法三维力学波形曲线图，不但可向我们提供每种被测手法作用"力"的大小、周期、频率等力学数据，以及"柔和、深透"等表示手法性状与作用力方向的客观指标；而且可通过对每个具体手法图的分析，来揭示其动作技巧的秘诀。例如，在图 6 的垂向曲线上，可以看到在一个㨰法周期的波形中，除了有一个明显的外摆波外，紧接其后的还有一个在力值上约为其 2／3 的内摆波。这说明，在一个㨰法动作周期中，不但在向外摆动时要加力，而且在向内摆动时也有一个力的作用，这样一个周期的㨰法动作，对人体可造成一大、一小 2 次较强的力刺激，因此，较其它手法而言，㨰法的治疗刺激量较大，力学信息丰富，这可能就是㨰法推拿在治疗痹、痿、瘫、麻等病症方面，具有一定优势的

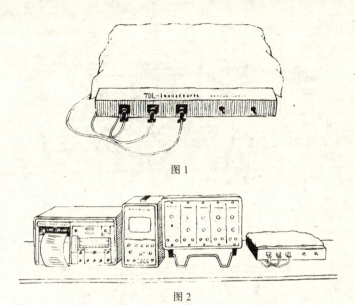

图 1

图 2

原因。再如，内功推拿的主治手法——平推法，从动作外形看，主要是以手掌在施术部位用力作来回的推擦，所以，初学者往往在操作时，只注意在水平方向上用力动作。但是，从图7所提供的平推法三维动态力曲线图来看，其垂、纵、横三向力的比值约为1：0.3：0，从而为我们揭示了平推法的技术诀窍在于：手的掌力主要是指向施术部位的垂直方向，从而达到"施术在外，力透其内"的效果。

　　总之，此项研究在继承、整理当代名医手法经验，提供手法刺激量与临床疗效的关系，发展充实传统推拿学内容，改革传统推拿手法教学方法，深入研究手法的动作原理及作用机制等方面，均具有广泛的实用价值与重要的学术意义。

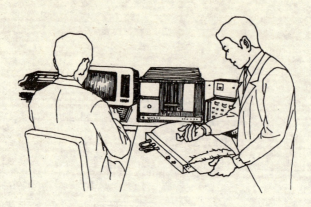

图 3

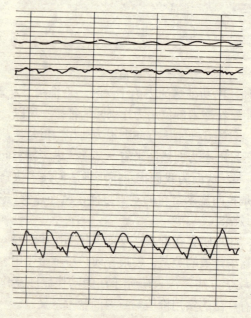

图 4

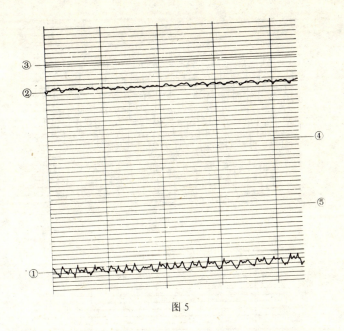

图 5

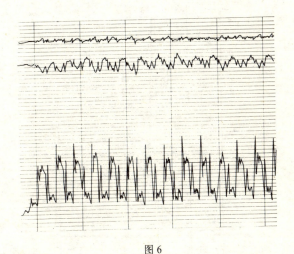

图 6

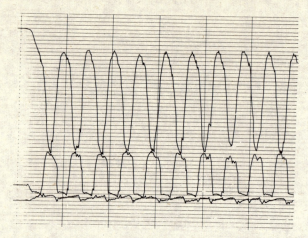

图 7

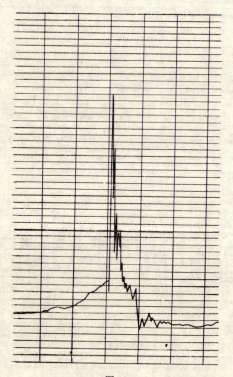

图 8

上篇 成人推拿

1 成人推拿简介

在古代，推拿并无成人与小儿之分。但是自明代以来，由于推拿在治疗小儿疾病方面的发展，在手法、刺激量、用穴、治法乃至适应症等方面，逐步形成了一套主要适合于小儿生理、病理特点的小儿推拿疗法。为了有别于小儿推拿今人提出了"成人推拿"这一名称。现将成人推拿临床须知分别说明如下：

1.1 手法与用穴特点

成人推拿的手法，无论何种流派，其常规操作与小儿推拿的相比，共同的特点是：着力面积与动作幅度较大，刺激量较重，比较适合于在成年人体表的十四经循行线、穴位及躯干、四肢特定部位上操作使用。小儿推拿的一些主要手法，如旋推法、指推法、运法等，多适宜于在手指及手掌部位的小儿特定穴位上操作，且刺激量也小，故成人推拿时一般不采用。但是，成人推拿的手法及其以用体穴为主的治疗方法，只要对手法的刺激量进行适当的调整与控制，同样可以用来治疗小儿的内外科疾病。

成人推拿的治疗形式，主要是运用手法在患者体表"推穴道，走经络"其临床用穴，主要是选择分布在人体躯干与四肢的十四经外行线的十四经穴、经外奇穴及阿是穴等。在临诊时，医生根据病人的年龄，性别，体质，病情与施术部位等各方面的情况，辩证取穴与选择手法，并将选择的手法与穴位按一定的规律与顺序，搭配、组合成一个推拿治疗处方，来进行具体的操作治疗。其配穴组方的规律与方法和针灸疗法一样，或局部取穴，或邻近取穴，或远道循经取穴，或俞、募穴相配，或原络主客配穴，或用子母补泻法，或采用子午流注原理组方，或以痛为输局部治疗，等等。

1.2 常用推拿介质

许多推拿手法，如擦法、摩法、平推法、指推法等，在临诊实用时要配合介质。可发挥其含药物的效力，增强手法的作用，提高疗效；同时又具有润滑作用，便于手法操作，保护受术者的皮肤，防止造成破损。

目前，在成人推拿常用的介质中，除各种传统的外，还有许多用现代工艺与配方制成的介质。现简介如下：

1. 滑石粉：一般在夏季使用，有润滑作用，在多汗部位运用手法时，局部敷以滑石粉可保护患者与医者的皮肤（图9）。

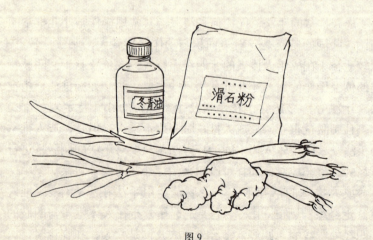

图9

2. 麻油：运用擦法时常在治疗部位上涂以少许麻油，不但可润滑皮肤，还可加强手法的透热效果。

3. 冬青膏: 将冬青油（水杨酸甲脂）与凡士林混合即成冬青膏。用擦法或揉按法时常用此膏加强手法的透热效应，并利用其祛风胜湿、活血止痛的药物作用（图9）。

4. 松节油、红花油、舒筋活络水等均可辨证选用。

5. 按摩乳: 由济南日用化工厂出品的栈桥牌按摩乳，是选用天然芳香油、中草药提取物以及表面活性剂等研制而成的一种新型推拿介质。药理与临床试验证明，按摩乳配合摩擦类手法应用于人体时，不但有润滑护肤作用，而且具有明显的活血止痛、消炎退肿与解除疲劳等医疗、保健作用。据有关报道: 应用按摩乳作介质，推拿治疗 150 例急性软组织损伤，治愈率可达 92%，与 60 例单纯用推拿手法治疗的对照组相比，治愈率提高 17% （P＜0.01），且平均治疗次数缩短 1.9 次 （P＜0.01）。故按摩乳是一种实用的推拿介质（图10）。

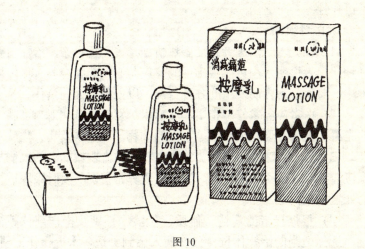

图 10

1.3 成人推拿临床须知

在推拿临床中，医患双方在施术前的准备工作，术中与术后的相互配合，以及基本的设施，是保证治疗安全、有效、无副作用，以及方便术者操作并使患者得到良好的医疗服务与心理安慰的必要条件。

1. 基本医疗设施

(1) 推拿诊疗室　要宽敞明亮、空气新鲜，温度适宜，一般室温要保持在 25℃左右，并用水方便。

(2) 推拿治疗床　要清洁整齐，平稳牢固，不要太高，也不能太低，一般以床面平术者的膝关节水平为宜。床不要靠墙，四周留适当空间，以便术者随时调整站立的位置，方便操作。

(3) 要准备好各种常用介质，并放在取用方便的位置。

(4) 治疗室内要备有各种大、小不同规格的治疗巾、治疗毯及软垫，以便施术时给患者铺、盖、靠、垫之用。

(5) 治疗室内要备有椅子、凳子，或可调节高度的凳子。

(6) 在治疗室的一面，要配有落地镜子数面，以供患者在进行医疗性练功时之用。

2. 医者须知

(1) 在施术时，医者态度要热情诚恳、和蔼可亲，治疗前要详细向患者说明术中可能会出现的反应与必要的配合与合作；施术中，要耐心解释所发生的各种情况，以取得病人的信任。

(2) 医者应经常修整指甲，注意保护双手，务使双手皮肤柔软光滑，施术时要除去戒指等手上的饰物，以免伤及病人皮肤。

(3) 施术中，医者要精力集中，密切注意观察病人的表情与反应，细心体察手下的感觉，一旦发现异常情况，及时采取适当的处置措施。

(4) 根据患者的病情、体质、年龄、性别及操作部位等情况，选择适当的治疗体位，务使病人感到舒适，术者操作方便，治疗的部位应充分显露。

(5) 施术时，术者始终要注意自身的协调性动作，使意念、呼吸及手法动作协调统一；在需要用暴发力时，也不要长久屏息、憋气与勉强用力，以避免发生岔气、胸痛、胸闷及手部关节韧带劳损扭伤等自伤现象。

(6) 在作平推、擦等需要直接在患者肌肤上操作的手法时，必须将治疗部位充分裸露；在作一指禅推法、擦法等需要隔衣或治疗巾操作的手法时，局部的衣、巾必需平整，以免挡碍手法动作而影响疗效。

(7) 在配合针刺、热敷、红外线照射等治疗时，最好在推拿后进行。如先作上述治疗，则需在 2 小时以后再作推拿治疗。

(8) 施术时，要严格掌握好刺激量与被动运动的幅度，做到轻则达到一定的刺激阈值；重则在患者可以耐受及人体结构与病理条件、生理功能可以负荷的范围之内，切不可用暴力给患者造成不应发生的手法性损伤，如：过量的擦、按、点、揉会擦破皮肤，引起皮下瘀斑；猛烈的击、打、叩、压可能误伤而致骨折及内脏损伤；过度的扳、摇、牵引可造成韧带撕伤、关节半脱位，如在脊柱过量施术，可导致颈椎半脱位、椎动脉内膜撕裂及小脑、脑干梗死等可怕的医疗事故。

3. 患者须知

(1) 接受治疗时，要信任医者，遵循医嘱，做好一切准备工作，与医者密切配合。

(2) 治疗前不要做剧烈运动，不要饱食后马上治疗、也不要在空腹饥饿时治疗，一般要在饭后 1 小时进行治疗。在诊室治疗的病人，最好在候诊室休息 10 几分钟后方能接受治疗。

(3) 治疗前，要排空大、小便，脱去外衣，解除腰带，并主动向医者说明自己身体的现状，如：是否有外感、发热；治疗部位皮肤是否有破损、感染；妇女是否在经期或孕期等。

(4) 治疗时，要保持安静，全身放松，不要看书报或入睡，要注意体验手法刺激的各种感觉，及时向医者汇报治疗中的反应。

1.4 成人推拿的适应症

1. 伤科疾病：各种扭挫伤、关节半脱位、落枕、颈椎病、腰椎间盘突出症、腰椎后关节紊乱症、退行性脊椎炎、臀上皮神经炎、梨状肌综合症、第三腰椎横突综合症、肩关节周围炎、肩峰下滑囊炎、肱骨外上髁炎、桡骨茎突部狭窄性腱鞘炎、半月板损伤、腓肠肌痉挛、胸胁屏伤、肋椎关节紊乱症、颞颌关节功能紊乱症等。

2. 内科病症：胃脘痛、胃下垂、胃与十二指肠溃疡、头痛、失眠、哮喘、肺气肿、胆囊炎、高血压、心绞痛、冠心病、泄泻、便秘、糖尿病、胃肠功能紊乱症、阳萎、尿潴留、神经衰弱等。

3. 外科疾病：乳痈初期、褥疮、术后肠粘连等。

4. 妇科疾病：痛经、闭经、月经不调、盆腔炎、产后耻骨联合分离症等。

1.5 成人推拿的禁忌症

1. 急慢性传染病　如肝炎等。
2. 感染性疾病　如丹毒、骨髓炎、化脓性关节炎等。
3. 各种出血性疾病　如胃溃疡出血期、便血、尿血等。
4. 各种恶性肿瘤　结核病及脓毒血症等。
5. 烫伤与溃疡性皮炎的局部。
6. 外伤出血。
7. 妇女月经期及孕期的腰骶部与腹部禁用推拿。

2 成人推拿常用手法

　　术者以医疗为目的，用手或肢体的其他部分，按各种规范的技巧动作，在受术者体表的经穴与特定部位，进行操作的方法称推拿手法。手法是推拿藉以治病的主要手段，手法的质量及临诊时辨证选用手法的水平，可直接影响医疗效果。

　　古代与近代医学家，创造与发明了许多行之有效的推拿手法，可见之于文字的推拿手法就约有 110 种之多。但在实际应用中，一般常用手法只不过 20~30 种。每种特定的手法，都有一定的规范化的技术动作方式，亦即"动作结构"，其内容主要包括：术者全身的体位、呼吸、意念的支持与配合，手法动作的预备姿势，动作阶段，动作要领以及动作环节的角度，摆动幅度，频率，节律，周期，动作肌的分工及相互关系等等各个方面。

　　传统推拿学对手法动作技术的基本要求是：持久、有力、均匀、柔和，从而达到深透的目的。所谓"持久"，是指手法能按要求持续运用一定时间，亦即要求手法在一定的时间内动作结构保持不变，且保持稳定的动力型式；"有力"，是指手法必须具有一定的力量，这种力量应该根据受术者的体质、病情、年龄、部位等不同情况而增减，轻则要达到一定的刺激阈值，重则不能超过病人的耐受能力；"均匀"，是指手法动作要有节律性，速度不要时快时慢，压力不要时轻时重，"柔和"，是指手法要轻而不浮，重而不滞，用力不可生硬粗暴或用蛮力，动作变换要自然；"深透"，是要求手法在操作过程中，必须掌握一定的用力方向，使手法的动态作用力最后要深入体内，作用到一定的组织层次。即要直达病所而发挥推拿的治疗作用。当然，以上几方面决不是孤立存在的，而是密切相关，有机地联系在一起的。它是对各种推拿手法动作技术要领的总结，故反过来又在实践中作为指导手法训练的原则与衡量手法优劣的尺度。但是，由于每种手法的动作结构不一，故对某一种手法动作技术的具体要求也不完全一致，而是各有侧重。如一指禅推法，㨰法则要求以柔和为贵，要柔中有刚，突出一个"柔"字；而击点法则要求击点准确，用力果断快速而刚强，要刚中带柔，则强调一个"刚"字；摩法则要求不宜急，不宜缓，不宜轻，不宜重，以中和之义施之，又立意在"中和"。

　　学员在认真进行手法技能训练的过程中，不但要从总体上把握好各种手法的动作要领，还要细心体验每种手法各自的特点，才能使手法"形、神"兼备，从而达到"一旦临证，机触于外，巧生于内，手随心到，法从心出"的高度境界。

　　现将临床最常用的 20 种手法及其训练方法一一介绍如下。

2.1　一指禅推法

　　用拇指指端螺纹面或偏峰着力于治疗部位，沉肩，垂肘，悬腕，以周期性的肘关节伸屈，前臂内外摆动并带动拇指关节伸屈的联合动作，为一指禅推法（图 11）。

动作要领

　　动作时，手握空拳，食、中、无名、小指自然屈曲，不要用力捏紧，上肢肌肉放松，拇指在着力点吸定的基础上，自然着力，不要用强力下压，拇指要盖住拳眼。手法的压力、频率、摆动幅度要均匀，使产生的"力"以一定的节律，持续地作用于治疗部位上。手法的频率在 120—160 次 / 分之间。

适用范围

　　本法的特点是着力点面积小，作用力的压强大，深透性强，刺激量的大小可根据需要任意调节，给于受术者的是一种持续的节律性的柔和刺激。它适用于全身各部经穴与部位，可用来治疗内、外、伤、妇、儿及五官等各科常见病。以螺纹面为着力点的称螺纹推，特别适用于腹部及胸部，以治疗消化系统及妇科病见长；以拇指指端为着力点的叫中峰推，则擅长于治疗头痛、头晕、失眠，高血压、肝郁等内科病症；而被称为缠法的以指峰为着力点的小幅度，快节律（200—240 次／分）推法，对喉科及外科痈、疖等病的治疗，则有独特的功效；以拇指桡侧为着力点的偏峰推则适用于在头面部操作，故常用于治疗近视，鼻渊，鼻塞流涕，头痛，头胀，耳鸣，面瘫，三叉神经痛，牙痛等疾病。

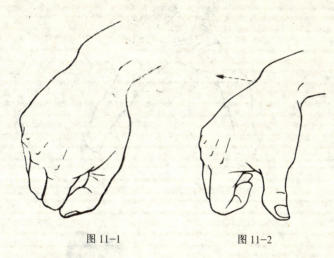

图 11-1   图 11-2

2.2 拿法

以拇指与食、中 2 指，或与其他 4 指，缓缓地对称性用力，将治疗部位挟持，提起，并同时捻搓揉捏，然后再放开，如此反复的提拿操作即为拿法（图 12）。

动作要领

本法动作时，拇指与其余 4 指各指间关节要伸直，以指面着力，不要屈指用指甲着力掐拿，腕、指关节要协调，并富于节律，提拿的劲力要深重，但加力过程要缓慢柔和，不要忽轻忽重，或突然用强力快速地捏放。

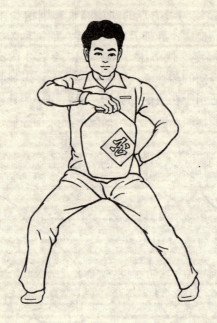

图 12-1

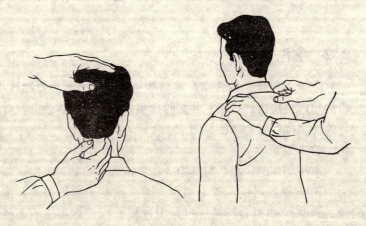

图 12-2

适用范围

本法刺激力较强，故病人会有明显强烈的酸胀感。它常施于颈项、肩背，侧腹部及四肢的肌肉、肌腱等各条索状的软组织，具有开窍醒神，发汗解表，祛风散寒，舒筋活血，解痉止痛等功效。临床施用时，根据施术部位与病情需要，可单手拿或双手拿。

2.3 按法

以指或掌着力，沿着与施术部位相垂直的方向，由轻而重，由浅渐深地缓缓用力按压，至一定深度后，稍作停留，或按揉几下，再慢慢地抬起术手，如此反复操作即为按法。按法以着力部位不同，可分为拇指按法，中指按法，掌按法与掌根按法等几种(图13)。

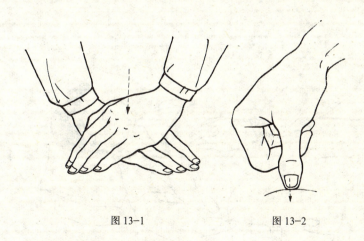

图 13—1   图 13—2

动作要领

操作时，术者要呼吸自然，发力时不要屏气，用力要平稳，要由轻而重逐渐加力至患者有酸、胀、麻、放射等"得气感"为度。每次按压的时间要掌握在 5—10 秒钟左右。在需要较大力度与反复多次操作时，最佳的具有省力效果的方法是：以双拇指或双掌叠按在治疗部位上，双臂伸直，反复地以上身向前略倾的动作，利用自身的重力在施术部位作自然支撑样的按压，而不要用手指或臂的主动用力来按压。

适用范围

这是一种由轻至中等程度刺激强度的手法，操作时，以患者产生得气感为度。指按法适用于全身各部穴位；掌按法常用于腰背及腹部。

2.4 摩法

用手掌或食、中、无名、小指掌面着力，在治疗部位上，以一定的节律沿顺时针，或逆时针方向作环形的抚摩动作的手法，称为摩法。以手掌着力称掌摩法；以4指掌面着力称指摩法（图14）。

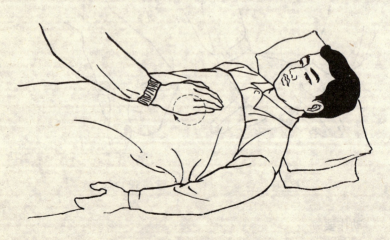

图 14-1

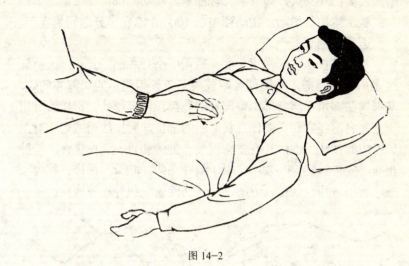

图 14-2

动作要领

摩法动作是沿圆环形轨迹进行的，用力要轻柔缓和，频率平稳适中。一般在 100—200 次／分左右。

适用范围

本法是推拿常用手法之一，主要适用于胸胁与脘腹部，具有疏肝理气，温中和胃，消积导滞，调节肠胃蠕动等功能，常用于治疗脘腹疼痛，食积胀满，胸闷气滞及胸胁迸伤等症。

2.5 揉法

用手指、掌根或大鱼际等在治疗部位作轻柔缓和的回旋动作的手法为揉法。因着力面不同，揉法可分为中指揉法、拇指揉法、掌根揉法、大鱼际揉法及肘揉法 (图15)。

动作要领

着力部位紧贴于治疗部位，肩、肘、前臂与腕关节协同，作小幅度的环旋转动，并带动该处的皮肤一起宛转回环，与其内层的软组织之间产生轻柔缓和的内摩擦。整个动作贵在柔和，揉转的幅度要由小到大，力量要先轻渐重，揉动的部位要吸定，不得在皮肤上摩擦与滑动。揉动频率在 100—140 次／分之间为宜。

适用范围

本法是推拿临床常用手法，适用于全身各部。其中，大鱼际揉多用于头面部，胸腹部及四肢关节急性扭伤后的局部肿痛处；掌根揉法多用于腰背部，臀部及四肢部肌肉丰厚处；指揉法可用于全身各部经穴和需要作点状刺激的部位；肘揉法则适用于对深层组织的按揉。本法具有宽胸理气，健脾和胃，活血化瘀，消肿止痛，安神镇静等功效，常用于治疗头痛，眩晕，面瘫，脘腹胀痛，胸闷胁痛，便秘，泄泻以及外伤性软组织肿痛等病症。

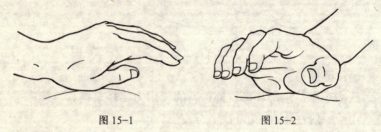

图 15-1   图 15-2

2.6 点法

用拇指或中指指峰，或用中指、食指或拇指屈曲后的近侧指间关节的突起部为着力点，沿着与施术部位相垂直的方向，以较重的力量按压患处的手法称点法。上述各种点法分别称为：中指点法，拇指点法与指节点法（图16）。

动作要领

术者在发力时，呼吸要自然，不可屏气，在加力阶段，用力要由轻而重，由浅及深，以受术者有较强烈的"得气感"但尚能耐受为度。不要用劲过重，以免造成皮下瘀血，或给患者以不可耐受的痛苦。

适用范围

本法是临床常用的一种点状的强刺激手法，由于其作用点小而集中，作用层次深，有类似针刺样的效果，故常用在肌肉或骨缝深处的硬结或压痛点，以使受术者有强烈的酸、麻、胀、痛等感觉，从而收到"以痛止痛"的功效。本法常用来治疗脘腹挛痛，肢体因顽痹、陈伤所致的疼痛以及麻痹、瘫痪等症。

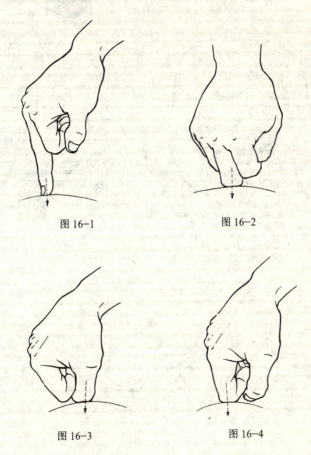

图 16-1   图 16-2

图 16-3   图 16-4

2.7 擦法

以手掌掌面、小鱼际或大鱼际处为着力面，在治疗部位沿直线进行往返摩擦的手法，称为擦法。擦法因着力面的不同而分别称为掌擦法，小鱼际擦法和大鱼际擦法（图 17）。

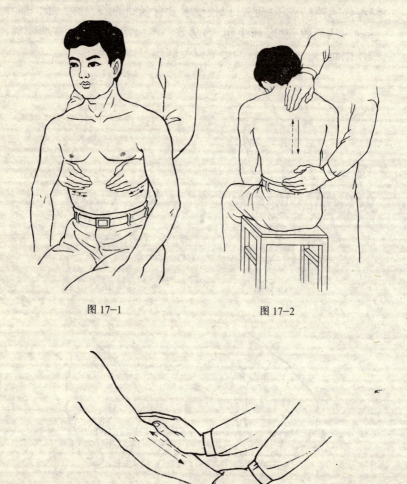

图 17-1   图 17-2

图 17-3

动作要领

擦法的动作幅度要大，使推擦的距离尽量拉长，而且，无论是沿人体上下直擦，或左右横擦，或斜擦，其动作在受术者体表的运动轨迹都要成直线。另外，在操作过程中，手的着力面要始终与施术部位的皮肤贴紧，并使施术路线全程均匀受力。用力要适中，不可用重力按压，以免擦伤皮肤。

适用范围

擦法与摩法一样，也是一种摩擦运动，所不同的是其动作运行的轨迹是直线，用力较摩法大，故有比摩法更明显的温热作用。临床也主要利用本法的"力"与"热"的作用来获取温经止痛，祛风散寒，消肿散结，行气活血等功效。临诊实用时，被擦部位要充分暴露，推擦的速度在开始 1—2 下时要缓和稍慢，以后可稍快，至局部发热为度。一般每次操作在 10 次以内，时间不宜长，以免局部过热发烫而起泡。本法在操作时，为防止擦破皮肤并帮助产热，往往需使用介质，如麻油、冬青膏、按摩乳等。

2.8 滚法

以手背尺侧 1／3—1／2 处为着力面，前臂作周期性的外、内摆动，同时，带动腕关节作屈、伸运动，使略弓成圆形的手背在施术部位上有节律地来回滚动的手法称为滚法（图18）。

动作要领

本法操作时，着力面要紧贴于治疗部位的皮肤，不能来回地拖擦与滑动；压力要均匀柔和，不能时轻时重或用重力硬顶；节律不能忽快忽慢。动作幅度：前臂约在旋前 45°至旋后 45°之间；腕关节约在屈 45°—伸 10°之间，手保持自然的屈曲姿势，无任何主动的捏拢与伸直的动作。肩带放松，自然下垂，肩关节处在前屈 30°—40°，并外展 30°左右的位置，肘关节自然屈曲成 90°—120°。滚动频率为 140—160 次／分。

适用范围

本法的特点是刺激面积大，作用力强，深透作用明显，除头

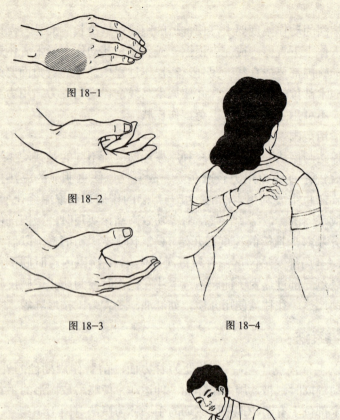

图 18-1

图 18-2

图 18-3

图 18-4

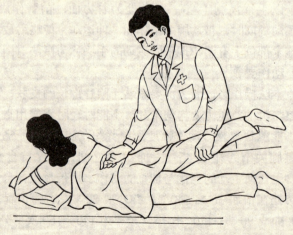

图 18-5

面部、前颈与胸腹部外，在全身各部均可使用，特别适用于腰背、臀及四肢肌肉较为丰厚的部位。如需加大刺激量，则动作时可调手势，以 2、3、4、5 掌指关节处着力来进行操作。它具有舒筋通络，祛风散寒，温经胜湿，活血化瘀，解痉止痛，松解粘连，滑利关节等功效。临床尤以治疗运动系统与神经系统的疾病见长。擦法是推拿临床使用率最高的手法之一。

2.9 振法

用中指端或手掌为着力点，以前臂伸、屈肌群小幅度、快速地交替收缩，使所产生的轻柔振颤持续地作用于人体的手法为振法（图19）。

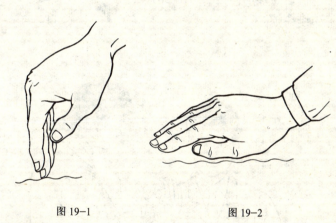

图 19-1　　　　　　　　　　　图 19-2

动作要领

不要主动用力按压着力点，前臂的肌群收缩要使手产生垂直方向的振动运动，振动频率约在 8—12 次／秒之间。术者要集中精力，气沉丹田，呼吸调匀，并用意念将气沿术手的掌侧导引至掌中劳宫穴或中指端，做到以意领气，以气生力，以力发振。整个动作自然，流畅，协调，统一。绝不可憋气，用强力硬屏发力。

适用范围

本法适用于全身各部，特别常用于头面部与胸腹部，具有镇静安神，明目益智，温中理气，消积导滞，调节肠胃蠕动等功能，故对失眠，健忘，胃肠功能紊乱等症的治疗效果尤为显著。

2.10 搓法

术者用双手掌相对用力，对被挟持的肢体作快速的来回搓擦，并同时作上下往返的移动为搓法（图20）。

动作要领

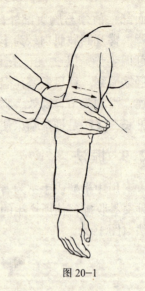

图 20-1

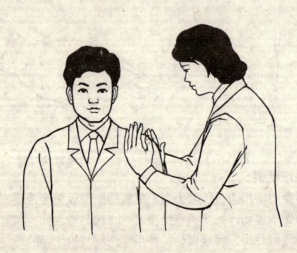

图 20-2

操作时，术者取马步，上身略向前倾，双手用力要对称，搓动要快而幅度均匀，上下移动要平稳而稍慢。

适用范围

本法是推拿常用的辅助手法之一，常用于上肢与胁肋部，也可用于腰与下肢，作为治疗的结束手法，具有调和气血，理顺关节筋腱，放松肌肉的功效。

2.11 抹法

用双手或单手拇指指面，紧贴于治疗部位，沿直线轻轻地作上下或左右的反复摩擦手法为抹法（图 21）。

动作要领

本法操作时，用力要适中，不要用强力按压而使动作滞涩；又不可用力太轻而使手法飘浮。动作的频率要均匀。在同一直线上抹时，双手要一起一落交替进行；向左右分抹时，双手要同时动作。夏天出汗时，可用滑石粉作介质。

适用范围

本法常用于头面、颈项部。治疗头晕、头痛、面瘫、三叉神经痛及颈项强痛时，常用本法作主治或辅助手法。本法具有开窍镇惊，醒脑明目，舒筋活血等作用。

2.12 提拿法

用拇指与食、中 2 指，或拇指或其余 4 指相对用力挟持并向上提起患者的筋腱或肌束的手法为提拿法（图 22）。

动作要领

本法是一种提法与拿法相结合的复合手法。动作要领与拿法相同，所不同的是，其向上的提持力较拿法为强。

适用范围

本法是一种刺激性较强的手法，具有兴奋神经，鼓舞阳气，发散壅蔽，祛风散寒等功效。对肌肉萎缩，神经麻痹，风湿顽痹、偏瘫等病症有明显的治疗作用。

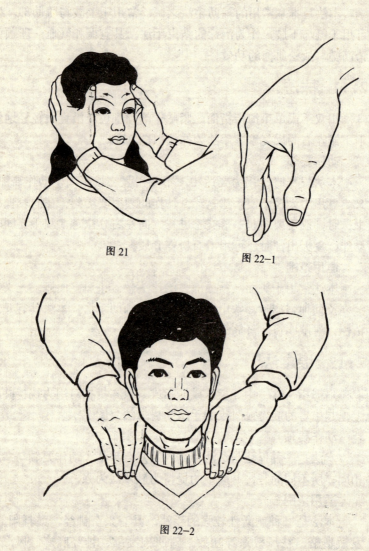

图 21

图 22-1

图 22-2

2.13 按揉法

术者在作按法的同时加上揉的动作，这种边按边揉的手法称为按揉法。

动作要领

本法是一种按法与揉法的复合手法。动作要领兼有这两种手法的特点。常用拇指、中指或食指操作，也可用食、中、无名指3指同时着力操作称为三指按揉法。如在穴点上需作比较深重的按揉时，可用双手拇指指面，一个在下按压住穴位；一个在上重叠按住下一个拇指的背侧，双手同时用力按揉称为双指重叠按揉法。

适用范围

本法刚中带柔，柔中有刚，给人一种重实有力，柔和舒适的刺激，具有安神镇静，祛瘀散结，解痉止痛等功效，适用于全身各部位的经穴或阿是穴。单指按揉法适用于头面及四肢，3指按揉法常用于胸腹部，双指重叠按揉法宜在腰臀部肌肉较丰厚处。

2.14 膊运法

以前臂尺侧上1/3屈肌肌腹处为着力面，在治疗部位上作摩擦或揉动的手法为膊运法（图23）。

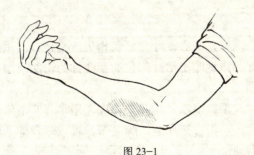

图 23-1

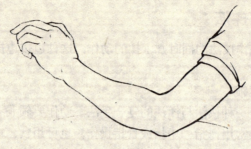

图 23-2

动作要领

本法的预备姿势是：术者一般取坐位，肩部放松，不要抬肩，上肢向前自然伸出，屈肘约 90°—100°，前臂呈完全旋前位，手掌向下，手指在自然功能位动作，肘关节在 90°—160°之间作节律性的伸屈运动，使着力面在治疗部位上产生摩运或揉动的效应。此间，术者要正坐，上身略向前倾，但要防止将上身完全趴伏在治疗部位上，以免使动作滞涩。

适用范围

本法较指摩或掌摩的着力面积大，压力也稍重，故适用于腰背、臀、大腿等部位以及其他需要在较大面积上作摩运或揉动手法的场合，也可用于腹部；对扭挫伤，腰脊症及坐骨神经痛等病症较好的疗效。

2.15 击法

用拳背，掌根，掌心，小鱼际，指尖或桑枝棒（用桑枝制作的治疗棒）有节律地叩击治疗部位的手法称为击法（图24）。

动作要领

拳击法时，手握空拳，腕关节伸直，用拳背叩击体表；

掌击法时，手指自然屈曲，腕关节伸直或略背伸，用掌心或掌根击打施术部位；

小鱼际击法，又称侧击法或切打法。操作时，手、掌及腕关

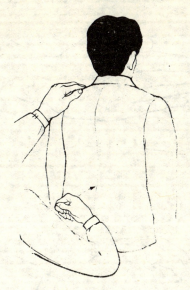

图 24-1

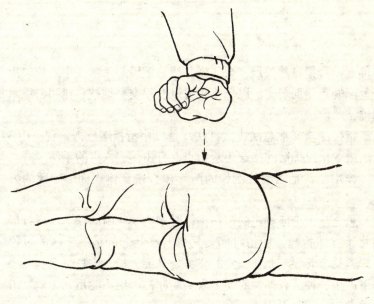

图 24-2

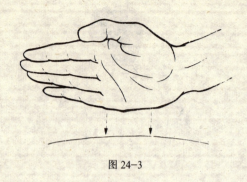

图 24-3

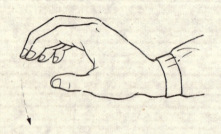

图 24-4

节伸直，拇指自然外展，余4指并拢，前臂与手掌在中立位，用小鱼际的尺侧面着力，以单手也可以双手交替地按节律叩击施术部位。

指击法，又称总法或点打法，是以中指指端或拇、食、中3指，或5指捏拢后的指端为着力点，打击体表穴点的手法；

棒击法，是用桑枝制作的治疗棒打击身体表面治疗区的方法。

总之，无论何种击法，在操作时用力要果断而快速，击打后要将手立即抬起，叩击时间要短暂，在抬起的前臂下落的过程中，腕关节既要控制住一定的姿势；又要放松，击打时手腕顺势向下，用一种富有弹性的劲力来实施叩击，绝不能用死力来打击受术者，击叩时不能使病人有任何痛感。

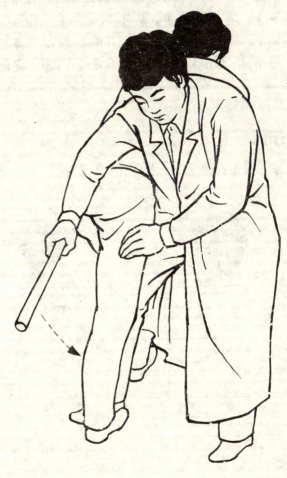

图 24-5

适用范围

　　拳背击法常用于大椎穴及腰骶部；掌击法常用于头顶前囟与百会穴；小鱼际击法适用于腰背与四肢部；指击法常用于头面、胸腹与四肢经穴；棒击法可用于头顶、肩背、腰骶及四肢部。本法具有舒筋通络，活血化瘀，调和气血等作用，对风湿痹痛，麻木不仁，肌肉痉挛、瘫痪及肌肉萎缩等病症有明显作用。

桑枝棒制法：用细的新鲜桑枝 12 根（直径约 0.5 厘米左右）去皮阴干，每根用桑皮纸卷紧，并用线绕扎，然后把桑枝合起来先用线扎紧，再用桑皮纸层层卷紧并用线绕好。外面用布裹紧缝好即成。要求软硬适中，具有弹性，粗细合用，直径4.5—5 厘米，长约 40 厘米。

2.16 拍法

用虚掌拍打体表的方法，称为拍法（图25）。

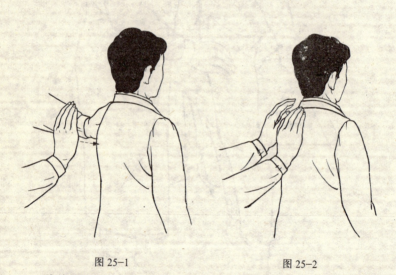

图 25-1　　　　　　　　　　　图 25-2

动作要领

本法操作时，要求 5 指并拢，手指伸直，2、3、4、5 掌指关节略屈，使掌心内凹而成所谓的"虚掌"。拍打时前臂先抬起，在向下落时，手腕顺势而下，与击法一样，以一种富有弹性的巧劲，用虚掌拍打在施术部位上。

适用范围

本法主要用于肩背、腰骶与大腿部，轻拍亦可用于胸腹部。强而长时间的拍打具有镇静止痛，活血祛瘀，解痉及强壮等作用；轻而短时间的拍打有清脑健神，兴奋神经，调理肠胃、宽胸理气等功效。常用于治疗各种风湿痹痛，陈伤劳损，新伤血瘀，肌肉萎缩，知觉减退，肠麻痹，胸闷胸痛及气功偏差大动不已等病症。

2.17 抖法

用双手握住患者的上肢或下肢远端，用力作连续的小幅度的上下擅动为抖法（图26）。

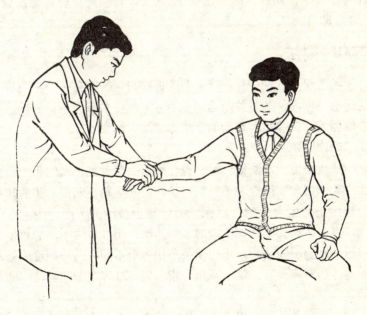

图26

动作要领

本法操作时，术者取马步势，上身略向前倾；双上肢自然前伸，曲肘约130°—160°之间；用两手握住腕部或踝部，将患肢伸直；抖上肢时将患肢固定在外展 45°—60° 位；抖下肢时，将患肢抬起至约离床面 30° 处；缓缓用力做连续不断的小幅度上下抖动。动作时，固定患肢的双手不要捏得太紧，要使被抖动的肢体放松，不可将其牵拉得太紧，抖动的幅度要由小而大，频率要快。

适用范围

本法主要用于四肢，常与搓法配合使用，作为治疗最后的结束手法，有放松肌肉，调和气血的作用。本法也可用在腰部，操作时将患者双下肢提起，用强力牵拉抖动，使产生的振动力直达腰部。此法又称为抖拉法，常用来治疗腰椎间盘突出症等，有较好的疗效。抖动肢体时每次做 10 几次；抖拉腰椎时，每次做 3—4 次即可。

2.18 摇法

术者双手分别握住治疗关节的近端与远端，在关节生理许可的运动范围内，顺着关节运动轴的方向，使关节作前后屈伸，左右侧屈或环转等被动运动的手法称摇法（图 27）。

动作要领

一般来说，本法操作时，握在被摇关节近侧上端的手为固定手，其作用是使治疗关节得到保护，使其运动不随摇动力的作用而超出正常生理范围，以保证力传导至被治关节而产生治疗效应。握在运动关节远侧下端的手称为动作手或主力手，它根据关节运动轴的不同结构，用力使关节作各个不同方向与幅度的被动摇动。如对肩、肘、腕、掌指、指、膝、趾等关节的摇法，即是如此。

如果运动关节可用自身的体重固定在床上或令助手固定，则术者可将双手在关节远侧下端用作动作手而摇动治疗关节，如腕、颈椎、腰椎等关节的摇法。

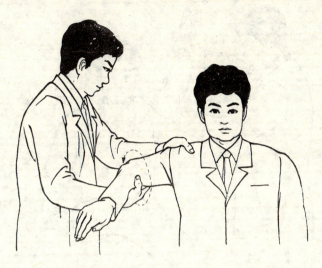

图 27-1

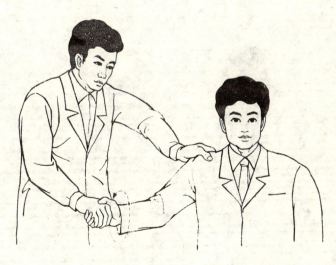

图 27-2

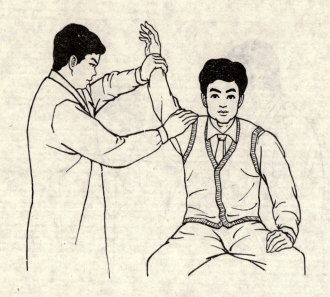

图 27-3

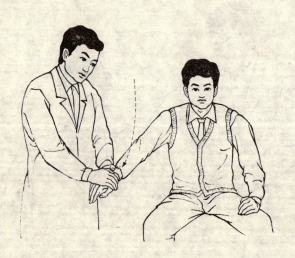

图 27-4

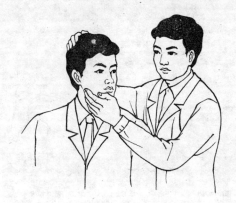

图 27-5

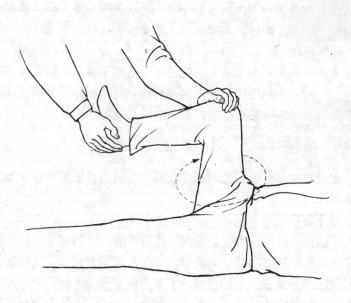

图 27-6

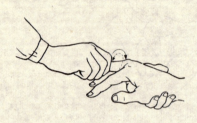
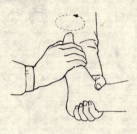

图 27-7   图 27-8

整个摇法双手动作要协调，用力要平稳、缓和，摇动幅度要由小渐大，不得超越关节运动的生理范围。当关节处在粘连等病理状态，而关节运动度明显缩小时，摇动的幅度要在病人能耐受的前提下，循序渐进，逐步扩大，切莫操之过急。

适用范围

本法是关节被动运动一类的手法，适用于颈椎、腰椎及四肢等关节。对关节粘连，强直，运动功能障碍，屈伸不利等症，具有滑利关节，解除粘连，增强关节活动功能等作用。

2.19 扳法

术者在被治疗关节的两端作相反方向的用力来扳动肢体的手法为扳法。

动作要领

本法操作时，术者必需掌握人体关节的运动解剖学特征，要对诸关节的结构，运动轴的数目，方向，运动方式，运动幅度及其影响因素等知识，了如指掌，才能把握正确的手法位置，使动作合理，做到省力，安全，无痛与有效。由于各类关节的解剖学特征不一，故其手法的动作要领也各异。现将临床最常用的几种扳法分别介绍如下：

1. 颈项部扳法

(1) 颈椎斜扳法：受术者端坐，头略向前屈约 30°，术者一手抵握住受术者的枕部，另一手抵握住下颏部，动作时，先将头向一侧旋转至最大限度（约 45°左右）。再两手同时用力作相反方向的扳动（图 28）。

(2) 颈椎定位斜扳法：受术者端坐，头前倾 30°，术者在其背后，用一肘部托住其下颏部，前臂将其头抱住，手则扶住其枕部；另一手拇指按在施术颈椎的棘突旁，余 4 指按于肩上，先肘部用力，将头旋转至最大限度（约 45°左右）。然后，作一个快速的小幅度的旋转牵拉动作扳动颈椎，同时另一手的拇指朝相反方向用力，将患椎固定并拨正（图 29）。

2. 胸背部扳法

(1) 扩胸牵扳法：本法是主要作用于胸肋关节的手法。操作时，令受术者端坐，两手手指交叉扣住，置于项部。术者在其背后双手握住受术者两肘部，并用一侧膝部顶住其背部。动作时，先嘱受术者自行挺胸并两肘后伸作扩胸动作，待其自主动作到功能位时，术者两手趁势作一个小幅度的快速动作，将两肘向后扳动，同时，膝部稍用力向前顶推其后背而完成扩胸牵扳动作（图 30）。

(2) 胸椎对抗复位法：令受术者取坐位，两上肢上举 180°。术者站在其身后，甲手向前握住其前臂下端近肘关节处，乙手拇指在后顶住患部脊柱。动作时，先嘱受术者挺胸，同时，术者顺势用甲手向后扳动其双上肢，乙手向前用力推按患者棘突，使其复位（图 31）。

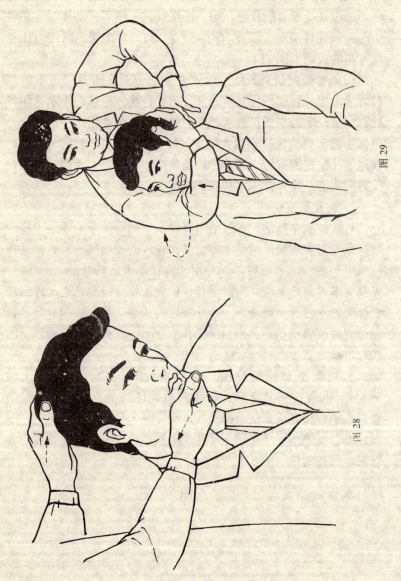

图 29

图 28

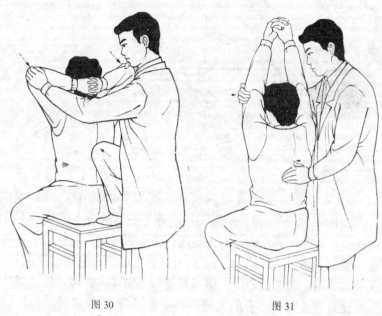

图 30   图 31

3. 腰部扳法

(1) 腰椎斜扳法:

A. 侧卧位腰椎斜扳法: 受术者侧卧位, 在下面的腿伸直, 上面的腿屈髋屈膝, 在上面的上肢放在身后, 下面的上肢自然地放在身侧。术者甲手抵住患者肩前部, 乙手抵住臀部或髂前上棘部。动作时, 甲手将其肩部向身后方向推; 乙手将骨盆朝其腹侧推转, 如此将腰椎旋转至最大限度后, 再双手同时相反用力, 作一个小幅度的快速的推压动作, 即完成本法 (图 32)。

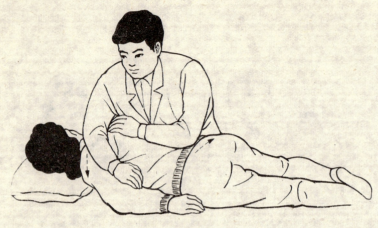

图 32

B. 仰卧位长柄式腰椎斜扳法：受术者仰卧位，侧上肢外展，同侧下肢屈髋 90°，屈膝；左侧上肢自然放在体侧，下肢伸直。术者站在其左侧，右手按压住受术者右侧肩前部，左手握住其膝部（图 33-1）。动作时，术者右手将其右肩紧压在床面，左手将其右腿向左侧牵拉，使其骨盆随之向左侧旋转，旋转至最大限度时（此时受术者的大腿约与床面平行），左手将所握持的下肢向下做一个快速小幅度的推压动作（图 33-2）。向右侧斜扳时，术者站在受术者左侧，其动作与手势均与上述相反即可。

C. 坐位腰椎斜扳法：受术者端坐，术者用腿挟住其一侧下肢，一手抵住其近术者侧的肩后部，另一手从受术者另一侧腋下伸入抵住肩前部，两手同时用力使其上身旋转以扳动腰椎（图34）。

（2）腰椎旋转复位法：受术者端坐于无靠背的方凳上（以向右侧旋转为例）。助手用双膝与双手将其左下肢固定。术者站受术者右后侧，左手拇指按抵于受术腰椎棘突的右旁，右手从受术者的右侧腋下穿过，把握住对侧的颈肩部。动作时，嘱受术者向前弯腰；待弯至最大限度时，术者右手用力将其上身板向右侧，

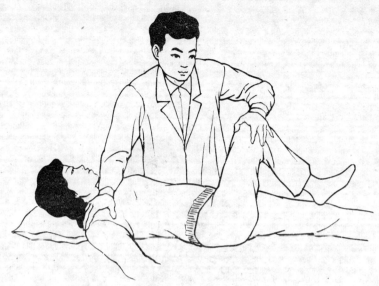

图 33—1

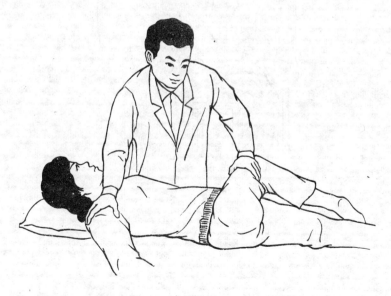

图 33—2

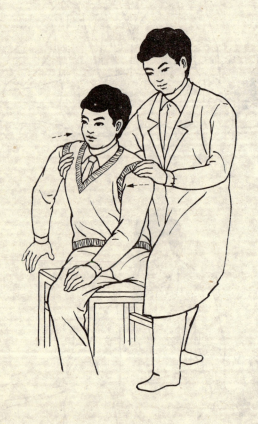

图 34

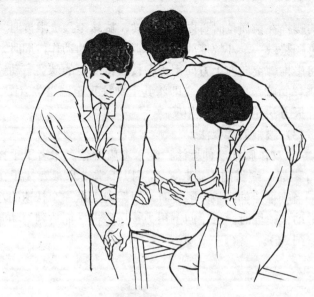

图 35-1

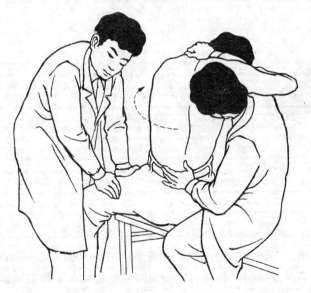

图 35-2

使其腰椎在前屈位时再向右侧旋转；旋转至最大限度时，术者右手再顺势做一个小幅度的快速牵扳与旋转的动作；同时，左手拇指将患椎棘突向左上方向用力推按；待手下的棘突有动感或出现"喀嚓"的响声后，右手立即将其上身扶正至端坐位（图35）。左侧旋扳方法相同，方向相反。

（3）腰椎后伸扳法：

A. 双腿腰椎后伸扳法：受术者俯卧位。术者甲手托住受术者两膝部，缓缓向上提起，乙手以手掌或掌根处按压在腰部患处，当腰椎后伸到最大限度时，甲手向上做一个快速的小幅度的托举动作，同时，乙手向下用力按压患椎，而达到扳动腰椎的目的（图36）。

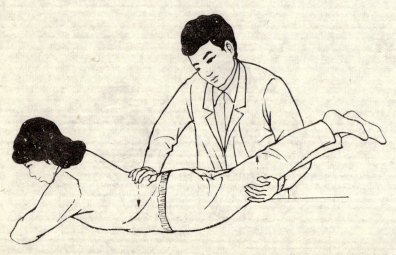

图 36

B. 单腿腰椎后伸扳法：受术者取俯卧位，术者站在其左侧，用右手把握住受术者的右膝部，左手掌根按压住腰部患椎的棘突上。动作时，先将右腿慢慢向上提起，左掌根紧压患椎，使腰椎后伸至最大限度时，右手再向上做一个快速的小幅度的提拉动作，同时左手掌根向下用力快速推压，使腰椎产生一个过伸动作，以扳动患椎使其复位（图37）。也可抬举左腿使腰椎后伸，其动作与抬右腿后伸腰椎法相同。

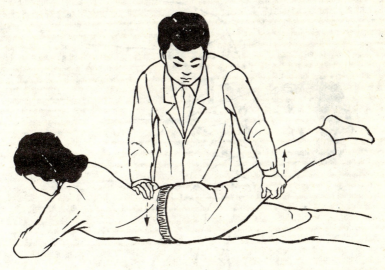

图 37

4. 肩关节扳法

（1）外展扳肩法：受术者端坐。术者在其患侧取下蹲位，将患肢的前臂部或肘部放置于右肩上，双手按压在患肩上端。动作时，术者慢慢站起，使肩关节外展，展至最大限度时，突然起立至肩关节外展90°的水平。同时，双手向下用力将肩关节紧压固定，使应力传至肩关节，以解除关节的粘连，恢复肩关节的运动功能（图38）。

（2）前屈、后伸扳肩法：受术者端坐，术者甲手握患肢前臂下端或肘部，乙手按住肩后部。动作时，先将患肢慢慢前屈，或后伸，至最大限度时，甲手突然用力向前屈或后伸方向扳动患肩关节，同时乙手将肩部固定并用力从相反方向与甲手扳肩的力量对抗，以加强传递到肩关节的应力，而达到扳肩的目的（图39、40）。

· 561 ·

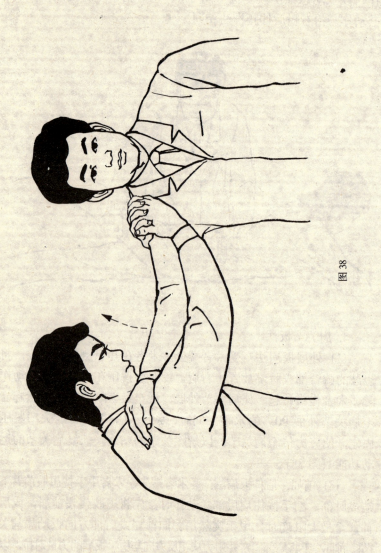

图 38

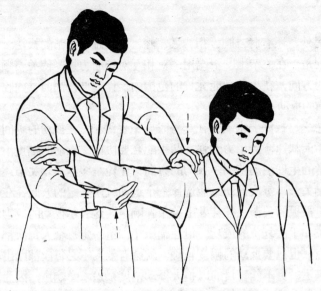

图 39-1

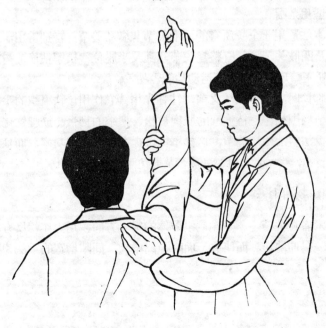

图 39-2

另外，还有肘、腕、指、髋、膝、踝、趾等关节的扳法。其施术原则是：在关节上、下端用一对相互对抗的力量，使关节顺着运动轴的方向，在生理功能允许的范围内，作过伸、屈曲、内收或外展方向的扳动。

总之，扳法要求动作在起势时要稳妥缓和；在扳动的瞬间则必须果断而快速，且用力刚强；两手配合要协调；扳动的幅度不得超越正常的生理活动范围；扳动的方向，无论是多运动轴关节还是单运动轴关节，每次扳动只能选择一个运动轴所限定的方向。在作扳法时，被扳的关节往往会发出关节弹响声，这表示扳动的应力已传递到位和手法复位的成功。但在临床中，不一定每个人每次都会有此效应，但只要扳动的幅度正确，就会有效。不必每次都以出现响声为满足，更不能盲目的以扩大扳动幅度来追求弹响声，因为，这样往往会由于过度的牵拉而造成关节、韧带不必要的损伤。

适用范围

本法适用于全身所有的运动关节与微动关节，特别常用于颈、腰椎及四肢关节。具有整复关节紊乱及半脱位，松解粘连，滑利关节，矫正畸形，恢复关节运动功能等功效。

临诊时，在作扳法之前，往往先用其它作用于软组织的手法，在关节周围操作，待痉挛的肌肉放松、挛缩的韧带、筋腱软化后，再用扳法整治罹病关节，这样不但可提高扳法的成功率，而且能使术者省力，受术者也可少受痛苦及避免手法造成的创伤。

2.20 拔伸法

术者在关节上、下端，沿肢体的纵轴方向，用力作相反方向的牵拉，引伸动作，而使关节面的距离增大，间隙增宽的手法为拔伸法。

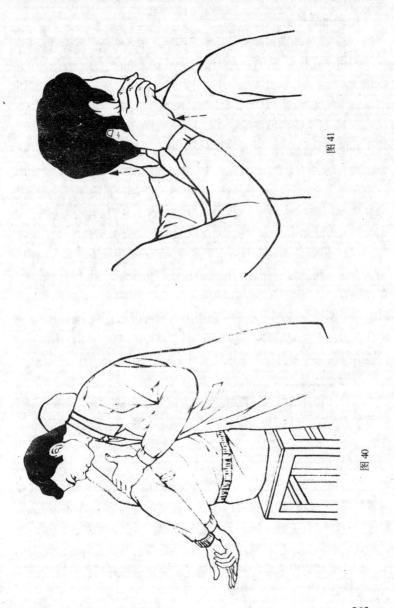

图 41

图 40

动作要领

1. 颈椎拔伸法

(1) 坐位颈椎拔伸法：受术者端坐。术者站在受术者背后，用双手拇指顶在枕骨下方，掌根托住两侧下颌角的下方，并用两前臂压住受术者两肩。动作时，两手用力向上将头部端起，同时两臂向下压肩作相反方向用力（图41）。

(2) 低坐位颈椎拔伸法：受术者端坐在无靠背的矮凳上。术者位于其侧方取马步势，用肘部将受术者的颏部托起，并用上臂与前臂，将其头部紧紧抱住，另一手托扶住其枕部（图42-1）。动作时，术者上身挺直，两手环抱，将受术者头部挟紧抱住，令受术者全身放松，然后从马步势站直，将受术者上身提起，使其离开矮凳，利用其自身的重量，完成对颈椎的牵引（图42-2）。

(3) 仰卧位颈椎牵引法：受术者仰卧，不用枕头。术者在其头侧取坐位，两足分别踏地，用双膝顶住两侧床腿，上身略向前倾，脊柱挺直，左手在下垫在其枕部，右手在上抓握住下颏部。动作时，左手紧托住枕部与右手一起用力将头部握固，两上肢伸直，腰背部发力使上身向后仰伸，并带动两手将受术者的身体在床面上滑行拖动，利用患者自身的重力完成对颈椎的牵引（图43）。

2. 腰椎拔伸法

(1) 俯卧位腰椎拔伸法：受术者俯卧，令助手固定两腋下（或嘱受术者两手拉住床头边缘），术者两手握紧受术者小腿下端。动作时，令受术者全身放松或咳嗽一声，此时术者与助手同时相对用力，拔伸腰椎（图44）。

(2) 背势腰椎牵引法：术者与受术者相背而立，用两肘挽住受术者肘弯部。动作时，术者用臀部抵住受术者需要牵引的腰椎或腰骶部，令受术者咳嗽一声，术者趁其咳嗽的瞬间，弯腰、屈膝、挺臀将受术者背起，使基双足离地面，然后做有节律的伸膝，挺臀动作，颤动或摇动受术者的腰部，使受术者的腰椎在后伸拉时受到其下半身自身重量的牵引（图45）。

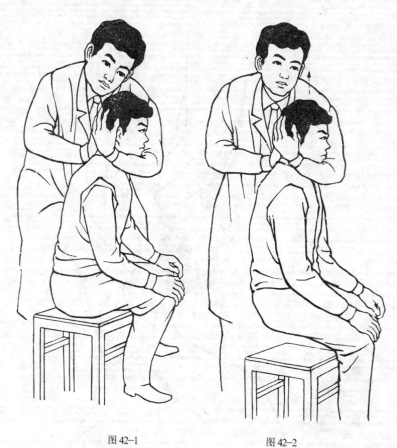

图 42-1 图 42-2

（3）肩关节拔伸法：受术者取坐势。术者用双手握住其前臂下端，令助手固定受术者身体。动作时，术者与助手缓缓地相对用力拔伸肩关节（图46）。

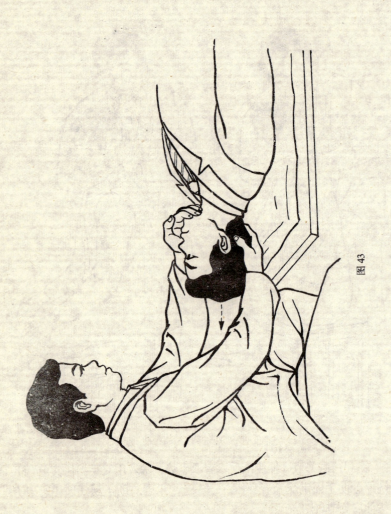

图 43

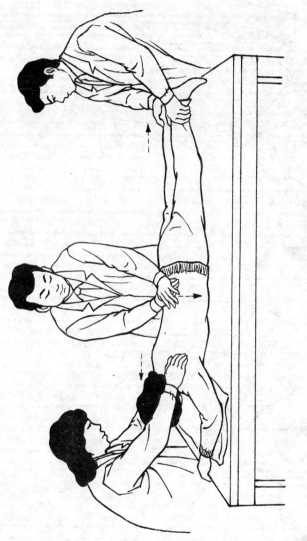

图 44

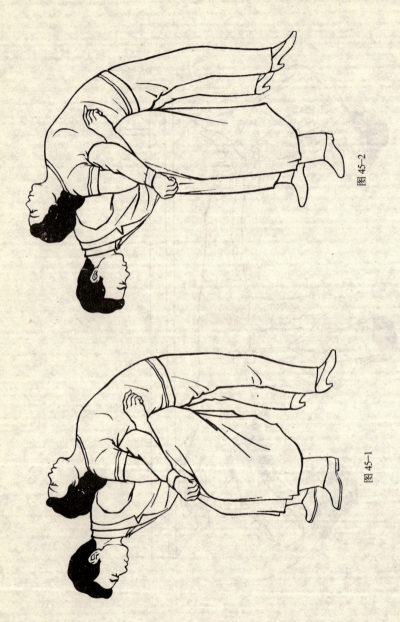

图 45-2

图 45-1

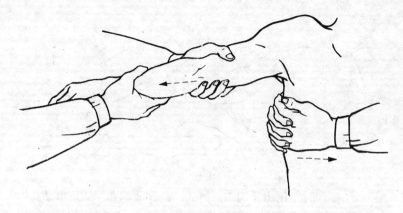

图 46

　　另外，还有肘、腕、指、髋、膝、踝、趾等关节的拔伸法，其操作方法是：术者用一手抓握住被拔伸关节的近侧端，另一手把握住其远侧端，两手同时作反方向的对抗用力，牵拉关节，使其间隙增宽（图 47、48）。

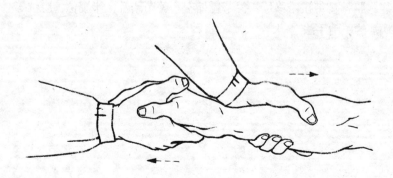

图 47

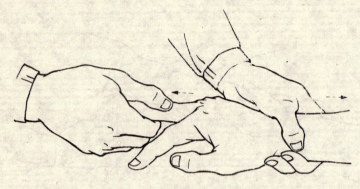

图 48

　　本法操作时，用力要均匀，持久，动作要缓和，切忌粗暴。作用力的方向要沿受术关节的纵轴进行，对畸形、僵直的关节要慎用本法。

　　适用范围

　　本法适用于颈椎，腰椎及四肢关节，有理筋，复位，增宽关节间隙，解除神经挤压，松解粘连等功效。是颈椎病、腰椎间盘突出症、肌腱韧带扭错移位、关节囊缩窄，关节紊乱、半脱位、脱位等病症的主治手法之一。

3 手法的练习方法与步骤

作为一个推拿专业工作者，不但要熟练掌握各种手法的动作技能，而且要有胜任日常繁重治疗任务的能力，这就要求推拿医生的身心具备特有的专业素质。这种素质的获得，一方面靠推拿练功，而更重要的则是进行严格的手法练习。特别是一些动作结构复杂，操作技巧难度比较高的手法，如一指禅推法、擦法、摩法、振法等，更须长期反复练习，才能运用自如，得心应手，在临床上发挥治疗作用。故中医推拿学特别重视与强调手法的专业训练，并在实践中创造、总结出一套行之有效的训练方法。初学者在认真练功的同时，必须严格按照手法基本训练的方法与步骤，日积月累，循序渐进地进行刻苦锻炼，才能练成精湛的手法技能与全面的专业素质。

手法基本训练的步骤主要分米袋练习，人体练习与常见病操作常规练习三个阶段，现将每个阶段的练习方法与要求简介如下：

3.1 米袋练习

除关节被动运动手法之外的所有手法，都先要在米袋上进行练习。米袋制法是：先缝 1 个长 25 厘米，宽 16 厘米的布袋，内装约 4 / 5 的优质粳米，用洗净的黄沙代替亦可，然后将口袋缝合，外面再做一个布质外套，以便于换洗，布套一端留有线绳的扎口。开始时，米袋可扎得紧一些，以后逐渐放松（图 49）。

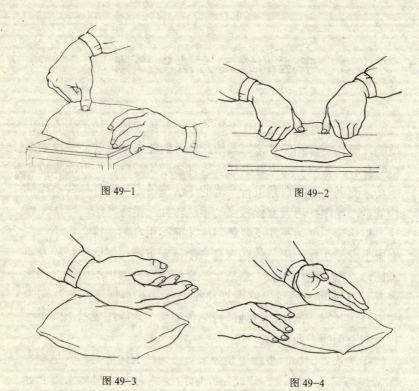

图 49-1

图 49-2

图 49-3

图 49-4

将米袋端放在桌上，练习一指禅推法、摩法、揉法、振法等手法时，学员应取坐位，练习擦法时可取站位。操作时，必须按照每种手法的动作结构，从预备姿势到动作要领，包括着力点的位置，每个运动关节的角度，摆动幅度、频率以及全身配合的姿势，呼吸，意念等，进行规范化的严格训练。指导教师要及时指出并纠正学员的错误动作。

开始练习时，主要精力要放在"动作是否正确"上，不要急于加力，因为在动作不正确的情况下，一味地加重手法的压力，不但有碍于正确动作的获得，而且有发生自伤的可能。只有在动作方式规范的前提下，才能达到手法的"最佳力学状态"，力量也就会自然地产生。

练习过程中要注意左、右手的交替练习。

另外，在米袋练习的初始阶段，一般先练习各种手法的定点操作技能，亦即所谓的"吸定"功夫，以后再练习走线操作的技能。此时沿米袋的长轴线由下而上，由上而下往返地边操作边缓缓地作直线移动。这两种技能的锻炼，可为日后在人体操作时"推穴道、走经络"的功夫打好基础。

总之，通过米袋练习，学员能掌握主要手法的规范动作结构与高度娴熟的操作技巧。在达到了这个目的后，即可进入第二阶段的人体练习。

3.2 人体练习

为了进一步获得在人体上进行手法操作的技能与体验，为临床应用打好基础，还要进行第二阶段人体手法练习的训练课目。在人体上进行手法练习的方法有两种：一种是将各种手法，在其所适用的人体部位上选择有关的经络与穴位，进行单一的手法练习；一种是将适用于人体各部位的多种手法，根据人体各部位的形态结构特点与经络、穴位的配布规律，按一定的线路与次序、编排组合成一组手法操作常规套路，来进行手法的综合练习。

3.3 常见病操作常规练习

本阶段手法练习的内容，主要是对临床中多种常见病推拿治疗的操作常规逐一进行练习。通过此阶段的学习，学员不但能比较熟练地掌握治疗每种常见病的手法，其中包括在一般人体练习阶段中没有涉及到的治疗各种疾病时所专用的特种手法；而且还可以了解与初步掌握推拿临床辨证取穴与组方的规律。所以这是正式进入临床之前的一个十分必要的训练环节。

4 十四经与常用腧穴

联属十二脏腑的十二经脉，与奇经八脉中的任、督二脉，合称为十四经。有关十四经及常用腧穴的学术内容，是全部经络学说与腧穴学说的主体部分。在推拿医疗实践中，它是最有实用价值的、最重要的基础理论。因为在推拿临床工作中，从对疾病的辨证、诊断，推拿配穴处方，手法选择及手法动作的操作等，无不遵循经络学说的指导。所以，学习推拿者必须首先掌握十四经及常用腧穴的基本内容。否则，动辄出错。

4.1 十四经概述

1. 十二经脉

由于十二经脉是经络系统的主体，故又称"正经"。它们分属十二脏腑，每一条经都分别和一个脏或腑相连，并以其所连脏腑命名。连于心脏的经脉称为"心经"；连于大肠的经脉称为"大肠经"……。凡是属脏的经脉又总称为"阴经"；属腑的经脉又总称为"阳经"。另外，阴经与阳经根据在上肢、下肢的分布，又有手、足三阴经、三阳经之分。

十二经脉在体表的分布规律是：阳经主要分布在上肢的外侧面、下肢的外侧面以及背部；阴经主要分布在上肢的内侧面、下肢的内侧面及腹部（其中足阳明胃经在躯干部的经脉例外，分布在腹侧）。其中手三阴经从胸部起始，循行至手；手三阳经从手起始，循行至头部；足三阳经从头部起始，循行至足部为止。足三阴经从足部起始，循行至腹部而终。

十二经脉通过支脉和络脉的沟通衔接，在脏与腑之间形成 6 组"属络"关系，相应地在阴、阳经之间形成 6 组"表里"关系。阴经属脏络腑，阳经属腑络脏，再通过同名的手足经的交接，构成了十二经脉的循环传注：始于肺经、终于肝经，又复于肺经，如此循环，周而复始，如环无端，使人体气血得以周流不息。十二经的全称，表里关系及流注衔接规律列表如下。

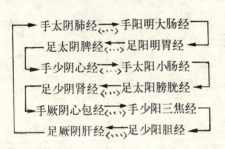

十二经脉的生理功能，主要表现在沟通内外，运行气血和调节平衡等 3 个方面：

经络内属脏腑，外络肢节，将人体的五脏六腑、四肢百骸、皮肉筋脉及五官等组织与器官紧密地联系成为一个有机的整体。"经"有"途径"的意思，是经络系统中直行的主要干道；"络"是"网络"的意思，是"经"以下的各级分支，它们纵横交叉密布全身。人体的气血就在这个系统中运行，将多种营养物质周流不息地传注输布给全身各部的组织、器官，从而保证人体正常生理功能得以维持。通过经络的纵横联系与整体调节，人体各部相互配合，相互协调，从而完成抚御致病因素侵袭和保卫机体的正常功能的任务。

机体在病理状态下，经络又是病证的反应系统与疾病的传变途径。内脏的疾病可通过经络反映到体表，在患某些内脏疾病后，往往在体表的某一特定部位上出现压痛、过敏等病理反应，例如肾病腰痛，胃病背痛等。体表的损伤和疾病也可以通过经络系统，由浅入深地影响到体内多层次的组织器官。某一脏器的疾病如不及时防治，也可通过经络的表里属络关系，使其它脏器受病。

2. 任脉与督脉

任、督二脉与冲脉、带脉、阳跷脉、阴跷脉、阳维脉、阴维脉总称为奇经八脉。它们和十二正经不同，既不直接属脏腑，亦无表里相配。其生理功能主要是对十二经脉的气血起调节作用。

任脉行于腹、胸正中，上至颏部。全身阴经的经脉均来交会，故称"阴脉之海"。有调节诸阴经气的作用。

督脉行于腰、背、项正中，上至头面。全身阳经的经脉均来交会，故称"阳脉之海"。有调节诸阳经气的作用。

八脉中唯任、督二脉各有其专属的腧穴，其余六经皆没有自己的穴位，而以正经的腧穴为本经的穴位。由于任、督二脉有上述的生理功能和腧穴作用，故与十二经一起成为推拿疗法的基础之一。

4.2 腧穴概述

腧穴是人体经络、脏腑气血输注出入与聚集的部位。腧穴有以下3种：凡是有一定名称和一定位置，按十四经排列的腧穴叫"经穴"；而虽有明确位置与名称，但未列到十四经系统的称"经外奇穴"。此外，还有概无具体名称，又无固定位置，而以压痛点或其他反应点定取的穴位称"阿是穴"或"天应穴"。

无论何种腧穴都与经络有密切关系，腧穴通过经络与脏腑及全身组织密切相关。它不但可以反映脏腑与组织的生理或病理变化，为临诊时辨证、诊断以及制定推拿穴位与手法组方提供依据，而且还是推拿手法的刺激点。因此，对腧穴进行手法刺激，就可调动相应经络的调节作用，以调节脏腑、气血的功能，激发机体内在的抗病能力，从而达到防治疾病的目的。

推拿临诊时，取穴正确与否直接影响治疗效果。临床取穴，必需采用一定的取穴方法，才能准确定位。常用的取穴法有以下几种：

部位	起　止　点	量法	寸数	说　　明	
头部	前发际至后发际	直量	12	如前后发际不明，则可以从眉心量至大椎穴作18寸。眉心至前发际作3寸；大椎穴至后发际作3寸。	
胸腹部	两乳头之间	横量	8	用于胸腹部取穴横寸	
	剑突端至脐中	直量	8		
	脐中至耻骨联合上缘	直量	5		
背部	两肩胛内缘之间	横量	6	用于腰背部取穴横寸	
上肢	腋前纹头至肘横纹	直量	9	上肢内、外侧通用	
	肘横纹至腕横纹	直量	12		
下肢	股骨大转子至膝中	直量	19	用于大腿	用于下肢前、外、后侧
	膝中至外踝尖	直量	16	用于小腿	
	耻骨平线至股骨内髁上缘	直量	8	用于大腿	用于下肢，内侧
	胫骨内侧髁下缘至内踝尖	直量	13	用于小腿	

1. 骨度分寸取穴法

将人体各部，规定成一定的长度与宽度，折成若干等份，每1等份为1寸。用这种方法来折量取穴，就叫"骨度分寸法"。本法适用于任何年龄，任何体型的人。各部分分寸见下表及图（图50）。

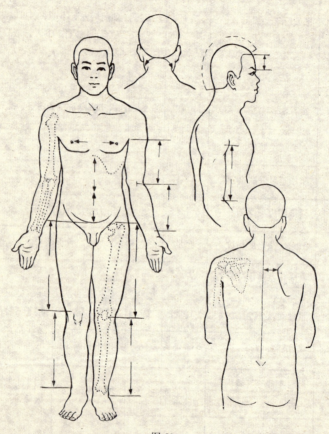

图 50

2. 指寸法

这是一种用患者手指测量取穴的方法，如患者身材与医者相仿，也可以依医生的手指来量取。一般以中指中节屈曲时两端纹头之间或拇指指间关节的横度为 1 寸；食指、中指、无名指、小指并拢时的近侧指关节之间的横度为 3 寸（图 51）。

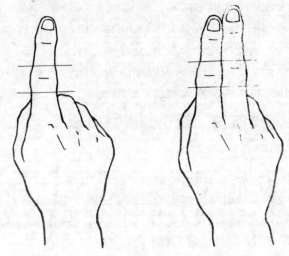

图 51-1

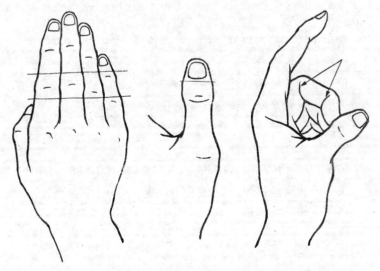

图 51-2

3. 解剖标志定位法

利用体表各种解剖标志为定穴依据，是最基本的取穴法。临床常用的大致可分为以下两种：

（1）定型标志：指不受人体活动影响而固定不移的标志，如五官、乳头、脐及各种骨节的突起或凹陷。

（2）活动标志：指需要采取相应的动作姿势才会出现的标志。如动作时肌肉的凹陷或隆起、肌腱显露、皮肤皱襞等。

4.3 十四经循行、常用腧穴及推拿手法

1. 手太阴肺经

本经起于中焦，内络大肠而属肺，其外行线自肺系横行浅出至中府穴，循上肢内侧桡侧缘，至拇指桡侧少商穴而终。从列缺分出的支脉，走向食指桡侧端与手阳明大肠经相联接互为表里。左右共 22 穴（图 52）。常用者如下：

中府
位置：前正中线旁开 6 寸，平第 1 肋间隙处。
主治：咳喘、胸闷、胸痛、肩背痛。
常用手法：一指禅推、按、揉、摩。

尺泽
位置：肘横纹中，肱二头肌腱桡侧。
主治：肘臂挛痛、咳喘、胸胁胀满、小儿惊风。
常用手法：按、揉、拿、一指禅推。

列缺
位置：以两手交叉，食指尽处，桡骨茎突上方，腕上 1.5 寸。
主治：头痛、口眼歪斜、半身不遂。
常用手法：按、掐。

鱼际
位置：第 1 掌骨中点，赤白肉际处。
主治：胸背痛、头痛眩晕、喉痛、发热恶寒。

中华全国中医学会常务理事
山东省卫生厅副厅长

张奇文

1990 年 3 月

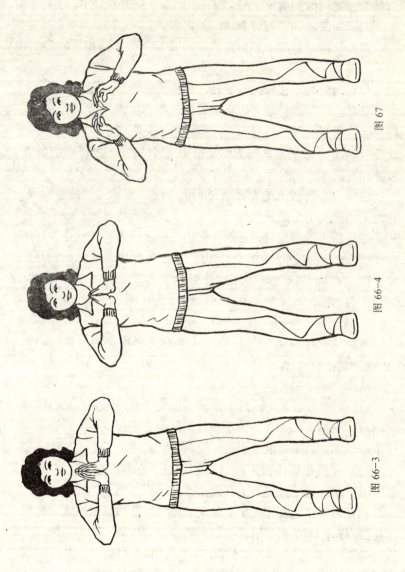

图 66-3

图 66-4

图 67

口唇微开，同时两臂侧平举，掌心向下，5指并拢。

(2) 两掌心向前慢慢合拢，指尖朝前。

(3) 徐徐将肘关节屈曲至90°，使腕、肘、肩相平，5指朝上。

(4) 两臂与手慢慢向内旋转，使指尖对胸与天突穴平。

要领：练习本势时，应全神贯注，各部肌肉放松，采用腹式顺呼吸，紧吸慢呼，鼻吸口呼，意守丹田，藏气于少腹。初练一次3分钟，1—2周后，每周酌量增1—2分钟，一般每次增至20分钟即可。

按语：本势久练能发展肩带肌肉与前臂旋肌的力量与耐力；并能锻炼腕关节的柔韧性，以使术者在手法操作时，增强肩部的悬吊支持能力，与前臂旋摆的持久力与灵活性。另外，当用在医疗性练功时，本势在动作 (1) 以后，也可改成以下练法：双手徐徐向前在胸前成抱球势，肩外展45°左右，5指微屈自然分开，掌心内凹，双手指端及劳宫穴相对 (图67)。

2. 摘星换斗势 (图68)

原文：只手擎天掌复头，更从掌内注双眸，鼻端吸气频调息，用力收回左右眸。

动作：预备姿势，立正。

(1) 右足向前外方向跨出，成丁字步，右足跟与左足内缘中点相对，间距约为1拳。两手同时动作，左手握空拳，屈肘向后靠于腰骶部；右手向前垂于右大腿内侧。

(2) 左腿屈膝徐徐下蹲 (屈约120°—160°左右)，同时，右足跟提起，足尖点地，上身保持正直，不可前倾后仰。

(3) 右手掌心朝下，5指握拢如钩状，自两腿间沿腹、胸中线缓缓举起，至头面部时，上臂内收，前臂外旋，钩手屈腕，呈肩前伸90°、屈肘90°、屈腕90°—100°的姿势，将右上肢停置于身体右侧。

(4) 钩手指端再尽量向外略偏，同时，头略向右上方抬起，双目注视掌心。

如练左手时，上述动作相反。

要领：屈膝下蹲时，膝不过足趾，全身重力主要落在后腿，前腿仅负体重 30% 左右。单手上举不要太高，以指尖离开头部约 1 拳为宜。5 指要捏齐，尽量令前臂与外旋指尖指向外侧，并尽力屈腕，将前臂与腕停置在产生酸、胀感觉的位置 10 秒钟左右。

然后，前臂与指尖回到中位停 10 秒钟左右，再向外旋转，如此反复练习直至规定的练功时间，即可收势。本势练时应神志专一。呼吸方法同韦驮献杵式，务使呼吸自然，旋臂发力时不得憋气屏息。初练 1 次 1—2 分钟，一周后每周每次增加 1 分钟，至 7 分钟后，每 2 周增加 1 分钟，一般每次练到 10—15 分钟即可。

按语：本势可增强下肢的支持能力；特别在发展胸大肌、三角肌、肱二头肌、前臂旋外肌及屈腕肌群的力量与持久力；拉长腕关节背侧韧带与前臂内旋肌，以发展其柔韧性与抗拉伸力。这对培养手法动作时肩部的持久支持力；一指禅推时悬腕的幅度与耐力；滚法时前臂内、外旋摆摆动的力度与速度，以及推拿医生长时间站立操作的工作能力等都十分重要。故本势在推拿专业练功中占重要地位，学习者一定要努力掌握，持之以恒，但要注意循序渐进，不可操之过急。

3. 倒拽九牛尾势（图 69）

原文：两腿后伸前屈，小腹运气空松，用力在于两膀，观拳须注双瞳。

动作：预备姿势，立正。

（1）上身向右转。

（2）右足向前跨出一大步成右弓步。上身正直，微向下沉，前腿曲膝 90°。

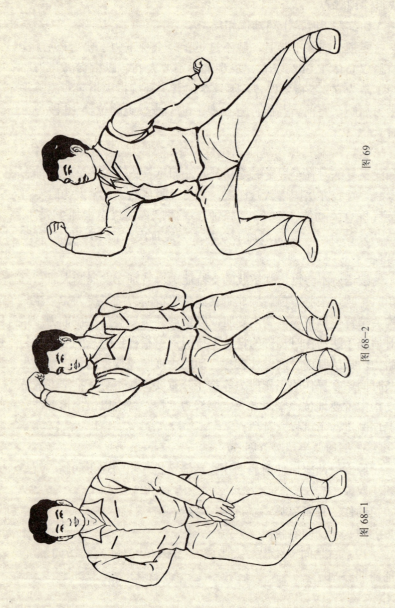

图 69

图 68-2

图 68-1

（3）两手握拳，前后伸出，拳心向上，两腕略屈，双肘屈曲140°—150°左右，前拳高不过眉，后拳平腰骶处。

（4）双目注视前手拳心，肘不过膝，膝不过足。前臂用力旋外，后臂同时用力旋内，前后两臂成绞绳状（称为螺旋劲）。含胸拔背、胸略内涵，藏气于少腹。

换步时向后转，上身转向左侧，动作左右相同。

要领：肩带肌肉始终保持放松，肩部不要抬起。两膀反复间歇用力，即双臂在作绞绳状拧旋时，在感到酸、胀、痛的位置停留10秒钟左右后，再间歇10秒钟左右发力。呼吸同上势。初练1次3分钟，1周后每周增加1分钟。一般增至8—10分钟即可。

按语：本势上要可发展前臂内、外旋肌的肌力、耐力与抗拉伸力，对㨰法、推法、擦法等动作的训练有很大帮助。

4. 三盘落地势（图70）

原文：上腭坚撑舌，张眸意注牙，足开蹲似踞，手按猛如擎，两掌翻齐起，千觔重有加，瞪睛兼闭口，起立足无斜。

动作：预备姿势，立正。

（1）左足向外横跨一步，两足与肩等宽，或略宽于肩。足尖微向内收。

（2）屈膝，臀部下蹲。同时，两手掌心朝上，自体侧沿胸徐徐上托与肩相平。

（3）然后，两手掌心翻转向下，缓缓下落，5指自然松开，如向下按物，至膝上悬空而驻，虎口朝里如握物状，上身稍向前俯。

（4）上身转为正直，前胸微挺，后背如弓，肩带肌肉松开，肩部不要抬起，肩关节外展约50度，肘尖指向外侧，前臂旋内，拇指外展，头项正直如顶物，双目直视，口唇微开，舌抵上腭，鼻息调匀。

要领：屈膝下蹲的深度，要视各人的负荷能力与练功基础而定，初练者可用高裆（约屈膝至 160°左右），以后渐渐可选用中裆（屈膝至 150°—140°左右）或转低裆（屈膝至 100°—120°左右）。下蹲时，上身始终保持正直，如正身坐在凳子上一样，不可前俯借力。屈膝时膝不可超过足尖。本势初练每次 1 分钟，以后每周增加 1 分钟，一般至 5 分钟即可。

按语：通过本势的锻炼，能使腋、臂的肌力与耐力充沛，抗拉伸力增强，下肢的持久支撑力发展，使手法动作时有一个稳固的下盘腿腰力量的支持而便于发力，且节省臂力。

5. 卧虎扑食势(图 71)

原文：两足分蹲身似倾，屈伸左右腿相更；昂头胸作探前势，偃背腰还似砥平。鼻息调元均出入，指尖着地赖支撑；降龙伏虎神仙事，学得真形也卫生。

动作：预备姿势、立正。

(1) 左足向前跨出一大步，屈膝 90°，右腿伸直用足尖蹬地，成左弓步。

(2) 两手向前 5 指撑地，掌心悬空，后腿足跟提起，头向上抬，双目向前平视。

(3) 前足收回向后伸直，将足背放在后足跟上，胸腹微收，躯干挺直，头向上昂起。

(4) 再全身后收，臀部向后突起，两肘挺直。然后，徐徐屈肘，头与躯干向前下方俯伸，如卧虎扑食之势，至头面部离地约 2 寸时，再缓缓伸肘，使头面与躯干向前上方慢慢抬起，接着再全身后收，臀部向后突起，成波浪形起伏往返动作。

要领：全部动作要缓缓进行，昂俯起伏动作过渡要自然，用柔和的悬劲与呼吸密切配合，在呼气时将上身向前慢慢推送，往返动作力求平衡，切勿屏气。换步时，左右相同。本势初练时，也可用 5 指与掌心同时着地支撑，在臂力与指力增强的基础上，再用 5 指着地，最后可用拇、食、中三指着地支撑则最佳。练习要量力而行，循序渐进。

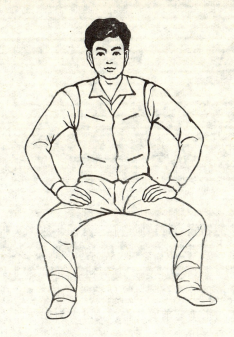

图 70

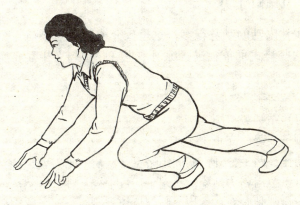

图 71-1

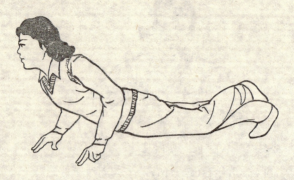

图 71-2

按语：本势能增强肩带诸肌、肱三头肌、肱二头肌的力量与耐力；特别是能发展手指的持久撑力与抗拉伸力，久练还能使手指的关节、韧带、关节囊等组织变得粗壮坚韧。这些素质的发展，能使术者在进行推、拿、点、按、擦、擦等手法操作时，发挥出强大而持久的指力与前臂的推拉力，并对防止手法时自身的运动创伤也有重要作用。

5.2 少林内功

少林内功的功势很多，这里仅介绍基本裆势与 4 个常用功势。这些势式可单独进行练习，也可联接起来相互变换进行锻炼。

1. 基本裆势

(1) 站裆势 (图 72)

预备姿势：立正。

动作：两足分开，其间距略宽于双肩，足尖朝里，双足成内八字。下肢用霸力站稳，头端平，目平视，呼吸自然，沉肩，挺胸，两肩胛骨向脊柱靠拢，腰间放松，少腹含蓄，臀部微收，两手叉腰，4 指在前，拇指在后待势。

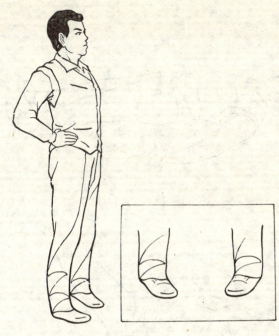

图 72

要领：霸力即双足以十趾用力抓地，同时，两足跟与大腿发力，使劲外旋，夹紧的用力方法。

(2) 马步势（图 73）

预备姿势：立正。

动作：两足分开，其间距较肩稍宽，两足成内八字，屈膝下蹲，膝不可向前超过足尖。头端平，目前视，挺胸直腰，臀部下沉不要向后突起，两手叉腰待势。

要领：下蹲的幅度分高裆、中裆与低裆（详见"三盘落地势"），可根据自己的身体与功力情况选择练习。

(3) 弓步势（图 74）

预备姿势：立正。

动作：两腿一前一后分开，两足之间距约较肩宽一倍；前腿屈膝，足尖向里，小腿约与地面垂直；后腿用劲挺直，足尖略外

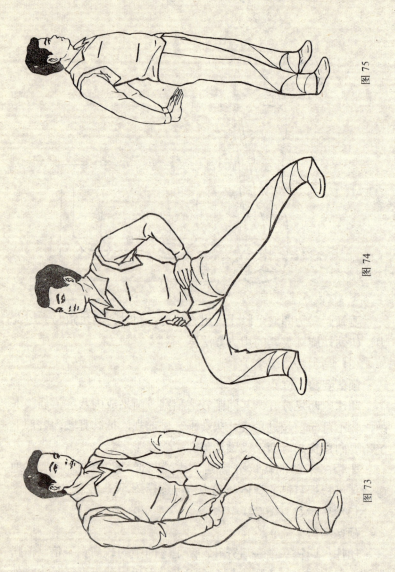

图 75

图 74

图 73

展。头端平，目平视，挺胸塌腰，蓄腹收臀，两手叉腰待势。

2. 少林内功常用功势

(1) 伸臂撑掌 (图75)

预备姿势：站势。

动作：站势数分钟后，叉腰的两手变俯掌 (掌心向下)，4指并拢伸直，拇指用力外展与4指约成直角，腕关节尽力背伸，双臂慢慢向后伸直，挺胸，两肩胛骨向脊柱夹紧，前臂用力旋前，使双手指尖向里，掌根朝外。肩部不要抬起，肩关节后伸约45°—30°，肘关节伸直。呼吸自然，以意运气，使气贯全身与四末。

要领：本势是少林内功主要的基础站桩功，练习时要注意"三直四平" (即臂直、身直、腿直；头平、肩平、掌平、脚平)。本势也可在马步势或弓步势的裆位上进行锻炼。初练从每次1分钟开始，以后根据情况慢慢增加练功时间，一般增至每次10分钟即可。

作用：本势久练能以意运气，练气生精，练精全神，使精神充沛，脏腑功能健全，并以气生劲，使劲力充实全身与四肢、增加臂、腰、腿部的力量与耐力。

(2) 前推八匹马 (图76)

预备姿势：站势。也可作马步或弓步势。两臂屈肘90°，掌心向上，拇指外展伸直与4指约成直角。

动作：

A. 蓄劲于双臂及指端，两臂徐徐用力前推，同时，慢慢旋内，使两掌相对，拇指向上、直至肘关节伸直，双臂与肩平齐。

B. 然后，再用力缓缓屈肘收臂，同时，双臂外旋，使掌心

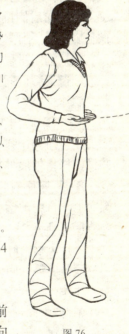

图76

朝上回到两胁。

要领：锻炼时，可按上述动作，来回推动 3—5 次，也可单臂动作，左右交替练习。呼吸与腿部用力方法与伸臂撑掌势同。

作用：久练能发展上肢运动时的下肢稳固的支撑能力与上下配合的协调功能，以利于上肢的发力与手法动作的顺利完成。

(3) 倒拉九头牛（图 77）

预备姿势：同上。

动作：

A. 两臂用力缓缓向前推进，同时，前臂慢慢内旋，至肘伸直时，两掌心向外，手背相对拇指向下。

B. 再变掌为拳，用力握紧，并徐徐曲肘收拳，同时前臂外旋，势如向后倒拉健牛状，至拳达两胁时，变拳为仰掌（还原至预备姿势）。稍作停顿后再重复上势动作，可反复 3—5 次。

(4) 霸王举鼎（图 78）

预备姿势：同上。

动作：

A. 两掌心向上，用力缓缓上举如托重物，过肩时双臂徐徐内旋，至肘向上挺直时，手指相对，掌心朝上，掌根朝外，4 指并拢，拇指外展伸直。

B. 蓄势片刻后，前臂渐渐旋外，翻掌使掌心与面相对，指端向上，自胸前蓄力而下，收回至腰胁两侧。稍待后，仍按上述姿势反复推举 3—5 次。

(5) 风摆荷叶（图 79）

预备姿势：同上

动作：

A. 仰掌向前上方徐徐用力推出，至肘伸直时，两掌在胸前交叉，左在右上或右在左上均可，两掌上下间距 1—2 寸。

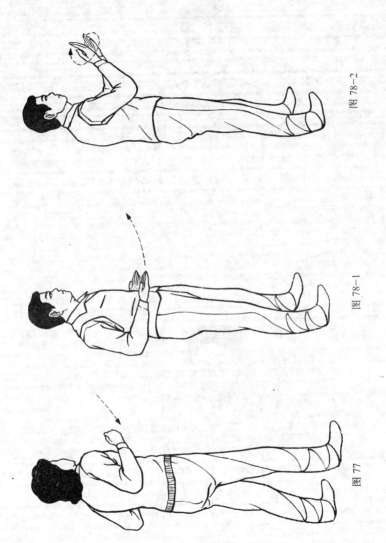

图 78-2

图 78-1

图 77

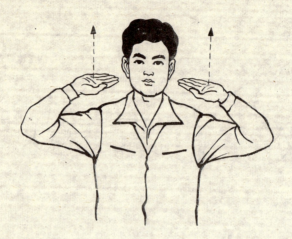

图 78-3

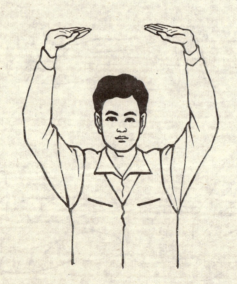

图 78-4

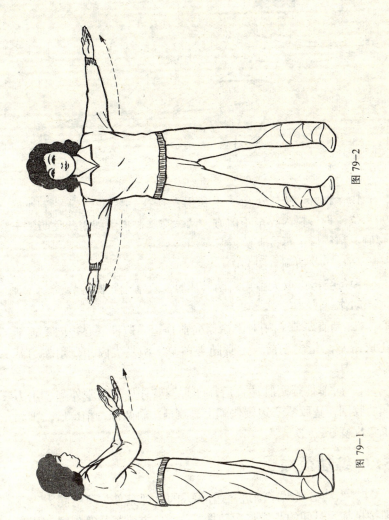

图 79-2

图 79-1

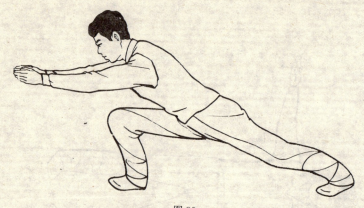

图 80

B. 两臂向左右分开，手掌仍保持托物状，至肩关节外展90°位，再慢慢内收至正前方，两掌交叉，再缓缓用劲收两掌至腰侧。稍待后，再按上势反复练习3—5次。

(6) 乌龙钻洞 (图80)

预备姿势：取大弓裆，两臂屈肘，直掌于腰侧待势。

动作：

A. 两直掌掌心相对，徐徐向前推运，边推掌心边向下逐渐化成俯掌，指尖朝前，上身随势前俯，两足尖内扣，用霸力站稳。

B. 向前推至两肘伸直后，即再双臂外旋，两掌外翻，用力屈肘收回，边收掌心边慢慢朝上，收至腰胁两侧。稍待后，再如上势反复3—5次。

5.3 练功须知

1. 练功必须循序渐进，根据各人的生理条件与负荷能力，合理按排练习时间的长短与运动量的强弱。并掌握从简到繁，从少到多，由弱渐强的原则。

2. 练功要持之以恒，每日坚持练功30分钟至1小时为宜，不可 3 天打渔 2 天晒网，时练时停。

3. 练功要功法专一，特别是初练者不能今天选练易筋经、少林内功，明天又练八段锦、大雁功。对于推拿学员必须以本章介绍的易筋经与少林内功为基本功法进行锻炼，待基本掌握，有了一定的功底后，方可再选练其它的功法。

4. 练功时要思想集中，心神合一，不开玩笑，不可屏气，不得勉强，蛮干，对练功中出现的任何问题如异常感觉、头晕、胸闷、胸痛、烦躁等情况，要及时求得教师的指导，以免发生练功偏差与损伤。

5. 练功的环境要保持安静，室内要光线充足，温度适宜，空气流通，但要避免寒风直接吹到身上。

6. 练功者的衣服宜宽松，不要穿得过多或过紧，不宜穿皮鞋或高跟鞋，要穿软底布鞋、球鞋或练功鞋。

7. 练功时间最好在早晨，练时不宜过饱或空腹；练功前不要剧烈运动；疲劳时不宜练功；练功完毕或中间休息时，应用干毛巾将汗擦干，穿好衣服，不可马上吹风或用冷水冲洗；不可吃生冷食物与饮料。练功后，要适当活动身体，以调和气血；可饮些温热茶水与营养饮料，以补充津液与养料。

8. 女子经期或孕期不宜练功。

（王国才）

6　成人常见病症治疗

6.1　感冒

感冒是四季常见的外感疾病，尤以冬春二季为多见，症状表现以头痛、鼻塞、流涕、恶风、发热等为特征。

病因病理：主要是由人体正气虚弱，气候突变，感受风寒或风热所致。冬季多属风寒，春季多属风热。

1. 风寒型：寒邪束表，毛窍郁闭，腠理不开，肺气不宣。

2. 风热型：风寒郁久化热，热郁肺卫，肺气失宣。

临床表现

1. 风寒型：恶寒发热，无汗、头痛，四肢酸痛，鼻塞，流涕，咳嗽，吐痰清稀，舌苔薄白，脉浮紧。

2. 风热型：身热，微恶风，汗出不畅，头痛且胀，咳嗽咯痰黄稠，咽痛，口干欲饮，舌苔薄黄，脉浮数。

治疗：

1. 治法：宣肺解表，风寒兼祛风散寒，风热兼疏风清热。

2. 手法：一指禅推法：抹、拿、按、揉。

3. 取穴：风池、风府、天柱、风门、肺俞、印堂、太阳、头维、合谷。

4. 操作：

(1) 推或按揉风府、风池、天柱、大杼、风门，反复5~7遍，穴位处操作时间略长。

(2) 推或按揉印堂、神庭、头维、太阳；印堂、鱼腰、太阳二线。

(3) 抹前额印堂至神庭及印堂至太阳二线，与头维、率谷，脑空，风池一线。

(4) 拿风池，项后大筋，肩井。

(5) 按揉风门、肩井、肺俞、最后拿肩井、合谷。

5. 加减:

(1) 风寒型加: 擦肩井、风门、肺俞，并用掌推法，将肩胛区推热。

(2) 风热型加: 推或按揉风府，大椎，掐揉合谷。

(3) 鼻塞不通加按揉迎香。

(4) 咽喉肿痛加掐少商，商阳。

(5) 咳痰不爽加: 揉天突、膻中。

6. 疗程: 每日 1 次,3 次 1 个疗程。

6.2 头痛

头痛是一种自觉症状,可见于多种急慢性疾病当中。

对颅内疾病中的脑脓肿,脑血管疾病急性期及颅内占位性病变,脑挫伤、外伤性颅内血肿的急性期不宜推拿。对其他疾病引起的头痛，一般均能通过推拿缓解症状，其中尤以偏头痛，肌收缩性头痛，感冒头痛，及高血压头痛疗效更为显著。

病因病理:

1. 劳逸失宜,起居不慎，六淫之邪乘虚而入，循经上犯，清阳受遏，而致外感头痛。

2. 暴怒伤肝;脾生痰浊，肾亏髓空。均可引起内伤头痛。

临床表现

1. 外感头痛: 头项强痛，发热严寒、遇风则剧、鼻塞流涕、舌苔薄白此为风寒头痛。头痛且胀，甚则头痛如裂、面红目赤、便秘尿赤、舌质红、苔黄，脉浮数，此为风热头痛。

2. 肝阳头痛: 头痛且胀，眩晕耳鸣，心烦易怒，失眠多梦、面红口苦，舌红，苔薄黄，脉弦有力。

治疗:

1. 治法: 疏风通络止痛。外感头痛宜散风祛寒止痛。内伤头痛宜平肝潜阳，活血化瘀，疏经活络。

2. 手法：推、拿、按、抹。

3. 取穴：印堂、头维、太阳、鱼腰、百会、风池、风府、天柱、肺俞、风门、合谷。

4. 操作：

(1) 患者坐势，医者站其背后，先推风池、风府、天柱等穴，时间约5分钟。

(2) 患者坐势，医者用一指禅，自印堂、鱼腰至太阳穴推5分钟，然后用按揉法，作用于角孙、百会等穴，约3分钟。

5. 加减：

(1) 风寒型头痛：加掐揉大椎、曲池、合谷。

(2) 风热型头痛：加按揉肺俞、风门。

(3) 肝阳头痛：加推桥弓，掐揉太冲。

6. 疗程：每日1次，6次1个疗程。

6.3 不寐

不寐又称失眠，其临床特点是初睡时难，睡时易醒，睡中多梦，严重者可通宵不眠。

病因病理

1. 思虑过度，伤及心脾，心伤则阴血暗耗，脾伤则无以生化精微，血虚难复，不能上养于心，致心神不安，而致失眠。

2. 饮食不节，肠胃受伤，宿食停滞，或积为痰热，壅遏于中，致胃气不和而不得安。其病理变化，总属阳盛阴衰，阴阳失交。

临床表现

1. 心脾不足：多梦易醒、心悸健忘，面色无华、四肢乏力，形体消瘦，精神不振，饮食欠佳，失眠或彻夜不眠，舌淡苔薄，脉细弱。

2. 阴亏火旺：头胀，耳聋耳鸣，心烦不眠，心悸不安，头晕健忘。

3. 胃中不和：失眠，脘腹胀满，不思饮食，呃逆，嗳气，睡不得安。

4. 病后虚弱：病后体虚不眠，面色㿠白，形瘦乏力，盗汗，自汗，睡后易醒。

治疗

1. 治法：实证宜疏肝清热,和中安神；虚证宜健脾益气，安神定志。

2. 手法：拿、抹、按、揉、搓。

3. 取穴：风池、风府、脑空、印堂、睛明、迎香、人中、承浆、角孙。

4. 操作

(1) 患者取坐势,医者站于患者背后，1 手扶向前额，另 1手 5 指张开，中指在督脉上，食指、无名指分别在足太阳膀胱区头部循行区，用 5 指拿法，自前发际至枕后部往返 3—5 次，随后拿风池、脑空，接着用两手拇指罗纹面交替抹颈部两侧胸锁乳突肌，自上而下 10～20 次。

(2) 患者取坐势，医者站于患者的正前方，两手拇指分别自印堂抹至神庭，按睛明，自攒竹抹至丝竹空，接着拇指分别按揉上穴 3～5 次，然后用拇指偏峰，自头维快速向角孙穴推去，交替进行按揉安眠二穴 1—2 分钟。

(3) 同上势，医者站于患者的左或右侧，1 手扶肩部，1 手擦胸部，左右往返，自上而下，随后换手擦背部。医者站于患者后，用双掌心擦两胁至热。

(4) 同上势，医者站在患者的前方，用右手拇指拿内关 50次，点揉大陵 50 次。

5. 疗程：每日 1 次，12 次 1 个疗程。

6.4 腹泻

腹泻，又称为"泄泻"，是指排便次数增多，粪便清稀，甚至泻下水样便。现代医学中由于胃、肠、肝、胆、胰等器官的功能和器质性的病变，如急、慢性肠炎等所引起的腹泻均属此范围。

病因病理

泄泻的主要病变在于脾胃与大、小肠。其致病原因是：外有感受外邪；内有饮食不节，脏腑虚表所致脏腑功能失调等；但主要在于湿邪困脾，脾胃虚弱，脾失健运、食物不能化为精微。水湿内生而致。

推拿治疗对脏腑虚衰或命门火衰而引起的久病久泄，有显著疗效。

临床表现

1. 脾胃虚弱：大便时溏时泄，完谷不化，反复发作，稍进油腻食物，大便次数明显增加，食欲不振、食后脘闷不舒，面色萎黄，精神倦怠、舌质淡苔白、脉缓弱。

2. 肾阳虚衰：黎明之前，脐周作痛，肠鸣而泻，泻后疼减、形寒肢冷、舌淡苔白、脉沉细。

治疗

1. 治法：健脾温肾,利湿止泻。

2. 手法：一指禅推、摩、按、揉、拿。

3. 取穴：中脘、气海、关元、天枢、足三里、脾俞、胃俞、大肠俞。

4. 操作：

(1) 患者取仰卧位，医者用轻揉缓和的按揉法，沿任脉的中脘、神阙、关元往返5—6次，然后逆时针方向摩腹，约3分钟。

(2) 取俯卧位，医生用擦法沿膀胱经，自上而下治疗,约2分钟，然后按揉肝俞、肾俞、脾俞、胃俞、大肠俞、以酌胀为度。

(3) 患者取仰卧位，下肢稍屈曲，医者用按揉法作用于足三里，约2分钟，再令患者取俯卧位，医者用1手拇指，自跟腱下方推至承山穴，并在该穴处重按，往返7～8次，然后，以同样的手法治疗另一侧。此法特别适用于单纯性消化不良引起的腹泻。

5. 加减

(1) 饮食不节加揉上脘。

(2) 肝气秉脾加揉肝俞、期门、章门。

(3) 脾肾阳虚加按京门、关元。

6. 疗程：每日1次，3次为1疗程。

6.5 胃脘痛

胃脘痛系指上腹部发生疼痛为主症的消化系统病症，包括现代医学所说的溃疡病，急慢性胃炎，胃痉挛，胃神经官能症，胆囊炎，胰腺炎，胆石症等。

病因病理

1. 病邪犯胃：外感寒邪，或过食生冷，寒积于胃，皆可使胃寒而作痛；或饮食不节，过食肥甘，内生湿浊，可发生热痛或食积痛。

2. 脏腑失调：肝气郁滞，失于疏泄，或由于脾胃素虚，劳倦过度，饥饱无度而致胃脘作痛。

临床表现

1. 寒邪犯胃：胃脘突然暴痛，畏寒喜温，局部得热则舒，口不渴，不喜饮，肠鸣泻水，苔白脉紧；食滞作痛：则症见胃部胀痛，嗳腐吞酸，吐后痛减，大便不爽、苔厚腻。

2. 脏腑失调：脾胃虚寒者表现为胃脘隐痛，泛吐清水，喜暖喜按，手足不温，大便溏薄，舌淡红，苔薄白，脉软弱或沉细，肝气郁结者表现嗳气，痛攻两胁，脉弦。

治疗

推拿对胃脘痛的治疗有显著的疗效。特别是脏腑失调而导致的胃痛，经一段时间的治疗，痛能消失。对急性胃痛者，在背部的压痛点或第 2 掌骨胃点，用较重的按法、揉法连续刺激 2 分钟左右即可使疼痛缓解。推拿对本病的治疗以理气止痛为临床通用之法，但是还需要进一步审证求因，辨证论治。如肝气郁滞者宜疏肝理气，脾胃虚弱者宜温中散寒，瘀血内停则宜活血化瘀。但胃及十二指肠溃疡出血期禁止推拿，以防大出血。

1. 胃脘暴痛的治疗

（1）取穴：阿是、肝俞、胆俞、脾俞、胃俞、足三里、内关，以及脾俞、胃俞附近的阿是穴。

（2）手法：按、揉、拿、振。

（3）操作：

A　病人取伏卧势，医者站在病人的右侧，以右手拇指循足太阳膀胱经，自上而下依次仔细触摸寻找脾俞和胃俞附近的压痛点，以右拇指面按压 1 分钟，再按揉脾俞、胃俞各 1～2 分钟，或待胃脘痛缓解而停止操作。

B　病人取仰卧势，医者坐于其右侧，以右手拇、食指掐拿双侧内关，足三里各 30～50 次，结束治疗。如果痛不止可以重复第一势，第二势，直至痛止。

（4）疗程：每日 1 次，3 次为 1 疗程。

2. 脾胃虚寒型的治疗

（1）取穴：上脘、中脘、关元、气海、膈俞、肝俞、脾俞、胃俞、足三里、内庭。

（2）手法：一指禅推法、按、振、摩、拿。

（3）操作：

A　患者取仰卧势，医者坐于患者右侧。先用轻快柔和的一指禅推法沿上脘、中脘、下脘，气海、关元反复操作 2—3 分钟。然后用右中指按在中脘穴上随呼吸起伏，逐步加重压力约 1

分钟。再按气海、关元各半分钟，摩中脘部 1 分钟。站立，用两手中指置腰部，拇指置脐旁天枢穴上，然后，双手拇指，中指相对用力拿 3～5 次，接用掌心置中脘作振法 2 分钟。

B 姿势同上，医者用右手拇指、中指相对用力拿足三里，内庭各 3—5 次，以局部酸痛为度。

C 患者取俯卧式，医者站其右侧，用一指禅推法，从背部足太阳膀胱经顺序而下，往返 4～5 遍，然后用适当的压力按揉肝俞、脾俞、胃俞、三焦俞，时间约 1～2 分钟。

(4) 疗程：每日 1 次，6 次为 1 疗程。

3. 肝气犯胃型的治疗

(1) 取穴：期门、章门、极泉、肩井。

(2) 手法：按、抹、拿、摩。

(3) 操作：

A 患者先取仰卧势，医者坐其右旁，用右手掌自肝区自上而下作摩法 2—3 分钟，然后按期门、章门各 1 分钟。

B 令患者端坐，两上肢上举抱头，医者站于患者身后，用双掌心自腋至髂前上嵴作抹法 40～50 次，拿极泉 3～5 次，拿肩井 3～5 次结束。

(4) 疗程：每日 1 次，6 次为 1 疗程。

6.6 中风偏瘫

偏瘫以半身不遂，口眼歪邪，语言塞塞等为主症，大多是由于高血压中风引起的后遗证，也可由其他脑部疾病，或外伤而引起。推拿能促进肢体功能的恢复，对本病具有不同程度的效果，早期治疗效果更显著。

病因病理

因风痰流窜经络，血脉痹阻，血瘀气滞，经脉不通，气不能行，血不能荣，故肢体废不能用；或因直接或间接的外力损伤脑部，使脑部骨碎膜破，血瘀阻络所致。

临床表现

单侧上下肢体瘫痪无力，口眼㖞斜，舌强语塞等。初期患者肢体软弱无力，知觉迟钝，活动功能受限，以后渐趋于强直挛急，日久患者肢体姿势常发生改变或畸形。

治疗

1. 治法：活血化瘀，行气筋舒。一般在中风发作后 2 周治疗。

2. 取穴：风池、肩井、肩髃、曲池、手三里、合谷、足三里；心俞、肝俞、肾俞、委中等。

3. 手法：一指禅推、㨰、按、点、捻、摇。

4. 操作：

(1) 患者取俯卧位，医者用㨰法施术于背部脊柱两侧膀胱经，自上而下 2 分钟，重点按揉心俞、肝俞、脾俞、肺俞、肾俞。然后用㨰法作用于臀部，大腿后侧，腘窝，小腿后面，重点按揉承扶、殷门、委中、承山、昆仑、太溪。以髋膝为重点，往返数次，作被动活动，如屈曲、内旋、外旋。

(2) 患者取仰卧位，医者坐于一侧，用㨰法在患侧上臂内侧，由前臂自上而下，以肩、肘、腕关节周围为重点，反复操作 3—5 分钟。在进行手法的同时，配合肩关节的外展，及肘关节的屈曲、继而进行腕关节屈伸活动及旋内旋外；然后用拇、食指，捻动其患肢的每个手指，以拇指为重点。

5. 疗程：隔日 1 次，15 次为 1 疗程。

6.7 痿证

痿证是指筋脉弛缓，软弱无力，因日久不能随意运动，出现肌肉萎缩，手足不用的一种疾病。临床上以下肢痿软较多见。在现代医学中，凡因运动神经系统或肌肉损害而引起的瘫痪，都属祖国医学痿证的范畴。例如多发性神经炎，脊髓炎，进行性肌萎缩，重症肌无力，周期性麻痹，肌营养不良症，癔性瘫痪和中枢神经感染的后遗症等。

病因病理

1. 感受风热：外受风热之邪，侵袭于肺，伤及肺之津液，筋脉失于濡润。

2. 湿热蕴蒸：湿热蕴蒸于内，则津亏无以利关节。

3. 肝肾亏虚：病体虚弱，房室过度，肝肾精气亏虚，而无以濡养筋脉。

临床表现

1. 肺热伤津：多在温病之后，肢体突然痿弱不用，证见心烦口渴，便秘尿赤，舌质红苔黄，脉细数。

2. 肝肾亏虚：多在久病之中，肢体渐见软弱，或下肢不用，肌肉削瘦，腰膝酸软，头晕目眩，脉细数。

3. 脾胃虚弱：大病久病之后，渐见下肢痿弱不用，神疲乏力，食少便溏，面色少华，舌淡，苔薄白，脉濡细。

4. 湿热阻滞：下肢痿 瘦 微肿，麻木不仁，胸脘满闷，身黄面黄，小便赤涩热痛，舌红，苔黄腻，脉濡数。

治疗

1. 治法：

养阴益胃，兼调肝、脾、肾3脏。

2. 取穴：肩髃，曲池，合谷，阳溪，髀关，伏兔，梁丘，足三里，解溪等。

3. 手法：擦、按、揉、点。

4. 操作：

(1) 患者取仰卧位，医者坐于一侧，左手握患肢，右手沿手阳明大肠经的肩髃、曲池、合谷、阳溪，用擦法，治疗3～4分钟，然后再用按、揉法在各穴施术1分钟，点各穴半分钟，做上肢的屈伸动作。

(2) 同上势，医者用擦法沿下肢胃经的走行方向，自上而下施术3—4分钟。然后按揉髀关、梁丘、足三里、解溪，约1～2

分钟。掐足趾的各趾甲根部及指间关节，捻各指，自上而下反复7～8次。

5. 加减：

(1) 肺热伤津者：加掐揉曲池、合谷、三阴交。

(2) 脾胃虚弱者：加揉脾俞、胃俞、手三里、足三里。

(3) 肝肾亏虚者：加揉肝俞、肾俞、悬钟、阳陵泉。

(4) 湿热阻滞者：加揉脾俞，丰隆。

6. 疗程：隔日 1 次，15 次为 1 疗程。

6.8 痹证

痹证是指气血为病邪阻闭而引起的疾病。

病因病理

当人体肌表经络受风、寒、湿之邪侵袭之后，气血为邪气所阻，经脉痹阻，气血不畅，引起肢体、关节、筋脉等处疼痛，酸楚、麻木、重着等症状。

临床表现

1. 风寒湿痹：四肢关节或腰背部疼痛，活动则疼痛加重，局部无红肿现象或兼有恶风，疼痛呈游走性或局部怕冷，得热则舒或肢体有沉重感。舌苔白腻，脉紧或弦。

2. 风湿热痹：关节红肿，疼痛，得冷则舒，疼痛拒按，关节活动受限，伴有发热，口渴咽干，舌苔黄燥，脉滑数。

治疗

1. 治法：风寒湿痹以祛风，散寒，利湿为主。风湿热痹以疏通经络为辅助治疗。

2. 取穴：肩井、曲池、合谷、环跳、阴陵泉、阳陵泉、鹤顶、昆仑、风池、大椎、肺俞、肾俞、大肠俞、小肠俞等。

3. 手法：擦、点、按、揉、擦。

4. 操作：

(1) 据病变所在关节而选择适当的手法治疗，然后用捻法、拔伸法。有活动障碍者，可配合作关节功能活动。

(2) 一般先用一指禅推法或撩法在患部周围的腧穴轻快柔和地操作 3～5 分钟，再逐步移到病变关节，最后按大椎 20～30次，拿曲池、合谷，各 5 次。

5. 加减：

(1) **热痹**：加掐揉大椎、曲池、合谷。

(2) **行痹**：加按揉百合、风府、风池。

6. 疗程：每日 1 次，12 次为 1 疗程。

6.9 高血压

在安静的状态下，收缩压 20kPa 或以上或舒张压为 12kPa或以上者，就是高血压。其主要表现有头胀、头晕等。高血压分为原发性和继发性两种。

病因病理

长期精神紧张或恼怒忧思，使肝气内郁，郁久化火，耗损肝阴，阴不敛阳，肝阳上亢；或由于年老肾亏，肾阴不足，肝失所养，肝阳偏亢；过度进食肥甘或饮酒过度，致痰湿内生，久而化热，灼津成痰，痰浊阻络，而致本病。

临床表现

头晕头痛且胀最为多见，耳鸣目眩，烦躁易怒，胸闷心悸，面红目赤，手指发麻，口干咽燥，便秘尿赤，舌红苔黄，脉弦数。

1. 痰湿中阻：头晕而重，头痛昏蒙，胸脘痞闷、泛泛欲呕，甚吐痰涎，舌苔白腻。脉弦滑。

2. 肝阳上亢：头晕头痛、面红目赤、口苦，性情急躁，易于发怒。

3. 阴阳两虚：眩晕头痛，耳鸣心悸，行动气急，腰酸膝软，失眠多梦，夜间多尿，舌淡或红，苔白，脉弦细。

治疗

1. 治法：平肝潜阳，化痰降浊。

2. 取穴：百会、四神聪、风池、肩井、桥弓穴。

3. 手法：按、揉、掐、拿。

4. 操作：

(1) 患者取坐位，医者用按揉法在百会处施术，然后掌摩头部，重按四神聪，约5～6分钟。再用拇指、食指捏拿风池穴，最后拿肩井数次。

(2) 患者伏卧位，医者用小鱼际擦法，沿背部膀胱经，自上而下施术，往返数10次。

(3) 患者坐位，医者站于一侧，一手扶患者头部，一手用食中指单程向下推桥弓穴，自耳后翳风，到缺盆连成一直线，反复治疗约5分钟，然后再治疗另一侧。

5. 加减：

(1) 头痛头晕甚者：加掐揉行间、神门、少海。

(2) 失眠神疲，面色萎黄者：加掐揉足三里、三阴交。

6. 疗程：每日1次，15次为1疗程。

注意事项

在推拿桥弓穴时应单侧操作，切不可双侧同时进行。

6.10 呃逆

膈下气逆上冲，喉间呃呃有声，声短而频，阵阵发作，难以自制。

病因病理

饮食不节，积于中焦，伤及脾胃，胃失和降，上冲而致；恼怒伤肝，肝失条达，气机不利，痰浊滋生，肝木克脾，挟痰上逆，胃膈气逆；或久病体虚，胃阴不足，胃失所养而致。

临床表现

1. 虚证呃逆：呃逆低微，面色苍白，食少困倦，气短心慌，语言无力，舌淡苔白，脉沉细无力。

2. 实证呃逆：呃声响亮，连续有力，胸胁胀痛，口臭烦渴，便结尿赤，舌苔黄，脉滑数。

3. 寒证呃逆：呃声低沉无力，气不得缓，得热则缓，饮食减少，口不渴，肢体不温，遇寒加重，舌苔白润，脉迟缓。

4. 热证呃逆，呃声响亮，口臭心烦，喜冷饮，口干舌燥，面红目赤，舌红苔黄，脉数。

治疗

1. 治法以和胃降逆为主。

2. 取穴：攒竹、鱼腰、缺盆、膻中、中脘、膈俞、胃俞、大肠俞、中魁、足三里、丰隆、内关。

3. 手法：掐、按、揉、摩、一指禅推。

4. 操作：

(1) 患者取仰卧位，医者坐于一侧，用双手拇指甲先掐双侧攒竹及鱼腰穴各1分钟。若呃逆止，用轻快柔和的一指禅推法在膻中、中脘各推1～2分钟，顺摩中脘3～5分钟，拿足三里，丰隆各3～5次。

(2) 患者取俯卧位，医者用右手拇指作一指禅推法于膈俞、胃俞，推3～4分钟，最后用中指，重点前穴各3～4次，按揉大肠俞，20～40余次。

(3) 患者取坐位，医者用左手握患者左手使其中指屈曲，用拇指甲掐其中第2指间关节桡侧中魁穴1分钟；拿缺盆3～5次，内关3～5次，结束治疗。

5. 疗程：每日1次，3次为1疗程。

6.11 癃闭

癃闭是指排尿困难，甚至小便闭塞不通的一种病症。

病因病理

其发病主要是由于膀胱和三焦气化失常，与肺脾肾三脏功能失调有关。肺热壅盛、膀胱湿热，肾阳不充，肺肾气虚，小便传送无力；跌打损伤，瘀血凝聚，也可引起本病。

临床表现

1. 膀胱湿热：小便不利，点滴不通，或量少而短赤，灼热，小便胀满，大便不畅，舌红，苔黄腻，脉濡数。

2. 肺热壅盛：小便不畅，或点滴不通，口燥咽干，烦渴欲饮，呼吸急促，舌红，苔黄脉数。

3. 肾阳虚亏：小便点滴不畅，排出无力，大便难下，下腹寒冷，腰膝酸软，面色㿠白，舌淡胖嫩，苔白，脉沉细。

治疗

1. 治法宜疏利气机，通利小便。

2. 手法：按、揉、推。

3. 取穴：利尿穴、丹田、三阴交、箕门。

4. 操作：

(1) 病人取仰卧位，首先嘱病人情绪稳定，医者站于一侧，用中指在脐至中极连线的中点，即利尿穴，作按法，由轻到重，逐渐加大压力，到病人能耐受的程度，轻压或中按即行排尿，就不必重按，待排尿停止，再将中指慢慢放开。如不排尿，加丹田穴 3—5 分钟。

(2) 患者同上势，下肢伸直，并稍外展外旋。医者先在患者的下肢内侧撒一薄层滑石粉，然后自膝内侧经箕门穴推向腹股沟处 1000 次，推后 10 分钟，令病人排尿。

(3) 拿三阴交 3~5 次，摇两踝关节各 5~10 次结束治疗。

5. 疗程：每日 1 次，3 次为 1 疗程。

6.12 便秘

便秘指大便秘结，排便困难、间隔时间延长。便秘的发生主要是由于大肠传导功能失常，粪便在肠内停留过久，水份过于吸收，而使粪质过于干燥所致。

病因病理

素体阳盛，嗜食辛热厚味，以致胃肠积热；或热病之后，余热留恋。耗伤津液，或年老体弱气血双虚，气虚则大肠传导无力，血虚则津少，而致便秘。

临床表现

1. 实秘；大便干结，小便短赤，面红身热，或兼有腹胀，口干心烦，或嗳气频作，胸胁痞满，纳减，苔黄燥，质红，脉滑数。

2. 虚秘：便秘或不畅，大便稍干，排便时努争，便后疲乏，甚至汗出气短，面白神疲，舌淡苔薄，脉弱，或小便清长，四肢不温，腰膝冷痛，或腹中冷痛等。

治疗

1. 治法：实秘宜清热润肠，顺气行滞；虚秘宜益气养血，温通开秘。

2. 手法：摩、按、揉、擦。

3. 取穴：天枢、中脘、神阙、气海、脾俞、胃俞、肝俞、大肠俞、八髎、长强、支沟、承山。

4. 操作：

(1) 患者取仰卧位，医者坐于一侧，先用掌摩法顺时针方向摩腹，约5分钟，然后用按揉法作用于天枢、中脘、神阙、气海，约2分钟。

(2) 患者取俯卧位，医者用小鱼际，自腰间向尾骨方向擦，约2分钟，再按揉脾俞、肾俞、大肠俞数次。

(3) 患者坐位，医者用掐揉法作用于支沟上巨虚，约3分钟，结束治疗。

5. 疗程：每日1次，6次为1疗程。

6.13 心绞痛

心绞痛是以胸骨后心前区出现阵发性或持续性疼痛为主的一种病症，属胸痹范畴。

病因病理

祖国医学认为本病的发生与年老体衰，肾气不足；或膏粱厚味，损伤脾胃；或情志不畅，气机郁结，气滞血瘀等因素有关。

临床表现

1. 气滞血瘀，心络受阻：阵发性心前区刺痛、痛引肩背，胸闷憋气，呼吸困难，舌质暗、舌边尖有瘀点，脉沉涩或结。

2. 胸阳不振：胸闷憋气，阵发性心痛，心悸气短，呼吸困难，面色苍白，体倦乏力，畏寒肢冷或自汗，夜寐不安，食欲不振，小便清长，大便稀薄，舌淡胖嫩，苔白润或腻，脉沉缓或结代。

3. 阴阳两虚：胸闷心痛、夜眠有时憋醒，心悸气短，头晕耳鸣，食少，四肢倦怠无力，腰酸肢冷，手心发热，小便频数，舌质紫暗，苔白少津，脉细弱或结代。

治疗

1. 治法：活血化瘀，行气通络。

2. 手法：摩、按、揉、点。

3. 取穴：云门、中府、乳根、期门、章门、极泉、厥阴俞、肺俞、心俞、肝俞、肾俞、命门、内关、大陵、涌泉。

4. 操作

(1) 患者取仰卧位，医者坐于左旁，用右手掌心摩中府、云门、期门、章门，自上而下5分钟，速度宜缓，宜轻，但要着实；再轻拿极泉3～5次。

(2) 同上势，医者左手握其左手，用拇指按揉内关、大陵各50次。医者站到患者右旁，按揉其右内关，大陵各50次。

(3) 患者取坐势或侧卧势，医者站其一旁，用一指禅推法，推肺俞、厥阴俞、心俞、肝俞、肾俞各100次。

5. 加减：

(1) 痰浊阻遏者：加揉足三里300次，脾俞、胃俞各300次。

（2）阴阳两虚者：加摩肾俞、命门各 300 次搓涌泉 300 次。再用掌心摩左上背部，相当于厥阴俞及心俞区 5 分钟，轻按两穴各 3～5 次。结束治疗。

6. 疗程：每日 1 次，15 次为 1 疗程。

注意事项

手法必须轻柔，治疗时不宜俯卧位，否则使胸闷，心悸加重。

6.14 胆绞痛

胆绞痛是消化系统疾病的常见症状，经常发生在急性胆囊炎，胆石症、胆道蛔虫症等疾病之中，属祖国医学"胁痛"范围。

病因病理

胆与肝相表里，与肝同具疏泻功能，以通降下行为顺；凡忧郁恼怒，使肝胆气郁，或饮食不节，脾胃运化失健，湿热郁结中焦，均影响通降之功，致胆气不利而痛。

临床表现

1. 气郁型：胁痛多为胀痛或绞痛或阵发性串痛，口苦咽干，不欲饮食，舌尖微红，苔薄白或微黄，脉弦紧。

2. 湿热型：胁部持续胀痛、或偶有阵发性疼痛，口苦，头晕，寒热往来，目黄身黄，小便黄浊或赤涩，大便秘结，饮食不佳，胃部有灼热感和嗳气等消化不良症状。

治疗

1. 治法：疏肝理气，活血化瘀。

2. 手法：按、揉。

3. 取穴：膈俞、肝俞、胆俞、鸠尾、章门、胆囊穴。沿背部膀胱经寻找阿是穴。

4. 操作：

（1）病人取俯卧势，医者站其一侧，用右手中指在背部足太阳膀胱经上仔细触摸，找出其背部压痛点，轻按之。同时，左手中指放在鸠尾穴，向上按 2～3 分钟。待痛止，再轻按膈俞、胆俞、肝俞各 3～5 次。

(2) 患者取仰卧势，医者坐于一侧，用右手中指按、揉章门、期门约 2～3 分钟，以轻度酌疼为度。

(3) 患者姿势同上，医者用双手拇指面分别重按两侧胆囊穴 50 次。

5. 加减：

(1) 恶心欲吐，加揉内关、中脘。

(2) 背部及肩胛部放射痛加揉肩贞、秉风、肩井。

(3) 大便秘结加揉天枢、神阙。

6. 疗程：每日 1 次，6 次为 1 疗程。

注意事项

1. 病人应安静休息，心情舒畅。

2. 注意体温变化，病情加剧时应及时配合药物治疗。

6.15 乳腺炎

乳腺炎多发生在产后哺乳期，初产妇最多。

病因病理

由于肝气郁结，胃热壅滞；复因乳头破损，凹陷，乳汁积滞，火毒之邪乘机入侵，致使经络阻塞，气滞血凝而发病。

临床表现

1. 肝郁型：乳房胀痛，有肿块，压痛，皮色不红，可伴有易怒、口苦、纳差等症状，苔薄白，脉弦。

2. 胃热型：乳房结块，红肿热痛，可形成乳房肿疡，发热恶寒，口干舌燥，大便秘结，舌苔黄，脉弦数或滑数。

治疗

乳痈治疗一般分初起，脓成，和已溃 3 个阶段，推拿治疗一般在乳痈初期尚未成脓时。

1. 治法：疏肝理气，消肿通络。

2. 手法：摩、抹、捏挤。

3. 取穴：乳根、乳中、期门、膻中、少泽、合谷、肝俞、脾俞，胃俞。

4. 操作

（1）患者取仰卧势，医者坐患侧旁，用一手大鱼际在肿块四周作揉法，速度快，手法轻重适当，揉5分钟，用双手拇、食指置肿块的四周，轻轻捏揉，用中指揉乳根，乳中、期门各1分钟。

（2）患者取坐势，医者相对而坐，在患处涂上滑石粉，医者用左手扶乳房，用右手的拇指、食指向乳头方向捏挤2分钟，捏挤时手法要轻快、熟练、有节奏感。此治法可使瘀积的乳汁排出，直至见到黄色乳汁为止。

（3）患者取俯卧位，医者站于一侧，用拇指面推肝俞、脾俞、胃俞穴各1分钟，再用拇指面按揉上穴各3~5次。

5. 疗程：每日1次，3次为1疗程。

注意事项

1. 保持心情舒畅，注意乳头清洁。

2. 哺乳期应按时哺乳，注意哺乳儿的口腔卫生，若有乳头皲裂应及时治疗。

3. 成脓后不采用推拿疗法。

6.16 痛经

痛经症状的特点是在月经前后或经期发生下腹部胀痛，腰膝酸软。严重者影响工作和生活。

病因病理

内伤七情，寒邪外袭，饮食生冷，均可引起气血运行不畅，而致痛经。

临床表现

1. 气滞型：经前或经期小腹作胀，疼痛拒按，经量少或经行不畅，乳房胀痛，头痛或偏头痛，舌红，脉沉涩。

2. 寒湿型：经前或经期少腹冷痛，遇寒则甚，经量少，色淡或暗红，有血块，苔白润而腻，脉沉紧。

3. 气血两虚型：经后小腹隐隐作痛，喜按，经量少而色淡，质稀，神疲乏力，面色苍白，舌淡苔白，脉沉细弱。

治疗

1. 治法：行气化瘀，温经散寒，补气养血。

2. 手法：一指禅推，按，摩，擦。

3. 取穴：素髎、关元、气海、肾俞、八髎、合谷、三阴交。

4. 操作：

(1) 患者仰卧位，医者用掌摩法作用于小腹部，约7~8分钟，以患者感到有热感为宜，然后按揉气海、关元3~5次，用中指按鼻尖素髎作揉法1分钟。

(2) 患者取俯卧位，医者先在八髎处用双手点按法，约3分钟，然后用小鱼际擦法作用于八髎部位，最后按压肾俞。

(3) 医者用掐法作用于合谷、三阴交，各约2分钟。

5. 加减：

(1) 气虚者摩腹用逆时针方向，气滞者用顺时针方向。

(2) 伴有恶心欲呕者，加推中脘、内关、膻中。

(3) 肝气郁滞者加按揉肝俞、期门。

6. 每日1次，6次为1疗程。

6.17 产后身痛

产后肢体酸痛，麻木不适，称"产后身痛"。

病因病理

产后气血虚弱，血不养筋；风寒湿邪乘虚而入，阻遏经脉，闭塞不通而致疼痛。

临床表现

1. 气血虚弱：四肢酸痛麻木、面色无华，舌淡苔少，脉细弱。

2. 外感风寒湿邪；肢体疼痛，游走不定，或着重肿胀，舌淡苔薄白，脉细数。

治疗

1. 治法：补养气血，温经散寒。

2. 手法：按、揉、掐、拿。

3. 取穴：肩井、脾俞、胃俞、肾俞、手三里、内关、外关、合谷、曲池、足三里、承山。

4. 操作：

(1) 患者取俯卧位，医者按揉脾俞、胃俞、肾俞约 3 分钟，在下肢再用轻柔的擦法自上而下擦 2～3 分钟，按足三里、拿承山 3～5 次。

(2) 患者取坐位，医者掐揉患者手三里、曲池、内关、外关、合谷、肩井穴约 5 分钟，拿肩井 2～3 次，结束治疗。

5. 疗程：每日 1 次，5 次为 1 疗程。

6.18 产后腹痛

产后小腹疼痛，称为产后腹痛。

病因病理

冲任空虚，气血虚弱，瘀血内结；气血虚弱、寒邪乘虚而入，瘀血内阻，而致病。

临床表现

1. 血虚型：少腹绵绵作痛，喜按，恶露量少色淡，头晕目眩，爪甲不荣，面色苍白，便秘，神疲乏力，舌淡苔薄，脉虚细无力。

2. 血瘀型：少腹疼痛拒按，得温则舒，四肢不温，恶露量少有瘀血，舌暗紫，苔白滑，脉沉涩。

3. 寒凝型：少腹冷痛，喜按喜温，四肢不温，恶露量少，舌黯淡，苔白滑，脉沉紧。

治疗

1. 治法：补益气血，活血化瘀，温经散寒。

2. 手法：摩、按、揉、擦。

3. 取穴：关元、石门、三阴交、大赫、脾俞、肾俞、命门、八髎、十七椎。

4. 操作：

（1）患者仰卧位，医者用摩法作用于患者小腹部，约5分钟。然后按压关元、石门、三阴交、大赫2分钟。

（2）患者俯卧位，医者用指揉法作用于脾俞、肾俞、命门、八髎、十七椎约5分钟。然后用掌擦法作用于八髎，以有热感为度。

5. 疗程：每日1次，7次为1疗程。

6.19　牙痛

牙痛是一个症状，现代医学认为多是由龋齿、牙髓炎、牙周炎等疾病引起。

病因病理

祖国医学认为过食辛辣肥厚之品，可使胃热内蒸，郁而化火，上攻而致牙龈肿痛；肾阴不足，虚火上炎，也可引起本病。

临床表现

1. 胃火牙痛：牙痛剧烈；口臭，便秘，舌苔黄腻，脉数有力。

2. 风火牙痛：痛甚且肿，形寒肢冷，脉浮。

3. 肾虚牙痛：隐隐作痛，时发时止，牙齿松动，脉细。

治疗

1. 治法：清胃泻火，疏风清热，滋阴泻火。

2. 手法：按、揉、掐、捏、拿。

3. 取穴：颊车、下关、内庭、合谷、外关、风池、太溪、行间。

4. 操作:

(1) 患者取坐位，医者站于一旁，左手固定头部，右手按颊车，下关2～3分钟，再揉2～3分钟。

(2) 姿势同上，医者用右手拿其合谷，若左侧痛甚，先拿右侧合谷1～2分钟，痛即能缓。

(3) 患者取坐势，双下肢伸平，医者掐其内庭、太溪或行间。

5. 疗程: 每日1次，3次为1疗程。

6.20 咽炎

咽炎的特点是: 咽干，咽痛，有异物感。

病因病理

外感风热，重灼肺系或胃系，郁热循经上犯，而致咽喉肿痛，此为实证；肾阴亏虚，虚火上炎，也可致咽痛，此为虚证。

临床表现

1. 实热型: 咽部疼痛、口燥欲饮、口臭龈肿，胃脘灼热疼痛，舌绛苔黄腻，脉滑数。

2. 阴虚型: 咽干喉痒，语言低微嘶哑，口渴喜饮，干咳无痰或痰少，舌红苔少或无苔，脉细数。

治疗

1. 治法: 清热利咽，滋阴降火。

2. 手法: 拿、揉、掐。

3. 取穴: 风池、天柱、人迎、廉泉、曲池、合谷、少商、商阳。

4. 操作:

(1) 患者坐位，医者位于后面，用左手扶住患者额部，右手拇指、食指在风池、天柱穴施用拿法，约4～5分钟，以患者感到分泌物增多为止，然后轻揉人迎、廉泉，约2分钟。

(2) 同上势，医者掐揉曲池、合谷、少商、商阳，治疗约5

分钟。

5. 加减：

(1) 肾虚牙痛加掐揉太溪、照海。

(2) 肺胃热盛，而致大便秘结者加掐揉丰隆、支沟。

6. 疗程：每 3 次为 1 疗程，每日 1 次。

（乔建君）

6.21　肱二头肌长头肌腱滑脱

　　肱二头肌长头肌腱起自肩胛骨盂上结节，向下跨过肱骨头，穿过肩横韧带和肱二头肌腱鞘的伸展部，藏于结节间沟的骨纤维管内。正常情况下该腱在肩关节活动时，只有纵向滑动而无左右移位运动。

病因病理

　　当由于先天性小关节发育不良，结节间沟内侧壁坡度变小；局部退行性变，骨质增生等原因所致肩横韧带松弛、二头肌长腱弛缓或延长，结节间沟底部沟床变浅；或者肩关节外伤而产生肩横韧带撕裂，胸大肌和肩胛下肌抵止部的急慢性撕脱时，如果上臂作过度的外展与外旋运动，就有可能将保护二头肌长腱的软组织撕脱，而使该腱向沟内侧移位；或自沟内脱出（图 81）；或该腱与肌联合附近的较粗部位嵌于腱管内而造成本症。

临床表现

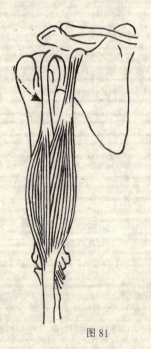

图 81

肱二头肌长腱滑脱，临床上多见有习惯性和外伤性2种。前者虽为慢性，但多因轻度外伤而致，且易经常复发。当急性外伤所致肱二头肌长腱脱位后，当即显示肩前部疼痛，肱骨呈内旋位，关节丧失外展、内收、外旋、内旋等各方面的功能活动，走路时伤肢不能前后摆动，以健手托住患肢前臂，保持肘关节屈曲位，以减少活动或上肢重量所造成的疼痛。

治疗

习惯性或外伤性肱二头肌长腱滑脱，采用推拿治疗，均有疗效。但前者治疗后多易复发，必要时应采用手术缝合；外伤性滑脱推拿效果较为理想。但由于肩关节脱位或肱骨颈骨折所致之肱二头肌长头腱脱位者，则需采取骨科整复疗法。

1. 治法：理筋整复，舒经活血。

2. 手法：一指禅推、揉、搓、拔伸等。

3. 取穴：肩髃、肩井、臂臑、曲池、手三里、外关、合谷等。

4. 操作：

(1) 患者正坐，医者立于患者对侧。右手4指放于患者患肩上部，掌心向下，拇指按放在三角肌前缘中部，即肱二头肌长腱外，并用力抵住肱骨颈部。左手握患肢腕部，使其掌心向前，肩外展至60度，前屈40度。

(2) 两手作对抗牵引，同时将患者前臂逐渐旋后，并把肩放回至40度外展位，使放下的前臂尽量旋后。此时，右手拇指用力向外上方推、按滑脱的肱二头肌长腱，同时左手将患肢作急剧旋前活动（图82）。

(3) 以拇指轻轻推、揉肱二头肌长腱处3～5分钟，然后以双掌在患肩周围作轻柔的搓揉手法。

必要时，可将患肢在内旋、内收位用三角巾悬吊2～4周，再作肩关节适当的运动练习，以免局部粘连。

5. 疗程：每日1次，3次为1疗程。

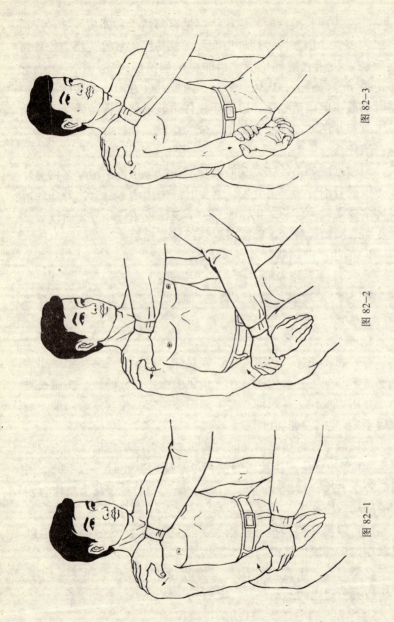

图 82-1

图 82-2

图 82-3

6.22 肱二头肌长头肌腱腱鞘炎

肩关节作外展、外旋活动时，肱二头肌长腱在其腱鞘内滑动的幅度最大。

病因病理

长期用力作肩部外展、旋外活动，使肌腱与腱鞘产生反复磨擦，引起炎症反应；或因突然牵扯而致损伤，使肌腱与腱鞘产生损伤性炎症，出现腱鞘水肿、变性、肥厚、粗糙与纤维变，在腱鞘与肌腱之间有时有纤维粘连，导致本病的发生。

临床表现

局部疼痛并向三角肌下放散，肱二头肌长腱处有锐利压痛，关节活动明显受限，肱二头肌舒缩时常能触及轻微的磨擦感，提物或使肱二头肌收缩时疼痛更为明显。

慢性劳损患者，压痛点局限于结节间沟处，肩关节活动除上臂外展再向后作背伸时疼痛外，其它方向的活动多不疼痛。

治疗

推拿治疗本病，对急性损伤而致者收效快且疗效显著，慢性劳损者，疗程较长。治疗期间，宜减少患肩活动，尤以肩部主动外展活动更不宜进行。

1. 治法：舒筋通络，散瘀止痛。

2. 手法：一指禅推、弹拨、揉、摩、摇、抖等。

3. 取穴：肩内陵、肩髃、肩井、臂臑等。

4. 操作：

(1) 患者取坐位，医者站或坐于患者患侧，以拇指指峰或罗纹面沿肱二头肌长腱到结节间沟处肩内陵穴行一指禅推法约3～5分钟。

(2) 再以拇指轻轻弹拨肱二头肌长腱20～30次；继以轻柔的拿法沿三角肌向下循上臂到肘部。

(3) 然后以双掌分别放于肩前、后作相对搓，约1～2分钟。最后环转摇动肩关节，顺时针和逆时针各 3 周。以抖上肢结束治疗。

亦可在肩部周围涂以冬青膏，以小鱼际沿结节间沟方向用擦法，以透热为度。若在患处配合热敷治疗，效果更佳。

5. 疗程：每日 1 次，5 次为 1 疗程。

6.23 冈上肌肌腱炎

冈上肌是组成肩袖的一部分，起于肩胛骨冈上窝，肌腱在喙突肩峰韧带及肩峰下滑囊下面，肩关节囊上面的狭小间隙通过，止于肱骨大结节上部。肌腱与关节囊紧密相连，增加了关节囊的稳定性。其作用主要是起动上臂的外展活动。

病因病理

长期反复的上肢外展活动易使冈上肌肌腱受轻微外伤，或导致肌腱的慢性劳损和退变等，产生无菌性炎症，致使本病发生。

临床表现

本病的主要症状为疼痛，外展活动受限和压痛。表现为肩外侧疼痛并扩散到三角肌附丽点附近。有时疼痛可向上放射到颈部，向下放射到肘部、前臂及手指；在冈上肌肌腱抵止点大结节处有明显压痛，肩关节伸屈活动一般不受限制，在肩部外展至 60～120 度范围时疼痛剧烈，甚者影响肩部活动，日久可有肩部肌肉萎缩。

治疗

本病以推拿手法治疗，疗效较好。急性期手法宜轻柔和缓，肩关节要适当制动；慢性期手法宜深沉。治疗的同时应配合适当的功能锻炼。局部宜保暖，勿受寒冷刺激。

1. 治法：活血化瘀，疏通经络。

2. 手法：一指禅推、按、揉、拿、平推、摇、抖等。

3. 取穴：肩井、秉风、曲垣、天宗、肩外俞、臑俞、臂臑等。

4. 操作：

（1）患者取坐位，医者站于患者患侧，患肢被动外展 30 度，使肌肉放松。医者一手托住患肢肘部，另一手拇指在肩峰下肱骨大结节顶部以一指禅推法并沿冈上肌行走方向往返推动 3～5 分钟。

（2）以拇指弹拨法与按揉法在患部交替治疗 3～5 分钟。

（3）然后在肩胛骨冈上肌处涂以冬青膏或其它推拿介质，以手掌根部或小鱼际行平推法，在平推的同时，以中指或食指端点按秉风、曲垣、肩外俞、肩髎等穴。平推以热感深透，点按以酸胀为度。

（4）捏拿肩井、三角肌 3～5 次。

（5）环转摇动肩关节顺、逆时针各 3 周。从肩部至腕部上下往复搓揉患肢 3～5 遍，最后以抖拉患肢结束手法治疗。

本病亦可配合局部热敷。

5. 疗程：每日 1 次，3 次为 1 疗程。

6.24 肩峰下滑囊炎

肩关节周围有许多滑液囊，其中最大者为肩峰下滑囊和三角肌下滑囊，前者位于肩峰的下面，后者位于三角肌的深面。两者的主要功能在于使肱骨大结节不致在肩峰突下面发生摩擦。

病因病理

肩部遭受直接或间接撞伤，使三角肌深层的滑囊损伤，造成急性的损伤性滑囊炎；慢性滑囊炎，大都是因滑囊变性引起。长期反复的肩部劳损，促使肩峰下滑囊退变，产生滑囊水肿、增厚的无菌性炎症，或发生滑囊壁内互相粘连，妨碍上臂外展和旋转及肩部的正常活动。

临床表现

肩外侧疼痛，常引向三角肌止端，上臂外展、外旋运动时，疼痛加剧。肩峰下压痛明显。急性期因滑囊臌胀，三角肌前缘呈圆形肿胀。初期肩部活动受限较轻，日久与腱袖粘连，而使肩部活动障碍。肌肉萎缩以冈上肌和冈下肌出现较早，晚期可出现三角肌萎缩。

治疗

急性期治疗手法宜轻柔，切勿用力按压患部，以免加重滑囊损伤；慢性期手法可适当加重。患者不要过分制动，急性期可作适当的轻度活动；慢性期则应进行适当的功能锻炼。患部宜保暖。

1. 治法：急性期宜消瘀止痛；慢性期宜活血化瘀，滑利关节。

2. 手法：一指禅推、揉、搓、平推、抖、摇等。

3. 取穴：肩髃、臂臑、肩内陵、天宗、曲池等穴。

4. 操作：

(1) 患者坐位，医者站于患者患侧，以一指禅推法施于三角肌部位，往复推动约3～5分钟。

(2) 继以平推法推上臂外侧及前后侧，推时涂以冬青膏或红花油，推至热深透为度。再以两掌相对搓揉上臂及前臂，上下往返搓3～5遍。

(3) 以拇指或中指端按揉天宗、肩髃、曲池、手三里、合谷等穴，以酸胀为度。

(4) 最后，轻轻环转摇动患肢，并以轻抖拉患肢结束手法治疗。

手法治疗后，可配合局部热敷，以促进炎症的吸收。

5. 疗程：每日1次，5次为1疗程。

6.25 肱骨外上髁炎

本病又称肱骨外上髁综合征、网球肘或肱桡滑囊炎，多发于中年人。

病因病理

肱骨外上髁为肱桡肌及前臂伸肌总腱附着部。如果前臂在旋前位腕关节经常作背伸性活动，其附着部位的软组织易因牵扯发生损伤，引起局部出血、粘连，甚至关节滑膜嵌入肱桡关节间隙而致疼痛。可因急性扭伤或慢性劳损引起，但一般无明显外伤史，多见于需反复作前臂旋转、用力伸腕的成年人，右侧多发。

临床表现

患者肘后外侧酸痛，尤其在旋转背伸、提、拉、端、推等动作时疼痛更为剧烈。同时，沿伸腕肌向下放射。局部可微呈肿胀，前臂旋转及握物无力。伸肌紧张试验和网球时试验阳性。

治疗

肱骨外上髁炎，采用推拿治疗，可收到较好效果，对病程短的患者可配合局部封闭疗法，疗效更佳，病程较长者，保守治疗无效时，可手术治疗。

1. 治法：舒筋通络，活血祛瘀。

2. 手法：一指禅推、揉、弹拨，擦等。

3. 取穴：曲池、肱桡关节间隙、手三里、外关、合谷等穴。

4. 操作：

(1) 患者坐位，医者坐于患者病侧。先以一指禅推法沿肱骨外上髁向前臂往返推 3～5 分钟。再在局部弹拨 5～10 次。

(2) 以右手（以推右侧为例）持腕部，使患者右前臂旋后位，左手用屈曲的拇指端压于肱骨外上髁前方，其它四指放于肘关节内侧，医者以右手逐渐屈曲患者肘关节至最大限度，左手拇指用力按压患者肱骨外上髁的前方，继之伸直其肘关节，同时医者左手拇指推至患肢桡骨头之前上面，沿桡骨头前外缘向后弹拨伸腕肌起点。

(3) 最后，在肘外侧涂以冬青膏或红花油，平推肱骨外上髁及前臂伸肌群，以热深透为度。左手握肱骨远端，右手握患者 4指，抖动前臂及肘关节结束手法治疗。

5. 疗程：每日 1 次，7 次为 1 疗程。

6.26 肱骨内上髁炎

肱骨内上髁炎又称"学生肘"，以青少年发病居多。

病因病理

肱骨内上髁是前臂屈肌总腱附着部。经常反复的屈腕、伸腕、前臂旋前，使前臂屈腕肌群牵拉，引起肱骨内上髁肌腱附丽处的积累劳损，产生慢性无菌性炎症；或因跌仆，腕关节背伸、前臂外展、旋前位姿势时，易使肌腱的附着点发生急性撕裂伤，产生血肿，继之纤维化，导致本病的发生。

临床表现

肱骨内上髁及其附近酸痛，尤其在作前臂旋前、主动屈腕时，酸痛更为明显，同时沿尺侧屈腕肌向下放射，屈腕无力。肱骨内上髁有明显压痛；尺侧屈腕肌及指浅屈肌有广泛压痛；抗阻力屈腕试验阳性。

治疗

1. 治法：舒筋通络，活血化瘀。

2. 手法：按、揉、弹拨、拿、搓揉等。

3. 取穴：小海、少海、外关等穴。

4. 操作：

(1) 患者坐位，以拇指从肱骨内上髁沿尺侧屈腕肌到腕部按揉，手法宜轻柔，同时配合腕部伸屈被动活动，使紧张的屈腕肌群放松。

(2) 随后在肱骨内上髁压痛点及其周围弹拨 2～3 分钟，再沿屈腕肌以轻快的拿法治疗，往返数次。

(3) 以两掌相对搓揉肘部及前臂，最后以抖拉前臂及肘部结束。亦可在肱骨内上髁处涂以冬青膏，擦摩局部，以热力深透为度。

5. 疗程：每日 1 次，7 次为 1 疗程。

6.27 腕关节扭伤

腕关节包括桡腕关节和腕骨间关节。可作屈、伸、内收、外展和环转运动。由于其活动范围大，而且活动频繁，极易发生扭伤。

病因病理

直接或间接暴力，引起腕关节周围软组织的损伤；亦有因腕关节超负荷量的过分劳累或腕关节长期反复操劳积累而引起本病。

临床表现

腕关节扭伤，有的具有典型明确的外伤史，有的无明显外伤史。

急性扭伤的症状，可见腕部肿胀疼痛，功能活动受限，活动时疼痛加剧，局部有明显压痛；慢性劳损腕关节疼痛不甚，无明显肿胀，作较大幅度活动时，伤处可有疼痛感，腕部常有乏力和不灵活感。

检查时，若将腕关节用力掌屈，在背侧发生疼痛，则为腕背侧韧带与伸指肌腱损伤；反之则为腕掌侧韧带或屈肌腱损伤。如果向各个方向均发生疼痛，且活动明显受限，则多为韧带和肌腱等的复合损伤。

治疗

腕部解剖结构复杂，损伤疾病繁多，临证时必须注意与桡、尺骨远端骨折，舟状骨骨折，月骨骨折或脱位，三角骨背侧撕脱骨折，舟、月骨无菌性坏死等相鉴别，若属上述情况者，宜采取骨科整复或手术治疗。推拿治疗腕关节扭伤，可收到良好效果。

1. 治法：舒筋活血，散瘀止痛。
2. 手法：一指推、点、揉、摇、拿、擦、拔伸等。
3. 取穴：少海，通里，神门，尺泽，列缺，太渊，合谷，阳溪，曲池。

4. 操作：

(1) 急性损伤，往往疼痛和肿胀较为明显，手法操作宜轻柔和缓。应先在伤处附近选用相应经络上的适当穴位，如在尺侧掌面，可选手少阴心经的少海、通里、神门等穴；在桡侧掌面，可选手太阴肺经的尺泽、列缺、太渊等穴；在桡侧背面，可选手阳明大肠经的合谷、阳溪、曲池等穴；在其他部位，选法同上。选好穴位后，用拇指点按揉法使之得气，即有较强的酸胀感，约1分钟，以疏通经气，促使经络气血畅通。

(2) 在伤处的周围，向上、下、左、右用一指禅推法，约3～5分钟，以散瘀活血，改善伤处周围的血液循环。同时配合拿法、弹筋，以缓解痉挛。

(3) 然后用摇腕手法，在拔伸的情况下，被动地使腕作绕环、背屈、掌屈、侧偏等动作，以恢复正常的活动功能。

(4) 最后，在腕部涂以红花油，以擦法擦之透热为度。

对肿胀明显者，可在治疗后用中药外敷。

急性损伤后期和慢性劳损，由于疼痛与肿胀较轻，运用以上手法时，要相应加重，活动幅度逐渐加大，以解除痉挛，松解粘连，改善关节活动功能。

5. 疗程：每日1次，3次为1疗程。

6.28　腕管综合征

腕管综合征是指正中神经在腕管内受到压迫所引起的手指麻木等神经症状。

病因病理

腕关节掌侧横行韧带与腕骨连接形成一"腕管"，它的背面由腕骨构成，掌面由腕横韧带构成。腕管内除有正中神经通过外，还有4根指浅屈肌腱、4根指深屈肌腱及1根拇长屈肌腱通过。当腕管内容物体积增大，腕管容积相对缩小时，就会挤压腕管内肌腱及正中神经而出现症状。引起腕管容积减小的原因有：①腕骨增生、骨折、脱位;②腕骨韧带增厚;③损伤或疾病引起腕管内容物（肌腱）肿胀。

临床表现

初期自觉手指麻木刺痛,睡眠中常因麻木刺痛而惊醒,但挥动患手后,症状即可缓解,麻木等症状主要在食指,其次是中指、拇指和无名指,小指不被累及。少数病人可见小指烧灼样痛;后期,病人出现大鱼际肌（拇指短展肌、拇指对掌肌）萎缩、麻木及肌力减弱,或拇指、食指、中指及无名指的桡侧一半的感觉消失。肌萎缩一般在 4 个月以后逐步出现,其程度与病程长短有密切关系。检查可见有症状的手指感觉减弱或消失,但掌部痛感仍存在。按压患肢大陵穴,症状加剧。

治疗

推拿治疗本病,只适应于因损伤或疾病引起腕管内肌腱肿胀而导致该病的一种类型,其它两种情况宜手术治疗。

1. 治法: 舒筋通络,活血化瘀。

2. 手法: 一指禅推、按、揉、摇、擦等。

3. 取穴: 曲泽、内关、大陵等穴。

4. 操作:

(1) 患者正坐,将手伸出,掌心朝上。医者坐位,一手托住患者腕背部,另手拇指点按揉曲泽、内关、大陵、鱼际等穴。

(2) 用一指禅推法在前臂至手沿手厥阴心包经往复治疗 3～5 分钟,重点推腕管及大鱼际处。手法宜先轻渐重。再用摇法摇揉腕关节及指关节。继之用擦法擦腕掌部,以达到舒筋通络,活血化瘀之目的。

(3) 捏腕法: 以右腕为例,患者正坐,前臂放于旋前位,手背朝上。医者双手握患者掌部,右手在桡侧,左手在尺侧,而拇指平放于腕关节的背侧,以拇指指端按入腕关节背侧间隙内。在拔伸情况下摇晃腕关节,然后将手腕在拇指按压下背伸至最大限度,随即屈曲,并左右各旋转其手腕 2～3 次（图 83）。

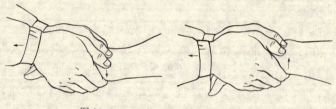

图 83-1   图 83-2

手法治疗后，以温经通络之药膏外敷腕部，并将腕部固定于休息位。症情缓和后，可配合中药薰洗。

5. 疗程：每日 1 次,10 次为 1 疗程。

6.29 膝关节侧副韧带损伤

内侧副韧带呈三角形，桥架于股骨内髁与胫骨内髁之间，其内面与内半月板的中后部的外缘密切相连。当膝关节伸屈活动时，韧带在股骨内髁上前后滑动。膝关节完全伸直与完全屈曲时，韧带均保持紧张。半屈位时,韧带松弛，关节不稳定，易受损伤；外侧副韧带起于股骨外上髁，止于腓骨头；韧带与半月板之间无联系，被疏松结缔组织相隔。屈膝时，此韧带松弛,伸至150 度时，开始紧张，完全伸直时最紧张。

病因病理

当膝关节微屈时，内外侧副韧带都较松弛，膝关节的稳定性较差，突然受到内翻或外翻的应力，易引起内侧或外侧副韧带的损伤，而致本病的发生。

临床表现

内侧副韧带拉伤或部分撕裂时，一般有明确的外伤史，患者膝关节内侧疼痛、压痛，小腿被动外展时疼痛加剧，膝内侧有局限性肿胀，2～3 天可出现皮下瘀斑。膝关节内积血，内侧副韧带完全断裂时，可摸到断裂韧带的间隙。膝关节侧向试验阳性，并可见到膝关节的超关节外翻活动。X 线膝关节正位片可见内侧间隙明显加宽（与健侧对比）。若为韧带止点撕脱者，可见有小骨片撕脱。若合并十字韧带撕脱者，抽屉试验阳性。

治疗

推拿手法治疗本病，一般只适应于韧带拉伤及部分撕裂伤者。韧带完全断裂者，须尽早手术缝合或修补。

1. 治法：活血散瘀，消肿止痛。

2. 手法：点、按、一指禅推、揉、摩、平推等。

3. 取穴：损伤部位的阿是穴、血海、三阴交、阴陵泉、膝关、曲泉等穴。

4. 操作：

（1）患者仰卧，伤肢伸直并旋外，医者先点按血海、阴陵泉、三阴交等穴以疏通经络气血，缓解疼痛。

（2）以掌或大鱼际轻揉局部 3～5 分钟，再以拇指一指禅推法沿内侧副韧带作由轻渐重的上下推动 3～5 分钟。

（3）然后在局部涂以冬青膏或红花油施平推法，以热深透为度。

新鲜损伤肿疼明显者手法宜轻柔，陈旧损伤者手法相对较重。

外侧副韧带损伤临床少见，其临床表现及推拿治疗方法与内侧副韧带相似。

5. 疗程：每日 1 次，3 次为 1 疗程。

6.30 踝关节扭伤

踝关节是由胫、腓骨下端和距骨组成的屈伸关节。其关节囊前后松弛，两侧较紧，前后韧带较薄弱，内、外侧副韧带较坚强。

病因病理

当跖屈时，距骨后部进入踝穴，踝关节相对不稳定，此时若足突然向内或向外翻转，踝外侧或内侧副韧带则受到强大的张力作用而被拉伤。

临床表现

有急性扭伤病史，踝部出现明显肿胀疼痛，不能着地，内、外踝前下方均有压痛，皮肤呈紫色。外踝扭伤者，将其踝关节内翻则外踝部疼痛加剧。外侧关节囊及腓前韧带损伤时，肿胀主要在关节外侧和外踝前下方。内踝扭伤，可能伴有外踝骨折。因此，内、外踝均肿胀疼痛。

治疗

推拿手法治疗，对单纯的韧带扭伤或韧带部分纤维断裂者，疗效较好。合并骨折或脱位者，应尽早行骨科手术或复位术。

1. 治法：活血化瘀，消肿止痛。

2. 手法：点、按、一指禅推、揉、拔伸、摇等。

3. 取穴：踝关节周围阿是穴、足三里、阳陵泉、太溪、昆仑、丘墟、悬钟、解溪、太冲等穴位。

4. 操作：

(1) 患者仰卧，医者用点按法点按足三里、太溪、昆仑、丘墟、绝骨、解溪、太冲等穴，以疏通经络、缓解疼痛。

(2) 再以鱼际揉法揉局部 3～5 分钟，继以拇指推法由上而下在小腿及踝关节周围施术，以活血祛瘀，消肿止痛。

(3) 患者仰卧，医者以右手（以右侧为例）紧握患者右拇趾，并向上牵引，先外翻以扩大踝关节内侧间隙，同时以左手食指压入间隙内，然后仍在牵引下内翻足部，扩大踝关节外侧间隙，以左手拇指压入关节间隙内。使拇、食指夹持踝关节，右手在牵引下将患足左右轻轻摇摆，内翻 1～2 次。然后背屈、跖屈，同时夹持踝关节的食、拇指下推上提两踝，背屈时下推，跖屈时上提（图 84）。

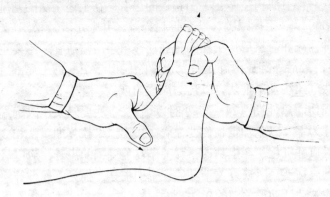

图 84-1

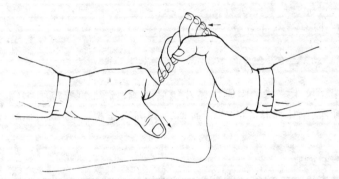

图 84-2

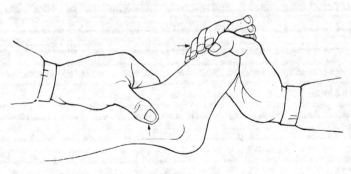

图 84-3

(4) 对伴有肌肉痉挛、关节粘连的患者，在上述手法的基础上，医者可以一手握跟腱、一手握住拇趾，并嘱患者放松踝部，先予拔伸、跖屈，然后作突然的背屈动作（手法需适宜，不要用力太猛），最后外翻或内翻足背，以解除肌肉痉挛，再于局部进行轻摩法、揉法及平推法，以热力深透为度。

在损伤的急性期（24～48 小时以内），手法要轻柔，以远端取穴治疗为主，以免加重损伤处血管破裂出血；恢复期手法相应加重，对血肿机化、产生粘连、踝关节功能受损的患者，应以较重手法剥离粘连，以恢复关节功能。牵引摇摆、摇晃、屈伸等法是常用的被动活动踝关节的手法。

亦可配合中药醺洗疗法。

5. 疗程：每日 1 次，3 次为 1 疗程。

6.31　踝管综合征

踝管位于踝关节内侧，是小腿后区和足底深部蜂窝组织间隙的骨纤维组织所形成的一条通道，管内有肌腱、通管和神经通过。

病因病理

由于足部活动突然增加或踝关节反复扭伤，使踝管内肌腱因摩擦而产生腱鞘炎，腱鞘肿胀。踝管内容物体积因此增大。但踝管为骨纤维管道，缺乏伸缩性，不能随之膨胀，因而形成踝管的相对狭窄，于是管内压力增高，由此产生胫后神经受压症状。另外，分裂韧带退变增厚，踝管内跟骨骨刺形成或骨折等原因，都可导致踝管狭窄，形成对神经、血管的压迫，而发生本病。

临床表现

早期常因行走站立过久而出现内踝后部不适感，休息后即可改善。随着病情的加重，上述症状反复出现，发作时间逐渐延长，病员有跟骨内侧和足底麻木感或蚁行感，重者可出现足趾皮肤干燥、发亮、汗毛脱落及足部肌肉萎缩。检查时轻叩内踝后方患者足部针刺感加剧；足极度背屈时内踝后方及足底部疼痛加重。

治疗：

推拿对因踝管内腱鞘炎、腱鞘肿胀而引起的疗效较好，而对分裂韧带退变增厚、踝管内跟骨骨刺形成或骨折等原因所致者，疗效较差，故宜手术治疗。

1. 治法：舒筋活血，散瘀止痛。

2. 手法：一指推、揉、弹拨、擦等。

3. 取穴：阴陵泉、三阴交、太溪、照海、金门等穴。

4. 操作：

(1) 患者仰卧，患肢外旋，医者点按所取诸穴继以一指禅推法于小腿内后侧，由上而下推至踝部，重点在踝管局部，沿与踝管纵轴向垂直方向推5～10分钟。

(2) 在踝管局部弹拨3～5分钟。

(3) 最后，顺肌腱方向用擦法，以透热为度。

在治疗期间，还可配合中药熏洗。

5. 疗程：每日1次，10次为1疗程。

6.32　跟腱扭伤

跟腱与其表层的深筋膜之间有一种腱围组织，其结构近似滑膜，共7～8层，各层之间虽有结缔组织联系，但互不粘合。跟腱腱围组织在踝关节屈伸过程中起润滑作用。

病因病理

因急性损伤或长期反复劳损，使腱围撕裂，渗血或变性坏死，都可导致腱围各层之间及腱围与跟腱之间产生粘连。

临床表现

临床的主要表现是跟腱疼痛。早期疼痛主要发生于活动开始时，一旦活动开后，疼痛反见减轻，但猛力跑跳时疼痛可加重。随着疼痛的加重，凡牵扯跟腱时都可引起疼痛。如上下楼梯、走路等。本病的压痛部位表浅，特别在捻动表面跟腱时疼痛明显。晚期可出现跟腱变性，其表面可摸到硬块，捻到时"吱吱"作响，跟腱失去韧性、缺乏弹性。局部增粗成梭形。患者足尖着地后蹬时，可引起抗阻力疼痛。

治疗

1. 治法：活血祛瘀，理筋通络。

2. 手法：一指禅推、捏、揉、拿、平推、摇等。

3. 取穴：太溪、复溜、承山、阳交、跟腱附近阿是等穴。

4. 操作：

(1) 患者俯卧，小腿及足踝部垫以软枕。医者坐于患者患脚旁，以一指禅推法从跟腱沿腓肠肌推至腘窝，往返推动 3～5 分钟，再以捏、拿法捏拿跟腱及腓肠肌，用力由轻渐重，以明显酸胀感为宜，自下而上，反复 5～10 次。

(2) 在跟腱及腓肠肌肌腹处，涂以冬青膏或按摩乳，行平推法，以热深透为度。

(3) 然后再以拇指重点推揉跟腱局部 3～5 分钟。局部以拇、食两指相对拿捻，腱围有硬块者，手法宜轻柔。

(4) 最后，令患者屈膝 90°，踝关节跖屈，使跟腱充分放松。医者一手握足背，一手在小腿后侧施以轻快柔和的捏拿法。随后，握足背之手将踝关节摇动，并慢慢加大幅度，使踝关节背屈。

推拿手法治疗后，可用洗药热敷、熏洗。

5. 疗程：每日 1 次，3 次为 1 疗程。

6.33 肩关节周围炎

肩关节周围炎中、老年人多发，又多为单侧发病，以肩关节疼痛和功能障碍为主要症状。

病因病机

一般认为本病的发生与气血不足，营养失调，风寒外侵于肩部或外伤劳损有关。现有人实验观察，本病与性激素水平有关。

临床表现

常无特殊原因而渐发肩部酸痛、无力和活动障碍。一般初发病时，以疼痛为主，多为酸痛性质，遍及肩关节周围，但常以肩关节前面为显著，有时可向前臂放射。疼痛昼轻夜重，至患者不能患侧卧位。患者经常保持着固定位置，突然碰及肩部或活动肩关节可引起肩部剧痛难忍。及至后期，往往疼痛症状逐渐减轻，肩部活动障碍的现象却日见严重。特别是外展和外旋及上举动作最为困难，内收和前屈动作也有障碍。外展时出现典型的"扛肩"现象（图85），梳头和穿脱衣服等动作均难以完成。严重时肘关节功能亦受限，屈肘时手不能摸肩。日久，三角肌等可有不同程度的萎缩。

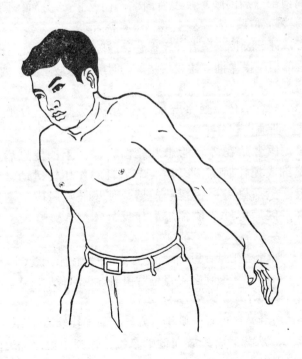

图 85

治疗

初期病人因疼痛较甚，可用较轻柔的手法在局部反复治疗，以疏通经络，活血止痛，加强局部肌腱及韧带的功能；晚期病人可用较重手法，如扳、拔伸、摇法以及肩关节的其它活动，以松解粘连，滑利关节，促使关节功能逐渐恢复。

1. 治法：疏筋通络，松解粘连，活血止痛。

2. 手法：一指禅推、点、按、拿、扳、拔伸、摇、抖等。

3. 取穴：肩内陵、肩髃、肩髎、臑俞、天宗、肩井、曲池、合谷等穴。

4. 操作：

(1) 患者仰卧或坐位，医者站或坐于患者患侧，用一指禅推法推肩前部（肩内陵）及上臂内侧，往返3～5分钟，同时配合患肢的被动外展、内收、上举、外旋等活动。

(2) 健侧卧位，医者一手握住患肢的肘部，另一手在肩外侧和腋后部用一指禅推、揉或㨰法，同时配合患肢上举、内收等被动活动。

(3) 患者坐位，拿捏肩井、点揉天宗、臑俞、肩髃、肩髎、肩内陵、曲池、合谷等穴。

(4) 医者站在患者的患肢稍前方，一手挟住患肩，一手握住腕部或托住肘部，以肩关节为轴心作环转运动，幅度由小到大。然后医者一手托起前臂，使患肢屈肘内收，手搭健肩，再由健肩绕过头顶到患肩，反复环绕5～10次，同时用另一手捏拿患肩。

(5) 医者站在患者患侧稍前方，一手握住患侧腕部，并以肩部顶住患肩前部。握腕之手将患臂由前方扳向背后，逐渐用力使之后伸（图86），重复3～5次。

(6) 医者站在患者健侧稍后方，用一手扶健肩，另一手握住患侧腕部，从背后将患肢向健侧牵拉，逐渐用力，加大活动范围，以患者能忍耐为度（图87）。

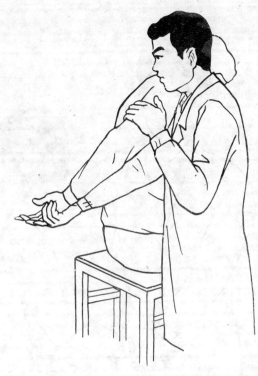

图 86

（7）医者站在患肩外侧，用双手握住患肢腕部稍上方，将患肢提起，边提边抖，向斜上牵拉。牵拉时要求患者先沉肩屈肘，再缓缓伸肘外展向斜上方上举。手法宜轻柔和缓（图 88）。

（8）前、后分别环转摇动患肩各 3 周，然后用两掌相对，从肩部搓至前臂，反复 3～5 遍，抖患肢结束治疗。

5. 疗程：每日 1 次，7 次为 1 疗程。

本病在治疗的同时，必须配合适当的肩部功能锻炼，方能受到较好疗效，及早康复。锻炼应持之以恒，循序渐进，根据患者具体情况可选下面几种方法：

（1）抬肩：弯腰，两上肢下垂，两手相握，两上肢向前摆动，幅度逐渐增大。

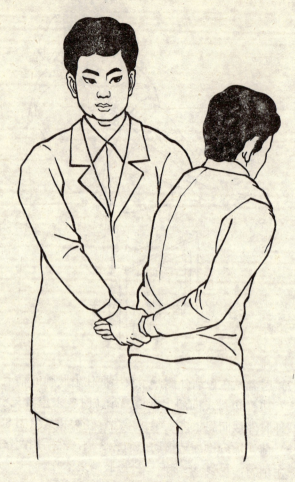

图 87

　(2) 肩外展：弯腰，两上肢下垂，向左右自然摆动，幅度逐渐增大。

　(3) 肩后伸：两足分开与肩同宽，两手在体后相握，掌心向外，用健手带动患手，尽力做后伸动作，身体不能前屈。

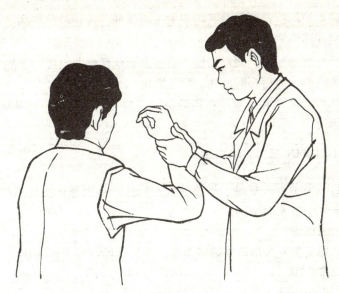

图 88-1

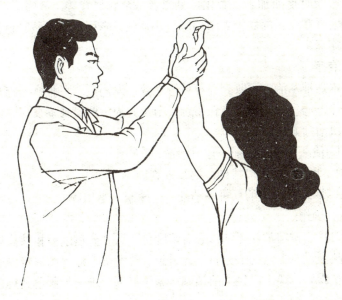

图 88-2

(4) 肩环绕：两足分开与肩宽，两臂伸直，作前、后环绕动作，幅度逐渐增大。

(5) 双手爬墙：面对墙壁，双手沿墙壁缓慢向上爬动，使上肢尽量高举、然后再回原处，反复数次。

(6) 内收外展：双手在颈后交叉，肩关节尽量内收及外展，反复数次。

6.34 肋椎关节紊乱症

肋椎关节紊乱症是一种急性突发病症，多因身体扭转不当，或因咳嗽、喷嚏而发病。

病因病理

肋椎关节发生滑膜嵌顿或关节发生轻微错位而引起本病。

临床表现

本症的症状较典型，即突感一侧胸肋部疼痛，咳嗽，打喷嚏及深呼吸时疼痛加重。查体可见患者呈含胸屈背势，呼吸浅促，压痛区常在受累的肋椎关节周围呈小片状，牵引患侧上肢时也常引起疼痛。

治疗

本病推拿治疗可收到立杆见影之效，发病后即可推拿治疗疗效最佳，病程较长者，易在错位关节及其周围产生炎症反应，需经几次治疗方能康复。

1. 治法：复位止痛，理气活血。

2. 手法：按揉、拔伸、摇、抖等。

3. 取穴：受损的肋椎关节处、阳陵泉、承山等穴。

4. 操作：

(1) 复位前放松手法：患者俯卧位，医者先后以拇指按揉患侧阳陵泉及承山穴约 5 分钟，此时患者胁背部疼痛逐渐减轻，肌紧张稍缓解，继之以轻柔的揉摩法施于局部，进一步缓解其疼痛及肌痉挛，约 5 分钟。

(2) 复位手法：

①扩胸顶背法：患者坐位，双手5指交叉放于颈后部。医者站其背后，两手分别握住患者两肘部，屈膝并将膝盖部顶在受累之肋椎关节处，两手轻轻向后扳肘扩胸，与此同时，膝盖前顶，嘱患者深吸气。扩胸与前顶两者应互相协调，用力轻柔和缓。一般2～3次即可。

②掌击法：患者坐位，术者站其侧前方，将前臂从前向后插入患者腋下，发力将患侧肩部提起，提起后嘱患者深吸气。术者趁其不备，用另一手掌根部自下而上地叩击一下患处，重复1～2遍。

③拔伸法：患者坐于低凳上，医者站在患者的患侧前方，双手分捏患侧手指，使其手掌向内。然后医者紧握患侧的手，由下向内而上地连续作圆形环转，幅度不宜过大。待患肢肌肉放松，运转自如时，突然用力向上提拔患肢。

(3) 结束手法：患者坐位，医者站于患侧偏前，令患者伸直患侧上肢，医者握住其手腕部，将患肢从下方经前方绕到后方，连续作环形转动10周左右，并嘱患者随患肢向前上举过程中吸气、绕后下落时呼气，然后双手握患者腕部牵拉、抖动患侧上肢结束手法。

5. 疗程：治疗1次，若不愈再按上法治疗。

6.35 颈椎病

颈椎病又称颈椎综合征。多发于中老年人。它是由于颈椎增生后引起的炎症刺激，压迫颈神经根、颈部脊髓、椎动脉或交感神经而引起的综合症候群。

病因病理

各种急、慢性外伤造成颈椎间盘、韧带、后关节囊等组织不同程度的损伤，从而使脊柱稳定性下降，促使颈椎发生代偿性增生。增生物直接或间接压迫神经和血管，因而产生症状；椎间盘退行性变化是本病的主要因素。

颈椎增生可发生在后关节、钩椎关节和椎体。由于增生部位的不同，可发生各种不同的症状。椎体前缘增生，一般无特殊症状。椎体后缘增生，使椎管前后径变窄，可出现脊髓压迫症状，称脊髓型颈椎病；钩椎关节侧方增生，使椎动脉受到压迫，称椎动脉型颈椎病；椎体侧后方、后关节前缘或钩椎关节后方增生，使椎间孔变小，可出现颈丛或臂丛神经受压症状，称神经根型颈椎病；后关节增生伴半脱位或对椎动脉的刺激，可出现交感神经症状，称交感神经型颈椎病。

颈椎增生而产生的症状，有两种情况：一是增生物直接压迫神经、血管；二是增生物对其周围软组织过度刺激而发生局部的损伤性炎症，炎性充血水肿，间接压迫神经、血管。

临床表现

1. 神经根型：由于退变增生的椎间小关节或钩椎关节刺激或压迫神经根所出现颈肩痛或颈枕痛及枕部感觉障碍等，或见颈部僵硬、一侧或两侧颈、肩、臂放射痛、并伴有手指麻木、肢冷、上肢发沉无力、持物坠落等症状。颈部活动呈不对称性限制，后伸或向患侧旋转时疼痛加剧。压顶 (Spurling) 试验、牵引试验、臂丛牵拉试验、棘突指压头后仰试验，转头加力试验均可为阳性，患者肩胛内缘、肩胛区或肩部可有反射性疼痛和继发性压痛点。

2. 脊髓型：由于椎体后缘增生、膨出的椎间盘和后纵韧带或肥厚的黄韧带突入椎管，压迫脊髓所致。可见上肢或下肢、一侧或两侧的麻木、酸软无力，颈颤臂抖，有不同程度的不全痉挛性瘫痪，如活动不便，步态笨拙，走路不稳，以至卧床不起，甚至呼吸困难，四肢肌张力高，腱反射亢进，浅反射减弱或消失，髌、踝阵挛和巴氏征阳性。多无颈部疼痛和运动障碍，脑脊液动力试验常为不完全梗阻。

3. 椎动脉型：又称缺血型，由于颈椎退变增生，使椎动脉扭曲，痉挛或受压，引起椎动脉供血不足所致。患者内耳和脑部缺血，表现为颈肩痛或颈枕痛、头晕、恶心、呕吐、位置性眩晕、猝倒、耳鸣、耳聋、视物不清等临床症状。上述症状常因头颈转动或侧屈到某一位置而诱发或加重。

4. 交感神经型：由于交感神经受到刺激而出现枕部痛，头沉，头晕或偏头痛，心慌，胸闷、肢冷，皮肤温度低或手足发热，四肢酸胀等症状，一般无上肢放射痛或麻木感，个别病人也可出现眼球后痛，视物不清，畏光，流泪、流涕、咽部异物感，胸前区痛，面部出汗等症状。

5. 前斜角肌型：由于颈 4、5 神经根受增生突出物刺激，引起前斜角肌痉挛，痉挛的肌肉压迫臂丛神经，出现前斜角肌综合征和颈 4、5 神经根受累的症状。

6. 间盘型：由于颈椎间盘退变、萎缩变化，刺激脑膜支末稍，引起颈、肩胛、背和肩部反射性疼痛。患者无神经根受累表现。

7. 混合型：同时表现为上述两型及两型以上症状。

颈部 X 线片示颈椎生理前凸消失或反向，颈椎侧弯，椎间隙变窄，椎间小关节、钩椎关节和椎体边缘硬化，椎间小关节间隙变窄，下关节突向后下滑移等异常征象。颈前屈、后伸位 X 线片可显示病变处椎体间的异常滑移。椎动脉造影对诊断椎动脉型有帮助。脊髓型患者蛛网膜下腔造影可见病变间隙有不全或完全梗阻影像。

治疗

推拿治疗本病，除骨性直接压迫外，均有一定效果，其中尤以神经根型、椎动脉型、交感神经型、前斜角肌型、间盘型效果较为显著。目前对颈椎病的治疗，推拿仍为首选治疗方法。但对脊髓型和伴有高血压及血管严重硬化的病人，不宜使用颈椎旋转复位法。其它类型使用本法时也应轻柔，切忌暴力。

1. 治法：疏筋活血，理筋整复。

2. 手法：一指禅推、按、揉、拿、拔伸、拔伸旋转、搓、平推、摇、抖等。

3. 取穴：风池、天柱、大椎、大杼、肩井、天宗、曲池、外关等穴。

4. 操作：

(1) 患者正坐，医者站于患者背后，先以拇指一指禅推法从风池穴向下沿颈椎棘突旁推至大杼穴。往返 5～7 遍，两侧交替。

(2) 以捏拿法，捏拿颈项部，重点在压痛点处，同时轻轻旋转颈项 2～3 分钟。

(3) 继以拇或食、中指端按揉天宗、秉风、缺盆、肩外俞等穴，后以双手捏拿肩井穴。再以食、中、无名指弹拨上臂内侧上 1/3 处，以拇指按揉曲池、手三里、外关等穴，环转摇动肩关节，抖上肢。

(4) 颈部拔伸：常用以下 3 种拔伸法：

① 患者仰卧，下肢伸直，上肢平放于体侧，医者坐于患者头侧，以双膝顶住床腿，一手放于患者下颌部，另手托住枕外隆凸处，以腰及上身后抑拔伸，边拔伸边轻柔摇动颈椎 2～3 分钟。在拔伸摇动的同时，可以柔和之力向左或右旋转扳动。可听到"咔嚓"响声。

② 患者坐位，医者站在患者背后，两前臂尺侧放于患者两肩部向下用力，双手大拇指顶在"风池"穴上方，切勿用力过猛，以免引起患者头晕等不适感。其余 4 指及手掌托起下颌部，并向上用力，前臂与两手同时向相反方向用力，把颈椎间隙拉宽，边牵边使头颈部前屈后伸及左右旋转。

③ 患者坐于低凳上，医者站于患者患侧，肘关节屈曲并托住患者下颌部，手扶健侧颞枕部，向上缓缓用力拔伸，并做颈部左右旋转活动；另一手拇指置于患处相应棘突旁，随颈部的活动在压痛点上施以按揉法。

伴有头痛、头晕等症者，除上述手法外，加分抹前额、眉弓，点睛明，分抹迎香、人中、承浆，扫散二侧颞部，合颞枕至项部。

5. 疗程：隔日1次，10次为1疗程。

6. 本病在推拿治疗的同时，应配合如下颈部功能锻炼方法：

(1) 坐位或站立，两手自然下垂（坐位时两手轻放于两大腿上），全身放松，头颈缓缓前屈至最大限度，如此反复20～30次。

(2) 坐位或站立，头颈先缓缓向健侧侧屈至最大限度，再缓缓向患侧侧屈至最大限度，反复20～30次。

(3) 坐位或站立，头颈先缓缓由正中位向健侧、后方至患侧复原位，如此环转20～30周，再向相反方向环转20～30周。

(4) 可用自制颈椎牵引托（托住下颌及枕部），坐于凳上牵引，头勿前屈、后伸及左右侧屈，宜保持正中位。牵引重量为3～5公斤，每次牵引半小时，每日1～2次。

6.36　落枕

落枕多于晨起时发病，临床上以急性颈部肌肉痉挛、酸胀、疼痛、颈不能活动为主要症状。

病因病理

多因睡眠时枕头高低不适，或睡卧姿势不良，或睡卧颈肩部当风等因素，使一侧肌群在较长时间内处于过度伸展状态，以致发生痉挛，肌纤维炎。亦有少数患者因颈部突然扭转不当，或肩扛重物时使部分肌肉扭伤或发生痉挛所致。

临床表现

患者颈项部多为单侧胸锁乳突肌或斜方肌痉挛、僵硬、疼痛为主要表现。头向患侧倾斜，下颌转向健侧，颈部活动明显受限，疼痛重者可牵及头部、上背部及上臂部。患处有明显压痛。

治疗

推拿治疗落枕，有良好疗效，一般 1～2 次可愈，病程越短，疗效越好。

1. 治法：舒筋活血，通络止痛。

2. 手法：一指禅推、按、揉、摇、拿等。

3. 取穴：阿是、风池、风府、肩井、天宗等穴。

4. 操作：

（1）患者坐位，医者站于患者患侧后方，先以轻柔的一指禅推法，在患侧颈项部及肩部推，另一手托患者下颌部，轻轻摇动，边推边摇。

（2）待摇动幅度渐大，肌肉渐放松时，摇至颈微前屈，托下颌之手迅速向患侧加大旋转幅度（一般在功能位基础上加大 5°），另一手轻轻向健侧推相应颈椎棘突。两手手法应协调一致，轻柔灵活，旋转幅度以患者能忍受为度。

（3）最后，拿风池、风府、肩井、按揉天宗，平推肩背部至发热，结束手法治疗。

5. 疗程：每日治疗 1 次，3 次为 1 疗程。

6.37　腰椎小关节紊乱

病因病理

外力或腰部活动不当导致腰椎小关节的解剖位置改变——关节错位或滑膜嵌顿而致本病。

临床表现

大多数患者无明显外伤史，多于弯腰或腰部左右侧屈或旋转时突感腰部疼痛，随即不能活动，咳嗽、打喷嚏疼痛加重，无下肢放射性疼痛。亦有因咳嗽、打喷嚏而致发病者。检查时有明显固定的压痛点，腰部活动明显受限，痛侧肌紧张痉挛。局部叩击痛，无明显下肢压痛，双下肢活动不受限。X 线腰椎片无骨质及椎间隙异常改变。

治疗

推拿治疗腰椎小关节紊乱症，有手到病除之效。若病发后即治疗，1次可愈。

1. 治法：理筋整复，行气止痛。

2. 手法：按、揉、斜扳、拔伸等。

3. 取穴：委中、承山、腰部阿是等穴。

4. 操作：

(1) 患者俯卧，医者站或坐于患者痛侧，以一手拇指轻按揉痛点，使其肌肉放松，同时以另一手拇指按揉痛侧承山或委中穴，以解痉镇痛，行气活血。

(2) 患者侧卧位，患侧在下伸直，健侧在上并屈曲，行斜扳法。扳时医者一肘部压患者臀部向前下方，另一肘部压患者肩部向后下方，拇指按住痛处相应棘突，向相反方向用力斜扳，可听到"咔嚓"响声。然后，嘱患者用力蹬腿，顺患者下蹬之力牵引足踝部，蹬拉3次即可。此时患者感到腰部轻松，疼痛消失，再轻揉原痛点2~3分钟结束治疗。

5. 疗程：治疗1次，若不愈再按上法治疗。

6.38 急性腰扭伤

腰部为全身活动及传递上身重量的枢纽，是日常生活和劳动中活动最多的部位之一，在持重和运动中，腰部肌肉较易受到损伤。

病因病理

过度后伸与前屈，扭转弯曲超过了正常范围，负重过大或用力过度，姿势不正，以及跌仆或暴力直接打击，使腰部的肌肉组织受到剧烈的旋转、牵拉而卒然受伤，引起本病。

临床表现

多有明显的扭伤史，重者伤后随即出现腰部剧痛，活动受限，坐、卧、行、走均困难，咳嗽、打喷嚏及深呼吸时疼痛加重，轻者扭伤当时腰部疼痛不明显，经数小时或 1～2 天后，腰痛渐重，以至腰部不能活动。检查时可见，初伤时多有明显的局限性压痛点，无下肢放射性压痛及叩击痛，伤处肌肉明显紧张，痉挛，脊柱腰部侧弯。

治疗

推拿治疗急性腰扭伤疗效较显著，治疗期间应卧床休息，防止再度扭伤。疼痛剧烈者，手法治疗后可配合热敷。在手法治疗时，应选择患者肢体放松的自觉舒适的位置进行操作为宜，以避免肌肉紧张，并防止再度损伤。

1. 治法：活血散瘀，通络止痛。

2. 手法：揉、平推、擦、点按等。

3. 取穴：阿是、肾俞、委中、承山等穴。

4. 操作：

(1) 患者取俯卧位，医者站于患侧，先以拇指轻轻按揉痛点，同时以另一手拇指点按同侧承山穴，待腰部肌肉稍放松后，再以擦法施于两侧腰肌，由轻渐重，但不宜过重，以患者腰部疼痛不增加为度。

(2) 在两侧腰肌（以痛侧为主）涂以冬青膏，行平推法，以热深透至肌肉深部为宜。

(3) 患者仰卧位，屈膝屈髋，双手扶患者双膝部，轻轻转动腰髋部，结束手法。

5. 疗程：隔日 1 次，3 次为 1 疗程。

6.39 第三腰椎横突综合征

第三腰椎位于腰椎生理前凸的顶点，是腰椎活动的中心。其横突最长，故与腰背筋膜的深层接触更为紧密而且活动范围广泛，承受的杠杆作用力最大。因此附着于第三腰椎横突上的肌肉容易被磨擦或牵拉而致损伤。

病因病理

因负重物，或腰部扭转不当，或长期反复弯腰活动，致使附着于第三腰椎横突的肌肉、筋膜损伤，引起腰背肌肉紧张或痉挛，从而刺激或压迫脊神经后支的外侧支而发生腰痛，本病发生。

临床表现

多有不同程度的腰部扭伤史或劳损史。病人一侧腰臀部疼痛，并沿大腿向下放射到膝平面以上，弯腰及旋转腰部疼痛加重。检查时，第三腰椎横突尖端有明显压痛，并可触及粗硬的条索样硬块。晚期可见轻度腰肌萎缩。

治疗

本病推拿治疗效果较满意。初期手法宜轻柔，切忌手法粗暴、过重，否则会引起新的损伤。治疗期间，要避免或减少腰部的伸屈及旋转活动。

1. 治法：舒筋通络，活血散瘀，消肿止痛。

2. 手法：一指禅推、擦、弹拨、按揉等。

3. 取穴：患侧第三腰椎横突端的阿是、承山、阳陵泉等穴。

4. 操作：

(1) 患者俯卧，医者站于患者患侧，先以拇指按揉患肢承山、阳陵泉穴，使患者能忍受为度，以疏通经络，解痉镇痛。继以轻柔的一指禅推法在患侧腰三横突及其周围推 3～5 分钟。

(2) 以弹拨法弹拨条索状硬块，方向应与索状硬块垂直。用力由轻渐重，以患者能忍受为度。

(3) 在局部涂以冬青膏或其它润滑介质，行擦法，以热深透为度。

(4) 最后行后伸扳法及健侧斜扳法结束手法治疗。

术后可配合腰部热敷。

5. 疗程：隔日 1 次，3 次为 1 疗程。

6.40 慢性腰肌劳损

病因病理

本病起于长期反复地腰部劳损，或腰部肌肉急性损伤未作及时治疗或治疗不彻底，或反复损伤，或腰部受寒受湿造成腰部肌纤维慢性炎症。

临床表现

有长期反复发作的腰痛史，多呈酸痛，每因劳累发作或加重，弯腰及久坐、久立腰部疼痛。腰部压痛较广泛，多无固定压痛点，痛久病重者可触及痛性硬结，腰腿活动多无明显障碍。急性发作时各种症状均显著加重，并可有肌痉挛、腰脊椎侧弯，下肢牵制作痛等症状。

治疗

1. 治法：舒筋通络，温经活血。

2. 手法：擦、揉、点按、擦、拍击等。

3. 取穴：肾俞、命门、大肠俞、委中等穴。

4. 操作：

(1) 患者俯卧，医者站或坐于一侧，先以擦法施于两侧腰肌约5分钟，继以拇指或掌根自上而下按揉两侧骶棘肌5～10遍，重点按揉肾俞、大肠俞、秩边等穴，同时以另手拇指点按委中、承山穴。

(2) 在腰椎两侧涂以按摩乳或冬青膏，行擦法，以热深透为度。

(3) 拍击腰背部两侧骶棘肌结束手法。

5. 疗程：每日1次，7次为1疗程。

6.41 腰椎间盘突出症

腰椎间盘突出症又名"腰椎间盘纤维环破裂症"，多发于中青年，临床以第四、五腰椎间盘及腰五骶一椎间盘突出为多见。

病因病理

由于椎间盘本身的退行性改变或发育不全，加之腰部突然受到外力的冲击，或长期反复的劳损，导致椎间盘纤维环破裂，使髓核冲破纤维环而向侧后方膨出，引起对神经根或脊髓的压迫。腰部受寒湿侵袭可更进一步引起损害。

临床表现

1. 症状

(1) 腰腿疼痛：大多数患者有长期反复发作的腰痛病史。渐渐感觉疼痛向一侧下肢放射（双侧者少见），咳嗽、喷嚏引起放射性疼痛加重，亦有开始先表现为一侧小腿外侧或后侧疼痛或麻木，而后渐感腰部疼痛者。多欲健侧卧位，患侧屈曲在上。

(2) 腰部活动障碍：急性期腰部各方向活动均明显受限，随病情的缓解，腰部活动幅度渐大。

(3) 主观麻木感：病程较长者，常有主观麻木感。多局限于小腿外侧，足背、足跟或足拇趾。中央型髓核突出可发生鞍区麻痹。

(4) 患肢发凉：大部分患者，自觉患肢怕冷，皮温较健侧低。

2. 体征：

(1) 脊柱侧弯，腰椎生理前凸减小或消失，甚至后凸。

(2) 腰部压痛、叩击痛并向患侧下肢放射痛至足底，沿患侧坐骨神经分布区压痛明显。

(3) 直腿抬高试验及背屈加强试验阳性。

(4) 拇趾背屈或跖屈肌力减弱。

(5) 仰卧挺腹试验或屈颈试验阳性。

(6) 下肢后伸试验阳性。

(7) 膝或跟腱反射低下，小腿后外侧及足背皮肤感觉减退。

(8) X 线检查：多表现为腰椎生理弧度消失，腰椎侧弯，椎间隙变窄，并除外其它椎骨及关节病变。

(9) CT 检查：椎间盘向不同方向突出或膨出。

治疗

目前，腰椎间盘突出症的非手术疗法中，推拿仍为最有效的方法。

在发病及治疗期间，病人应注意卧硬板床休息，并注意腰部保暖，症状缓解后，应做适当腰部功能锻炼。

1. 治法：还纳复位，松解粘连，行气活血、通经散瘀止痛。

2. 手法：牵拉、斜扳、旋转、按揉等。

3. 取穴：腰部阿是、秩边、环跳、殷门、委中、承山、阳陵泉、解溪等穴。

4. 操作：

(1) 患者俯卧，医者站于患侧，以拇指按揉棘突旁压痛点 2～3 分钟，由轻渐重，同时点按患侧委中或承山、阳陵泉穴，待腰部肌肉稍松后，嘱患者患侧卧位，健侧在上，以拇指按住偏歪之棘突行斜扳法，可听到"咔嚓"响声。

(2) 患者仰卧位，双手握住患肢足踝部，抖拉患侧下肢 3 次。

按揉棘突痛点及委中、承山穴后，亦可行腰椎旋转复位手法，以调整腰椎后关节、牵拉神经根、扩大神经根管和椎间孔。

牵引可人工对抗牵引或牵引床牵引，牵引重量以超体重 10 千克为宜。牵引的同时按压棘突旁，促使髓核还纳。

对病久患者，经多种手法治疗效果不显著的，可行骶裂孔或椎间孔注药后牵引推拿术。即以 1% 利多卡因 20 毫升，地塞米松 10 毫克，注入相应椎间孔或骶裂孔后，再行对抗牵引、按压复位术。

5. 疗程：推拿治疗隔日 1 次，7 次为 1 疗程。

（管　政）

7 成人保健推拿

通过自己的双手，运用简单的手法在自身体表经穴与某些特定的部位进行推拿，以达到保健，养生与对某些疾病自疗目的的方法，称为"保健推拿"。由于保健推拿主要是采用自摩自捏自己给自己治疗的方式，故又称"自我推拿"。保健推拿，主要是因为自我手法的刺激，激发了自身的经穴系统而发挥治疗作用的。同时，自我手法的动作过程，本身也是一种主动的运动锻炼。所以，只要根据自身的具体情况，选择好治疗部位与经穴，循序渐进，持之以恒地进行自我推拿，一定会取得理想的保健，养生与疾病自疗的功效。人体各部常用的保健推拿方法及其作用介绍如下：

7.1 头面、五官部保健推拿

1. 头面部

操作

(1) 分推前额

从印堂至前发际正中之连线为中线，两手食指屈成弓状，以第二指节的内侧为着力面，自中线向前额两侧分别分推至丝竹空、太阳、头维穴处，约 40～60 次左右 (图 89)。

(2) 双抹两颞

以两手拇指螺纹面，紧按两侧鬓发处，由前向后反复用力推抹，约 30 次左右，以酸胀为宜 (图 90)。

(3) 按揉脑后

以两手拇指螺纹面或指端，紧按风池穴，先用力按压 10 余次，再作旋转按揉，随后再按揉脑空穴约 30 次左右，以酸胀为宜 (图 91)。

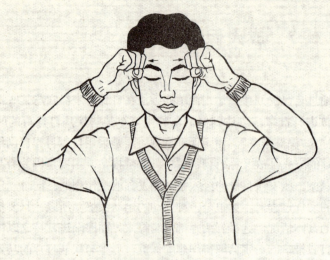

图 89

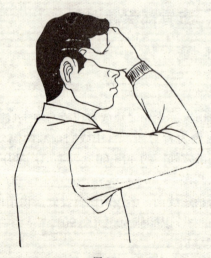

图 90

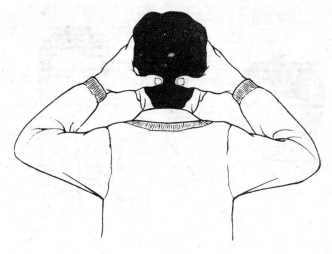

图 91

(4) 拍击头顶

人正坐，眼睛睁开前视，牙齿咬紧，用手掌心在囟门穴处作有节律的拍击动作，约 10 次左右（图 92）。

(5) 搓手浴面

先将两手搓热，随后掌心紧贴前额，用力向下擦到下颌，再沿下颌下缘向外至颊车，再向上经耳前、鬓角转推至前额中间，如此，反复旋转推摩面颊，每次约 20～30 遍左右，以面部有热感为宜（图 93）。

作用

上法对防治头痛、头晕、失眠健忘、神经衰弱、面瘫病症有效。

2. 眼部

操作

(1) 揉攒竹

以双手拇指螺纹面，分别按在双眉内侧头凹陷处的攒竹穴处，由轻而重反复揉约 20 次左右，以酸胀为宜（图 94）。

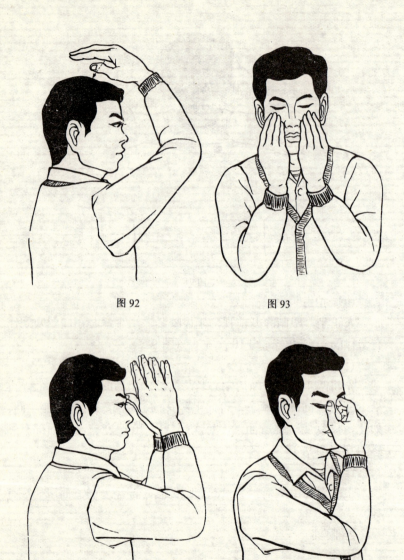

图 92　　　　　　　　　　图 93

图 94　　　　　　　　　　图 95

(2) 揉睛明

以右手拇、食 2 指螺纹面，按压在目内眦角上 1 分凹陷中之睛明穴，先用力向下按压，然后向上挤捏，如此一按一挤，反复进行，每次约 20～30 遍左右（图 95）。

(3) 按揉四白

以双手食指螺纹面，分别按在眼下眶正中下 1 寸处的四白穴，反复按揉 20 次左右，以酸胀为宜（图 96）。

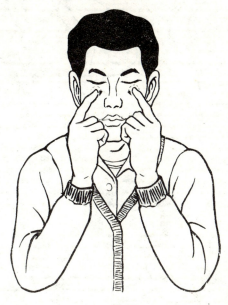

图 96

(4) 刮眼轮

双手食指屈曲，以第 2 指节的内侧面紧贴上眼眶的内侧端，自内向外推抹至眼眶的外侧端，然后再如此推抹下眼眶，如此先上后下，自内向外反复刮推约 20～30 次（图 97）。

(5) 熨眼

双目轻闭，先将两掌搓热，用双手掌根轻压热熨双目 30 秒钟，再轻轻揉动 10 余次（图 98）。

(6) 揉太阳

以两手拇指螺纹面紧贴双侧太阳穴处，反复按揉 30 次左右，以酸胀为宜（图 99）。

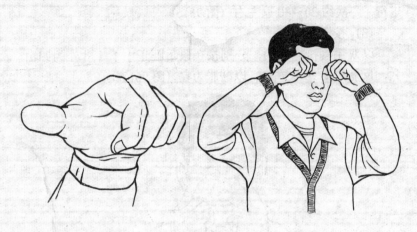

图 97-1　　　　　　　　　　　　　图 97-2

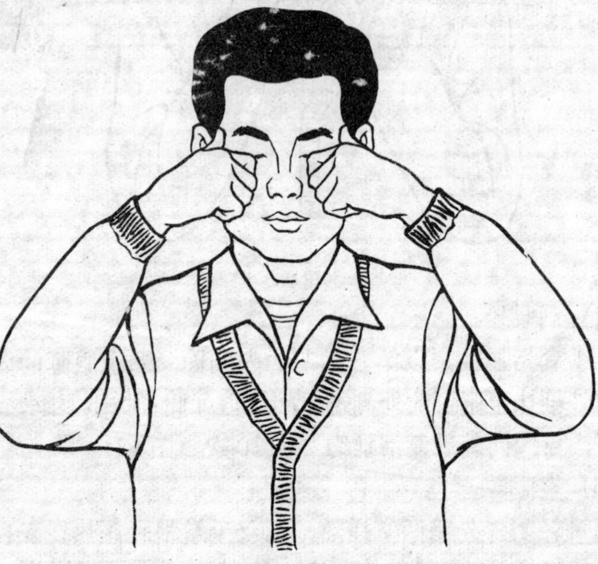

图 97-3

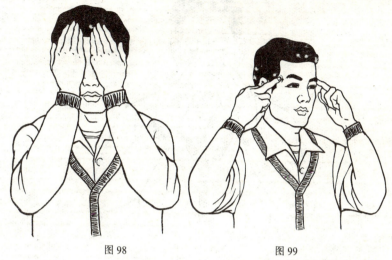

图 98 图 99

作用

上法可防治近视眼、视物不清、青光眼、视神经萎缩等各种眼病。

3. 鼻部

操作

(1) 按揉迎香

以两手中指螺纹面，按压在双侧迎香穴处，用力反复按揉30次左右，以酸胀为宜（图100）。

(2) 搓擦鼻旁

先将两手食指或中指掌面相对搓热，趁热在鼻翼两侧的鼻唇沟处，上、下搓擦，以热为宜，每次擦30次左右（图101）。

作用

上法对防治感冒、鼻塞流涕、过敏性鼻炎、慢性鼻炎、副鼻窦炎等病症有效。

4. 耳部

操作

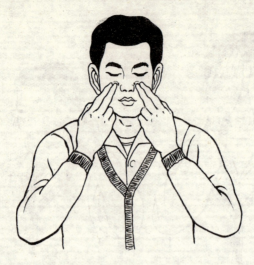

图 100

（1）按揉耳周诸穴

以双手拇指端，或中指端为着力点，分别按揉耳周围之耳门、听宫、听会与翳风等穴，每穴按揉 20 次左右，以酸胀为宜（图 102）

（2）摩擦耳轮

以双手拇指螺纹面与屈曲成弓状的食指桡侧面，轻轻捏住两侧耳轮，上、下反复摩擦 20～30 次左右（图 103）。

（3）鸣天鼓

以两掌心掩住两耳孔，掌根在前，手指指向耳后，用食指搭在中指上，向下弹击枕外隆凸两旁，使耳中隆隆作响，约 20 次左右（图 104）。

（4）搓擦耳前

以双手拇指桡侧，或食指掌面，紧贴在耳前，由上而下，由下而上的反复搓擦约 30 次左右，以热为宜。

作用

上法对防治耳鸣、重听、耳聋、中耳炎等病有效。

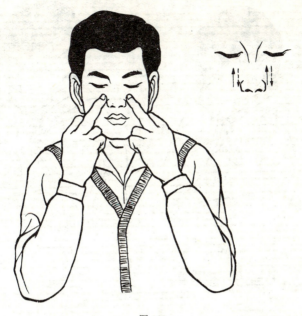

图 101

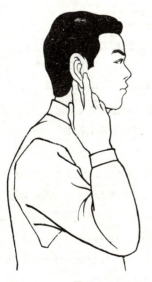

图 102

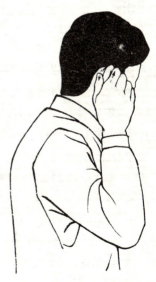

图 103

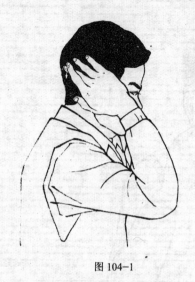
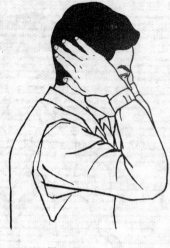

图 104-1   图 104-2

7.2 四肢部保健推拿

1. 上肢部

操作

(1) 按揉上肢诸穴

用拇指螺纹面，或中指指面先后按揉肩关节周围的肩内陵、肩髃、肩井穴，肘关节周围的曲池、手三里、尺泽、曲泽、少海、小海穴，前臂与腕关节周围的外关、内关、阳池、阳溪、合谷等穴，每穴按揉 20 次左右，以有酸、胀、麻等得气感为宜。左上肢诸穴由右手操作，右上肢诸穴由左手操作 (图 105)。

(2) 推擦上肢

先用一手掌心分别将对侧上肢的肩、肘、腕关节的前、后、内、外各面擦热，每面约擦 10～20 次左右，再沿经络循行方向，用一手掌心在对侧上肢的外侧，自腕背横纹外向上直擦至肩外侧之肩髃穴，再转向肩前方，沿上肢内侧向下直擦到腕内侧横纹处。如此在上肢的外侧由下而上，在上肢的内侧由上而下的反复推擦 30 遍左右，以擦热为宜 (图 106)。

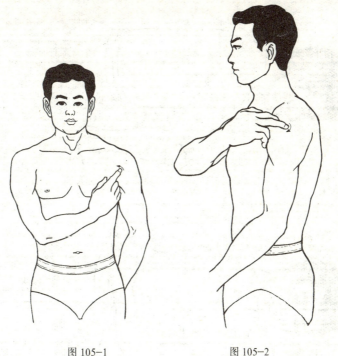

图 105-1   图 105-2

（3）擦捻掌指

先用一手之大鱼际，将另手之手背各掌骨间的肌肉分别擦热，再以拇、食 2 指，分别将另一手的各个指间关节一一揉捻（图 107）。

作用

上法可防治肩周炎、肩峰下滑囊炎、网球肘、腕部腱鞘炎等上肢各关节疾患，并有放松上肢肌肉，解除疲劳，增加上肢关节运动功能，预防职业性劳损等功效。

2. 下肢部

操作

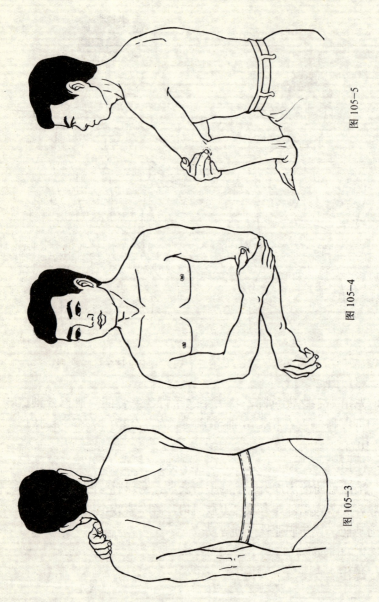

图 105—5

图 105—4

图 105—3

· 704 ·

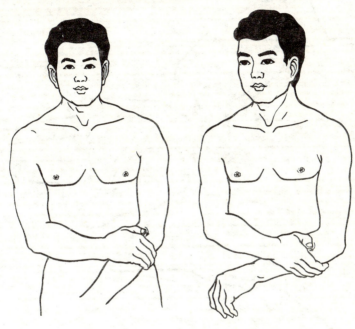

图 105-6 图 105-7

（1）按揉下肢诸穴

用拇指指面，或指端，或中指端，自上而下分别用力按揉居髎、环跳、伏兔、足三里、阳陵泉、承山、三阴交等穴，每穴按揉 20 次左右，以有得气感为宜（图 108）。

（2）按揉大腿

以两手掌根，自上而下，分别用力按揉大腿外侧，内侧与前侧肌肉 3～5 遍，以酸胀为宜（图 109）。

（3）按揉髌骨

下肢自然伸直，肌肉放松，以一手拇指指面及屈成弓状的食指桡侧面，拿捏并按揉髌骨（图 110）。

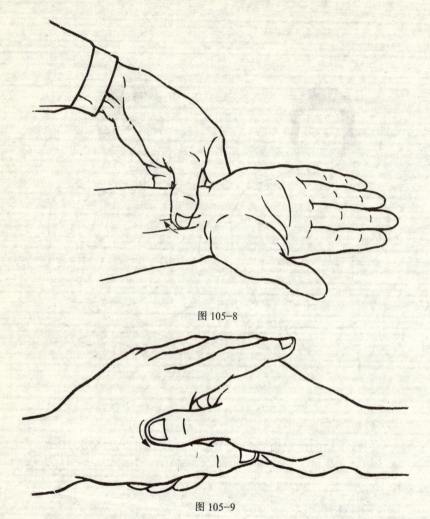

图 105—8

图 105—9

(4) 拿小腿

以一手拇指与食、中指指端，提拿捏揉腓肠肌，自上而下直至跟腱，用力柔和，每次操作 10 遍左右，以酸胀为宜（图111）。

(5) 拍击下肢

以两手掌心或掌根，自大腿根部起，从上而下，相对用力拍击下肢，直至小腿下端，约 10~15 遍左右（图 112）。

（6）擦涌泉

用一手小鱼际掌侧面，快速用力摩擦对侧足心之涌泉穴 30 次左右，以发热为宜，两足交替进行（图 113）。

（7）摇踝关节

正坐搁腿，一手抓踝上，一手握住足跖趾部，作顺时针及逆时针方向的旋转摇动踝关节，各约 20 次左右（图 114）。

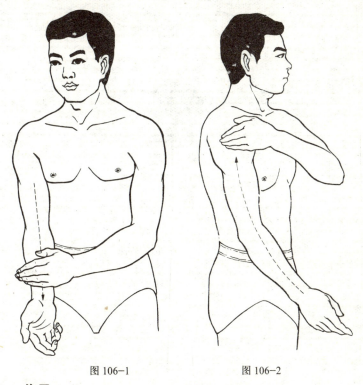

图 106-1　　　　　　　　　图 106-2

作用

上法对治疗臀上皮神经损伤、臀筋膜劳损、膝关节肿痛、腓肠肌痉挛、踝关节损伤等病症有效，并有放松下肢肌肉，消除疲劳，增强下肢各关节运动功能，预防各种职业性损伤等功效。另外，按揉足三里、三阴交、擦涌泉等法配合腹部及头部自我推拿手法，对胃肠消化系统、泌尿生殖系统与中枢神经系统有保健作用。

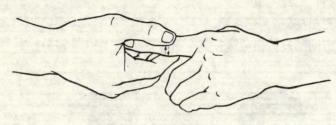

图 107

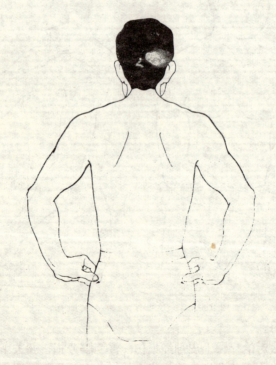

图 108—1

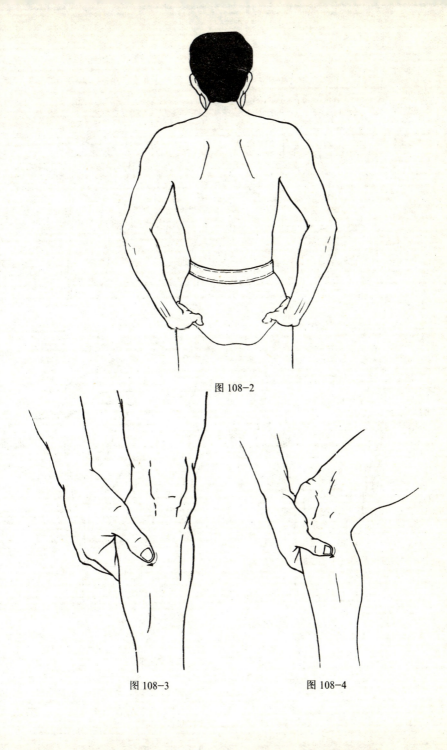

图 108-2

图 108-3

图 108-4

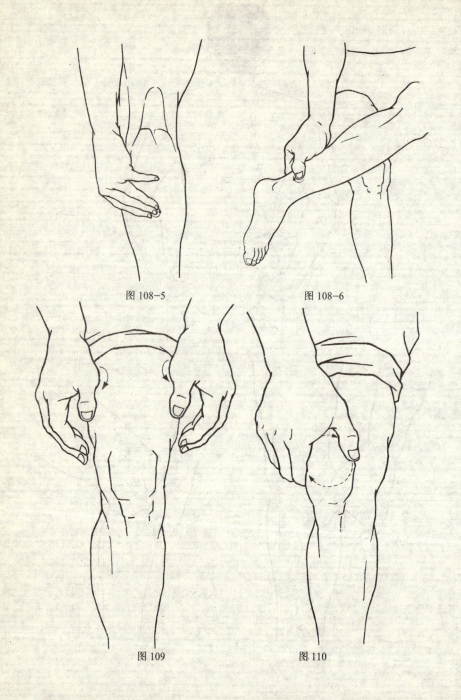

图 108-5

图 108-6

图 109

图 110

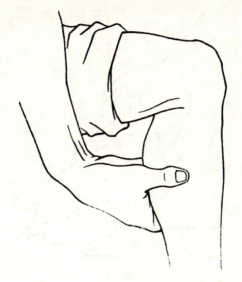

图 111

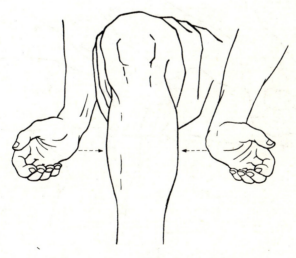

图 112

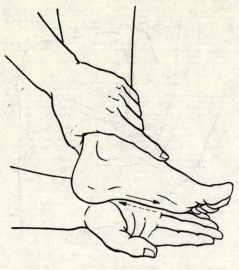

图 113

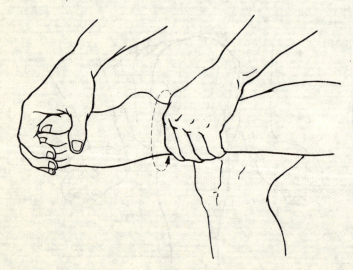

图 114

7.3 胸腹部保健推拿

1. 胸部

操作

(1) 按揉胸部诸穴及肋间

以一手中指螺纹面，先分别按揉膻中、中府、乳根、乳旁等穴，每穴 20 次左右，再自锁骨下肋骨间隙开始，从上而下，由内向外，用力按揉每个肋间隙，以酸胀为宜（图 115）。

(2) 拿胸肌

一手拇指紧贴胸前，食、中两指紧贴腋下相对用力提拿由胸大肌外侧组成的腋前壁，一提一拿并加以缓慢柔和的捏揉动作。每次操作 5 次左右（图 116）。

(3) 拍胸

以一手握虚拳，沿胸前正中线与两侧乳中线，自上而下，叩击胸部，在每条操作线路上叩击 10 次左右，叩击时不要屏气（图 117）。

(4) 擦胸

用一手大鱼际，或全掌紧贴胸部体表，横向用力来回摩擦 20 次左右，以发热为宜（图 118）。

作用

上法对岔气、胸痛、胸闷、咳嗽、气喘、气机不畅、心悸等病症有防治作用。

2. 腹部

操作

(1) 按揉腹部诸穴

用中指端，或大鱼际或掌根为着力面，分别按揉中脘、章门、天枢、气海、关元、中极等穴，每穴 20～30 次左右，以产生气感为宜（图 119，120）。

(2) 摩腹

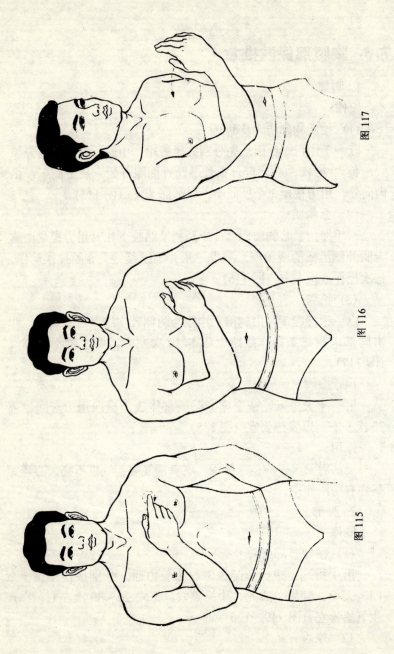

图 117

图 116

图 115

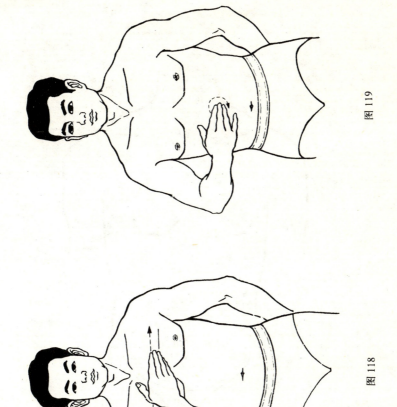

图 119

图 118

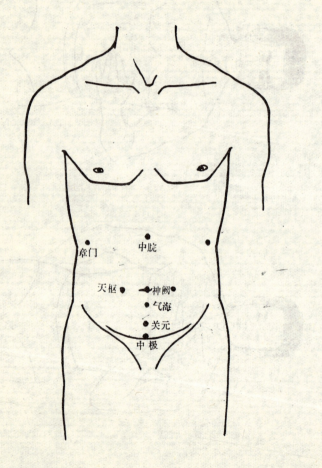

图 120

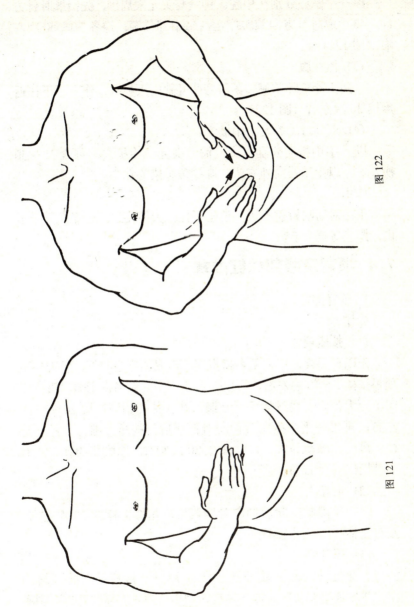

图 122

图 121

以一手掌心分别在中脘、神阙与关元穴周围，先沿顺时针方向，再沿逆时针方向旋转摩运，每个部位顺、逆各 30~50 次左右（图 121）。

（3）擦少腹

以两手小鱼际掌侧贴紧脐旁两寸处的天枢穴、作上、下往返摩擦 30 次左右（图 122）。

（4）点气海、关元、中极穴

以一手中指端分别点击气海、关元、中极穴，每穴 30~50 次左右，以生殖器向外有胀、麻等传导感为宜。

作用

上法对防治胃脘不适，消化不良，大便秘结，腹痛，月经不调，阳痿等病症有效。

7.4 项背及腰部保健推拿

1. 项背部

操作

（1）按揉项背

先以双手食、中、无名指指端，沿双侧风池向下，经天柱至项根按揉 5~10 遍左右，再以一手食、中、无名指指端，沿风府向下至大椎穴一线按揉 5~10 遍，在穴位处稍停按揉 20~30 次左右。再用一手中指向后伸向对侧背后，按揉大椎、大杼、身柱、风门、肺俞等穴，每穴按揉 30 次左右，以酸胀为宜。左右交替操作（图 123）。

（2）拍背

以一手虚掌，向后伸向对侧背后，拍打上背部 10 次左右。左右交替操作（图 124）。

（3）摩膏肓

上身挺直，两上肢外展 90°，屈肘，做肩关节的环转动作，并尽量增大向后的伸展幅度，利用肩胛骨的环转动作，刺激

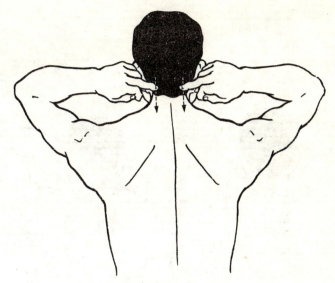

图 123-1

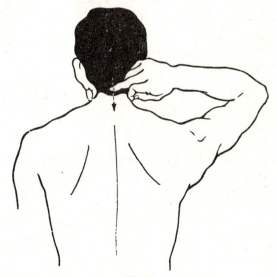

图 123-2

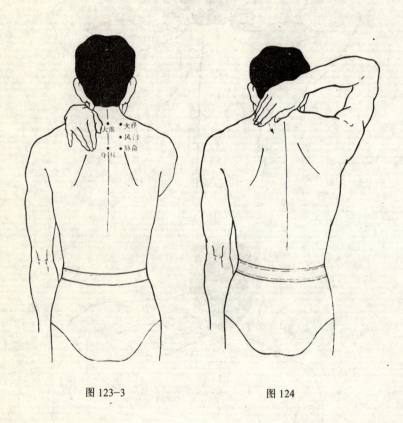

大椎 · 大杼
· 风门
· 肺俞
身柱 ·

图 123-3　　　　　　　　　　图 124

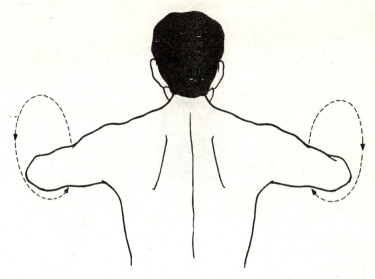

图 125-1

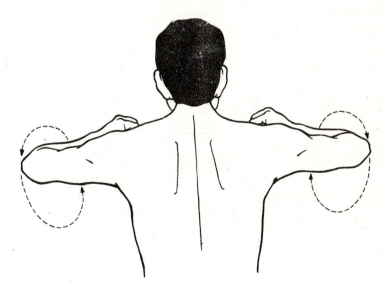

图 125-2

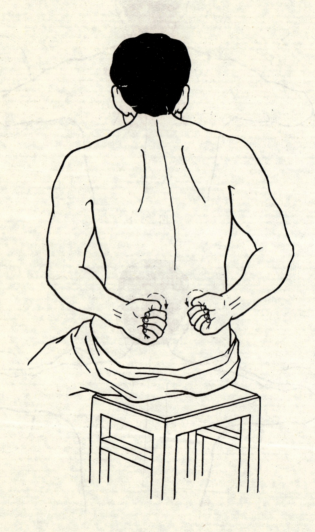

图 126-1

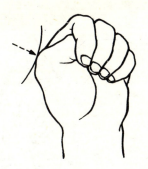

图 126-2

位于两侧肩胛间区的膏肓等穴区（图 125）。

作用

上法对防治背痛酸胀，颈椎病、落枕、咳嗽、哮喘、痰结、虚劳、胸闷、胸痛、心悸、心绞痛等病症有效。

2. 腰部

操作

（1）揉腰部诸穴

两手握拳，以食指掌指关节突起处用力，分别按揉肾俞、志室、腰眼诸穴，每穴按揉 30 次左右，以酸胀为宜（图 126）。

（2）捶振腰区

两手握拳，以拳眼处着力，自上而下，分别沿肾俞至膀胱俞一线，志室经腰眼至胞肓一线与命门至腰骶关节一线，叩击捶振腰部 5～10 遍（图 127）。

（3）擦腰

用两手掌根紧按腰部皮肤，自第二腰椎水平，向下至骶髂关节处，上下往返摩擦，以发热为宜（图 128）。

作用

上法对防治多种原因引起的腰部酸痛，无力、失眠、阳痿、

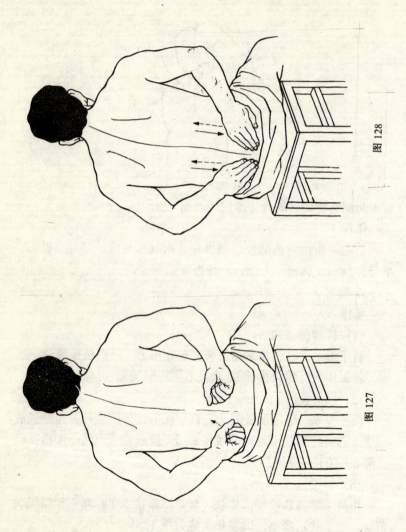

图 128

图 127

尿频、腰椎骨质增生、腰椎间盘突出症、腰肌劳损、月经失调、腹泻等病症和放松腰部肌肉，消除疲劳，增强腰部运动功能等有效。

以上介绍的各部位自我推拿法，在实用时可作为全身性的保健、养生法，按头面→颈项→上背→胸腹→腰骶→上肢→下肢的顺序，每天依次全套操作 1 遍至 2 遍，也可根据自己的身体情况，选做其中的一部分，如经常容易感冒的人，可重点做头面、项背及胸部的自我推拿，作为针对性的健康保健，如果从事某种职业，身体的某些部位容易疲劳，劳损而影响工作效率的人与好发职业病的人，则可选择其中相关的部位进行操作，以提高工作效率与防治职业病，如长跑运动员或经常取站姿工作的人，可每天在训练与工作前后做腰骶部与下肢部的保健推拿。又如伏案工作的脑力劳动者，可在每天工间休息时间与下班回家后，选做头面、颈项及腰背、上肢部的自我推拿，以消除腰背与颈项部由于长时间弯曲前倾位工作所造成的疲劳，并提高大脑的工作效率。另外，保健推拿，又可用作中、老年人许多常见慢性病的自疗与康复手段。运用时，应根据病情，选取有关部位的自我推拿方法，组成适合于该疾病的自疗推拿组方，每天进行自我推拿，如慢性腹泻者可按以下组方操作：按揉百会穴 50 次，摩脐周围 50 次，摩关元 50 次，擦少腹 30 次，按揉肾俞穴 30 次，摩擦肾区 50 次，点击关元穴 30 次，按揉足三里 30 次，按揉三阴交 20 次。再如糖尿病患者的自我推拿组方为：按揉中脘穴、关元穴各 50 次，摩中脘、神厥穴顺、逆各 30 遍，捶振肾区 30 次，摩擦腰部 30 次，按揉足三里 30 次。

（王国才　李华东）

下篇 小儿推拿

8 小儿推拿简介

8.1 概述

小儿推拿是祖国医学的重要组成部分，是以手法在小儿体表特定部位或穴位上进行操作为治疗手段的一门临床医学学科。

小儿推拿操作简便，不给患儿造成痛苦，对某些疾病疗效高，没有副作用。小儿推拿不但能治疗各类常见病和疑难病，并能预防疾病，因此它是一种前景广阔的医疗方法。

8.2 小儿推拿的有关知识

1. 小儿推拿的特点

(1) 整体观念，辨证论治

小儿推拿是在祖国医学整体观念的基础上，以阴阳、五行、脏腑、经络、营卫、气血等学说为理论指导，根据辨证论治的原则，在患儿体表运用各种手法来调整脏腑、营卫、气血，从而达到治疗疾病的目的。

(2) 经络学说

小儿推拿是通过经络"行气血通阴阳"的作用，来调整脏腑营卫的，也就是说是藉着经络来调整机体生理机能的。

2. 小儿推拿手法的补泻问题

凡能起到促进机体机能之发挥，补益人体气血阴阳之不足，治疗各种虚弱症候的操作方法，通称为补法。与补法相反，能治疗各种实证，起到清除肠内宿食、燥屎及其它有害物质，使从大便排出，使体内热毒通过泻下而得到缓解的手法，通称为泻法。

由于小儿的生理病理特点，对其用补法或泻法必须恰到好处，中病即止，切忌剧烈攻伐或一味补之。

手法的次数多少，操作力的轻重变化，如同用药的剂量一样重要。手法轻，时间长，可以达到补的目的；手法重，时间短，可以起到泻的作用。

推拿操作在具体穴位上有方向性，有的穴位向心方向是补，离心方向为泻；有的穴位向心方向为清，离心方向为补。同一个穴位不同的操作方向有不同的作用，这就说明推拿穴位具有双向调节作用。因此，只有掌握各种手法及手法在不同穴位上的不同刺激方向的具体作用，才能达到补虚泻实的目的。

本章中所用手法次数，以1岁小儿为实例，年龄越小，推拿次数越少，手法相应也轻；相反，年龄越大，体质越强，邪实越甚，推拿次数越多，手法越重。一般1岁左右的小儿用推、揉、摩等较柔和的操作方法，一个穴位300次即可，而刺激较重的掐、按、拿、摇等手法，治疗3～5次即可。总的操作时间1—3岁小儿需15～20分钟左右，6个月至1岁的患儿应5～10分钟左右，对新生儿的操作时间3～5分钟即可。

根据病情确定疗程，对病程长，慢性病，如厌食、哮喘、遗尿、瘫痪等，可以定为15次为1个疗程；对不愈者，可连续2～3个疗程；对病程短，常见病，多发病，一般3～6次为一个疗程；如不愈，可以连续1个疗程；在慢性病的2～3个疗程间，可暂停诊10～15天后再重新开始治疗。

3. 小儿推拿穴位的特点

小儿推拿除了运用十四经穴及经外奇穴外，还有许多特定的穴位，这些穴位不仅呈点状，还有线及面状。这些特定穴位分布在两肘、两膝以下者居多，运用这些穴位都可以主治五脏的疾病。

4. 注意事项

（1）小儿推拿的顺序

一般是先上肢，次头面，再胸腹、腰脊，最后是下肢。在上肢操作，一般不分男女，习惯于推拿左手（也可推拿右手），也可以根据病情的轻重缓急，或患儿体位而定顺序的先后，灵活应用。

（2）小儿推拿处方的组成

每张处方必有主穴、配穴的区分，确定主穴和配穴，对临床效果有密切的关系，因此，应认真学习，准确掌握。

（3）小儿推拿介质

这些介质如葱汁、姜汁、麻油、韭、蒜、白芥子、冰片、麝香等既有滑润的作用，又有疏经活络，通关开窍的作用。

5. 小儿的生理病理特点

（1）生理特点

主要是脏腑娇嫩、形气未充，年龄越小越显著。

肺主一身之气，但易于受邪，又不耐寒热，故称为"娇脏"。小儿脾常不足，往往导致肺气弱，而为"肺常不足"。

脾为生化之源，但小儿机体处于不断生长发育的过程之中，对营养物质的需要量大、致使脾胃负担相对较重。因此"脾常不足"就显得更为突出。

小儿的发育，抗病能力等均与肾有关，各脏之阴取资于肾阴的滋润，各脏之阳也有赖于肾阳的温养。小儿能否健康成长，与肾气的盛衰有密切的关系。小儿时期肾的功能和作用相对不足，故称为"肾常虚"。

总之，小儿无论在物质基础，还是功能活动方面，均属幼稚和不完善，这是小儿的生理特点之一。

小儿生理的另一个特点是：婴幼儿生机勃勃，发育迅速。从体格、智力以及脏腑功能诸方面，均处于不断完善和发展中。年龄越小，生长发育就越快，好比旭日之初生，草木之方萌。

（2）病理特点

小儿"肺常不足"，卫外机能未固，外邪每易由表而入侵袭肺系，最易引起流行病及咳嗽、感冒等病症。

小儿"脾常不足"，常为饮食所伤，易发生腹泻、呕吐、积滞、疳症等。

小儿"肾常虚"，肾虚无以资助它脏，脾虚不能滋养肾精，影响小儿生长发育，久之出现发育迟缓之症状。由于小儿脏腑娇嫩，形气未充，所以在患病之后，寒热虚实的变化比较明显，其传变速度也较迅速。

小儿病理的另一个特点是：由于发育迅速，活力充沛、脏气清灵、病因单纯（较少七情影响），容易趋向康复。

9 小儿推拿手法

9.1 推法

推法是医者用拇指螺纹面或偏峰（桡侧），或并拢的食中指螺纹面，着力于患儿身体表面应推的部位，进行单方向直线推动的方法。

动作要领

上肢放松，肘关节自然屈曲，术指对准接触面，用力均匀柔和轻快。以拇指螺纹面或桡侧面进行直推时，腕关节要作小幅度屈伸活动（图129-1）；以食中指并拢直推时，腕关节应作小幅度外展内收活动，使动作协调深透（图129-2）。本法推行方向必须呈直线状，以前推为主，回收时应稍微离开皮肤。本法频率每分钟240次。

适用范围

本法具有祛风散寒，清热止痛双重作用，且能通经活络。广泛适用于小儿的头面、上肢、胸腹、腰背和下肢部穴位。临床上常把此法作为清、补两法运用。如推大肠穴：自指根推向指尖为清，自指尖推向指根为补。

9.2 按法

按法是医者用拇指或中指顶端按压患儿身体某处和穴位的方法。

动作要领

拇指按时，医者左或右手握拳，拇指伸直，顶端按压穴位，食指屈曲贴靠住拇指面，以协助其发力（图130-1）；中指按时，医者以拇指面抵住中指远端指间关节掌面，中指顶端在穴位上按压（图130-2）。本法按压时用力必须缓和渐进，切忌粗暴。

适用范围

本法具有通经活络，开通闭塞，祛寒止痛作用。适用于全身各部和穴位。

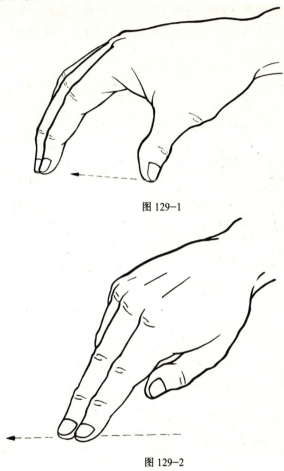

图 129—1

图 129—2

9.3 摩法

摩法是医者用指或掌在患儿身体某处摩动的方法。

动作要领

　　肩肘部放松，腕关节微屈，指掌自然伸直，平贴于施术部位，令其随同腕关节及前臂作盘旋摩动。指摩时，以中、食、无名指3指腹在穴位处作不断地环旋抚摩（图131-1）；掌摩时，用手掌环旋抚摩施术部位（图131-2）。用力宜协调柔和，频率可根据病情灵活确定。一般指摩法每分钟80次，掌摩法每分钟60~80次。

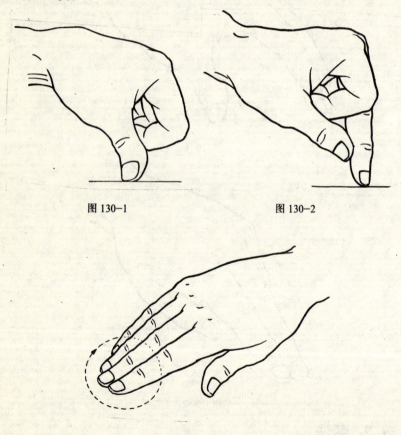

图130-1　　　　　　　　　　图130-2

图131-1

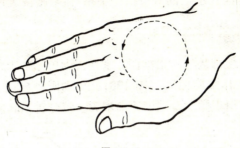

图 131-2

适用范围

本法具有舒气活血，消肿退热，消积导滞，温中健脾作用。在临床尚有逆时针方向摩为补，顺时针方向摩为泻；掌摩为补，指摩为泻；缓摩为补，急摩为泻等说法。本法对胃肠疾患最为有效。一般指摩法适用于头面等较小部位，掌摩法适用于胸腹胁肋等部位。

9.4 掐法

掐法是医者用手指甲在患儿某处或穴位上深深地间断掐压的方法。

动作要领

拇指伸直或微屈，指尖对准施术部位，其余 4 指并拢握成空心拳，贴靠住拇指，然后进行掐压（图 132）。掐压时缓缓用力，使指端掐入，切忌爆发用力。本法多在最后施行（急症例外），用力大小及持续时间长短，应根据病情及患儿反映适当掌握。

适用范围

本法具有定惊醒神，通关开窍作用。适用于头面部、手足部穴位，宜救治小儿急症、惊症。

9.5 揉法

揉法是医者用指面（拇指、中指）、掌根或大鱼际在患儿身体上揉动的方法。

动作要领

肩部及腕部放松，用指面、掌根或大鱼际贴于患处，以腕关节连同前臂作回旋揉动（图133）。揉动时，要用力吸住皮肤，并带动皮下组织揉动，幅度逐渐增大。每分钟160次。

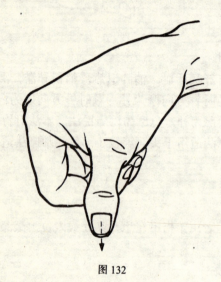

图132

适用范围

本法能消肿止痛，祛风散热；又可调和气血，理气消积。适用于全身各个部位。主治脘腹胀痛、胸闷胁痛、便秘泄泻等，对软组织急性损伤疗效尤显。

9.6 运法

运法是指医者用拇指或食、中指的正面，在患儿选定的部位上作连续地弧形或环形运动。

动作要领

指面一定要贴紧施术部位，但不可用力重滞。仅在身体表层施法，一般不带动皮下组织。运动时要缓缓而行（图 134）。频率为每分钟 160 次。

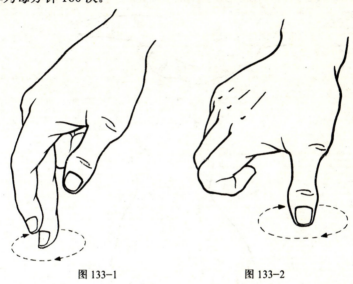

图 133-1   图 133-2

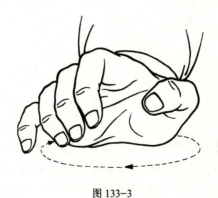

图 133-3

适用范围

本法能理气和血，舒筋活络。常用于小儿颞部及手部穴位。

如运太阳穴，运八卦穴等。

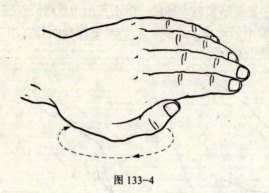

图 133-4

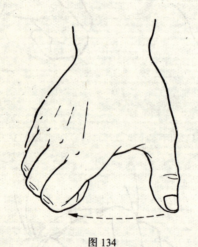

图 134

9.7 捏法

捏法是医者用手拿握住患儿身体某处部位、穴位，进行捏挤或提、拿捏、推综合的方法。根据适用部位不同，分为两种：

1 捏脊法：医者食指屈曲，以食指中节桡侧缘抵住皮肤，拇指端前按，拇、食指挟住皮肤，捻起并用力提拿，双手交替前移（图135）。因本法只适用于脊背部，故称捏脊法。

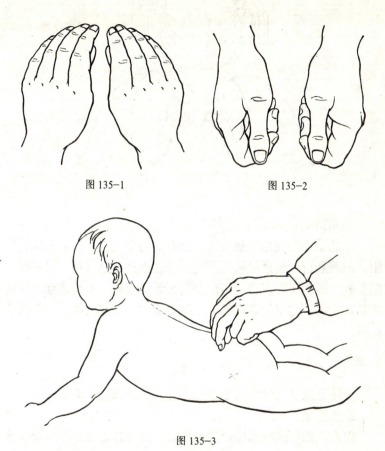

图 135-1

图 135-2

图 135-3

2. 捏挤法：是医者用双手拇指与食、中、无名指等指端，自穴位或部位周围向其中央捏挤的方法（图136）。

动作要领

用力要柔和，切忌粗暴及使用蛮劲。捏拿皮肤要把表皮及皮下组织一同捏提起。进行捏脊时，要从患儿腰骶部开始，直线向上至大椎穴处，每次施术约 3～5 遍。进行捏挤时，用力不可太大，以无显著痛感为度，缓缓捏挤直至局部皮肤红润充血为止。

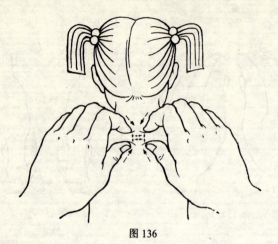

图 136

适用范围

本法是小儿推拿中最常用，最有效的手法之一，具有调和阴阳，健脾和胃；疏通经络，行气活血，泄热止痛作用。捏脊法功偏于补，适用于脊背部，治疗小儿积滞、腹泻、呕吐等症；捏挤法功偏于泻，适用于较小部位，如大椎穴、天突穴等，可以清热止呕。

9.8 分法

分法是医者同时用两手指面分推穴位或部位两侧的方法。

动作要领

以双手拇指螺纹面接触施术部位，自穴位或部位中央向两旁作"←o→"或"ͻoͼ"方向分推（图 137）。双手用力不可太重，动作应柔和协调。频率每分钟 100～120 次。

适用范围

本法具有调和阴阳，分理气血，消积导滞作用。可适用于面、腕、胸、腹、背等部位。

9.9 捣法

捣法是指医者用中指端或其屈曲的近端指间关节背面突起的

部分轻叩穴位的方法。

动作要领

单手操作，腕部发力，指端或指间关节突起部分着力，叩击轻巧有弹性（图138）。一般速度较慢，每分钟100次左右。

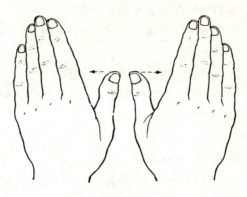

图 137

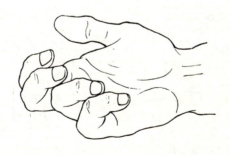

图 138

适用范围

本法能宁神定惊，舒筋通脉。常用于手掌、颅顶及浅表关节部位。

10 小儿推拿常用穴位

10.1 头颈部穴位

天门穴

位置：两眉间中点至前发际成一直线。

操作：用两拇指自下而上交替直推，称开天门（图 139）。

次数：30～50 次。

作用：发汗解表，镇惊安神，开窍醒脑，止头痛。

主治：风寒感冒，头痛、发烧、无汗、惊吓、精神萎靡等。

坎宫穴

位置：从眉头起至眉梢成一横线。

操作：患儿取仰卧位，医者坐在床头，先用两拇指掐按眉弓中点一下，再用两拇指桡侧面自眉心向眉梢作分推，称推坎宫（图 140）。

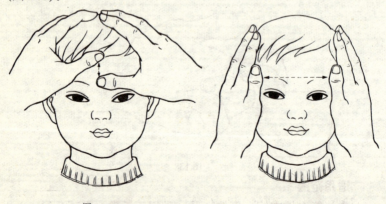

图 139   图 140

次数：30～50 次。

作用：发汗解表，醒脑明目，止头痛。

主治：感冒头痛，头晕，目赤痛，惊风，近视，斜视等。

太阳穴

位置: 眉及外眼眦连线中点, 眉后约 1 寸凹陷处。

操作: 患儿取仰卧位, 医者端坐在床头旁, 两拇指桡侧自眼向耳直推, 称推太阳。用中指端揉该穴, 称揉太阳或运太阳 (图 141)。向眼方向揉为补, 向耳方向揉为泻。

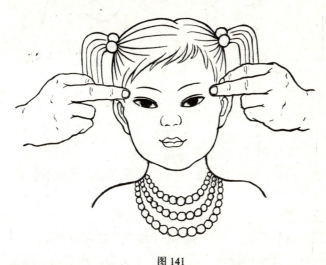

图 141

次数: 30~50 次。

作用: 疏风解表、清热明目、止头痛。

主治: 头痛, 发热, 恶寒无汗和次及近视, 斜视等。

耳后高骨穴

位置: 耳后颞骨乳突处。

操作: 患儿取俯卧位或端坐位, 医者站在患儿身后, 以两拇指或中指端作揉法或掐法, 称揉耳后高骨或掐耳后高骨 (图 142)。

次数: 揉 30~50 次; 掐 3~5 次。

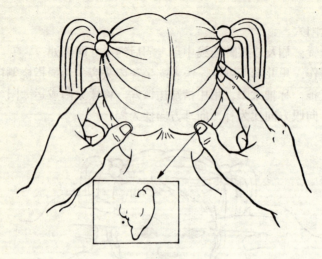

图 142

作用：发汗解表，止头项疼痛。

主治：头痛，惊风，烦躁不安，颈项疼痛，转侧不利等。

百会穴

位置：两耳尖直上，与鼻尖正中线在头顶部交点处。

操作：患儿取仰卧位，医者坐于床头旁。或患儿取端坐位，医者站于患儿身后，以左手扶住儿头一侧或前额处，以拇指按或揉，称按百会或揉百会（图143）。

次数：按 30～50 次，揉 100～200 次。

作用：安神镇惊，升阳举陷。

主治：头痛眩晕，惊风，惊痫，脱肛，遗尿等。

印堂穴

位置：两眉头连线的中点。

操作：患儿取仰卧位，医者坐在患儿右侧，以指端按之或揉之，称按印堂或揉印堂（图144）。

次数：50～100次。

作用：安神，开窍，止痛。

主治：前额痛，睡眠不安，鼻炎，近视，斜视等。

山根穴

位置：两目内眦之中，鼻梁最低凹陷处。

操作：患儿取仰卧位，医者坐于床右侧，以一手扶儿头，一手拇指甲掐，称掐山根；或以中指揉，称揉山根；以拇指食指相对捏，称捏山根（图145）。

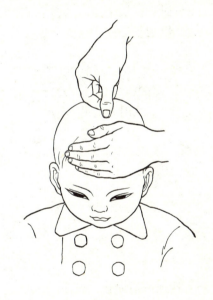

图143

次数：掐3～5次；揉30～50次；捏20～30次。

作用：开窍，醒目定神。

主治：惊风。

水沟穴

位置：鼻下唇上，人中沟正中线上 1/3 与下 2/3 交界处。

操作：患儿取仰卧位或端坐位，医者坐或站在患儿的一旁，以拇指甲掐之，继以揉之，称掐揉水沟（图 146）。

次数：3～5 次或醒后即止。

作用：开窍醒神。

主治：惊风，昏厥，口眼歪斜，抽搐，唇动。

承浆穴

位置：颏唇沟的中心。

操作：患儿取仰卧位或端坐位，医者站在患儿的右侧，以拇指甲掐，称掐承浆；以拇指面揉，称揉承浆（图 147）。

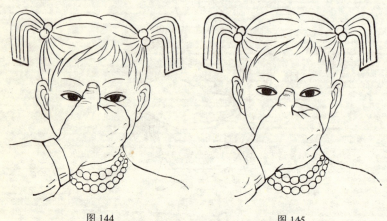

图 144　　　　　　　　　　　图 145

次数：掐 3～5 次或醒后即止。揉 30～50 次。

作用：醒神开窍，镇惊止痛。

主治：口眼歪斜，牙痛，中暑昏厥，癫痫等。

风池穴

位置：胸锁乳突肌与斜方肌之间，入后发际 5 分处，平风府穴。

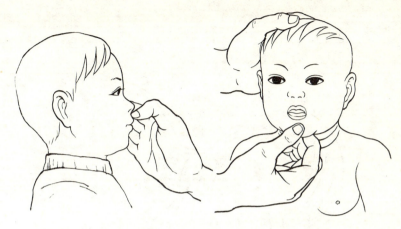

图 146　　　　　　　　　　　　图 147

操作：患儿取端坐位，医者站在患儿身后，用两拇指对准穴位用拿法，称拿风池（图 148）。

次数：5～10 次。

作用：发汗解表，祛风散寒。

主治：感冒，头痛，目眩，颈项僵硬疼痛，转侧不利，近视，斜视，小儿肌性斜颈。

牙关穴

位置：耳下一寸，下颌骨陷中。

操作：患儿取端坐位，医者站于患儿面前偏侧，用拇指按或中指揉，称按牙关或揉牙关（图 149）。

次数：按 5～10 次；揉 30～50 次。

作用：开牙关，止牙痛。

主治：牙关紧闭，口眼歪斜，牙痛及腮腺肿痛。

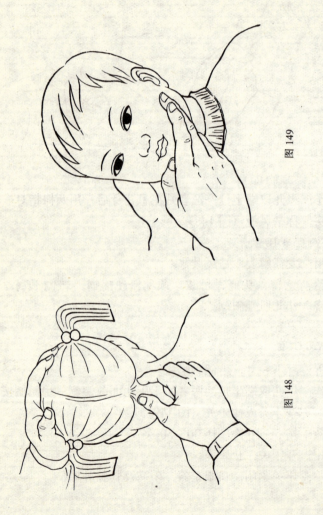

图 149

图 148

天柱骨穴

位置：颈后发际正中至大椎穴成一直线。

操作：患儿取端坐位，医者站在患儿背后一侧，用拇指或食中两指自上而下直推，称推天柱骨（图150）。

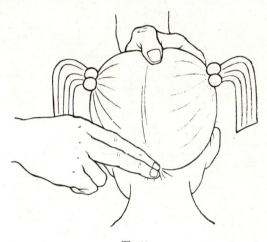

图150

次数：100～300次。

作用：降逆止呕，祛风散寒。

主治：恶心，呕吐，风寒感冒，头痛，项强，近视，斜视。

囟门穴

位置：前发际正中直上2寸，百会前骨陷中。

操作：患儿取端坐位，医者站在患儿左或右侧，以两手食中无名小指挟儿头，两拇指自前发际向该穴轮换推之（囟门未合时，仅推至骨缝的边缘），称推囟门。用拇指端轻揉本穴称揉囟门（图151）。

次数：推或揉各50～100次。

作用：镇惊安神通窍。

主治：头痛，鼻塞，惊风，衄血，烦躁不安等。

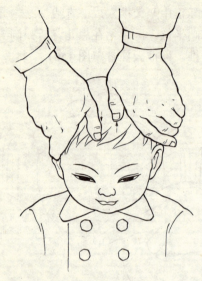

图 151

10.2　胸腹部穴位

天突穴

位置：胸骨上凹陷正中。

操作：患儿取仰卧位，医者站在患儿右旁，用中指端按或揉，称按天突或揉天突（图 152）。用双手拇食两指捏住局部皮肤，向中间挤，称挤捏天突。

次数：10～15 次。

作用：理气化痰，降逆平喘，止呕吐。

主治：痰壅气急，喘咳胸闷，咯痰不畅，食积停滞，恶心呕吐。

膻中穴

位置：前正中线，两乳头连线的中点（平第四肋间隙处）。

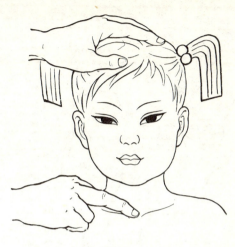

图 152

操作: 患儿取仰卧位或端坐位, 医者站于患儿右旁, 用两拇指桡侧面, 从膻中穴向两侧分推, 称分推膻中 (图 153); 以食中指指腹自胸骨端向下推之膻中穴, 称下推膻中; 以中指螺纹面在穴位上作揉法, 称揉膻中 (图 154)。

次数: 推揉各 100~200 次; 分推膻中 50~100 次。

作用: 宽胸理气, 宣肺止咳化痰。

主治: 胸闷胸痛, 咳嗽气喘, 痰鸣, 恶心呕吐。

乳根穴

位置: 乳下 2 分。

操作: 中指端揉, 称揉乳根。

次数: 20~50 次。

作用: 宽胸理气, 止咳化痰。

主治: 胸闷, 胸痛, 咳嗽, 气喘, 痰鸣。

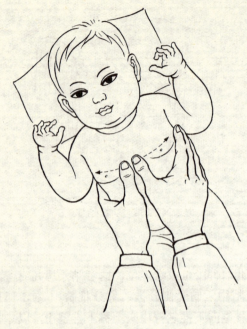

图 153

乳旁穴

位置：乳头外旁开 2 分。

操作：患儿取仰卧位或端坐位，医者用右手中指端揉，称揉乳旁（图 155）。

次数：20～50 次。

作用：宽胸理气，止咳化痰。

主治：胸闷，胸痛，咳嗽，气喘，痰鸣。

中脘穴

位置：脐上 4 寸处。

操作：小儿取仰卧位，医者以指端或掌根作按法或揉法，分别称按中脘或揉中脘；或以掌心或四指并拢作摩法，称摩中脘

（图 156）。

次数：揉 100～300 次；摩 5 分钟。

作用：健脾和胃，消食和中。

主治：食积，腹胀，腹痛，呕吐，泄泻，食欲不振，嗳气等。

胁肋

位置：以腋下两胁至天枢处。

操作：小儿取正坐位，以两手抱头，医者站立于小儿正面或背面，以两手掌从腋两胁下搓摩至天枢处，称搓摩胁肋（图157）。

次数：50～100 次。

作用：舒肝理气，化痰开积。

主治：食积，痰积，气积，胸闷，胁痛，痰喘，气急，疳积，肝脾肿大等。

神阙穴（脐）

位置：肚脐正中

操作：患儿仰卧，医者用中指端或掌根作揉法，称揉脐；用食、中、无名指作指摩法或掌摩称摩脐（图 158）。

次数：揉 100～300 次，摩 3～5 分钟。

作用：温阳散寒，补益气血。

主治：泄泻，呕吐，腹胀，腹痛，食积，便秘，肠鸣，脱肛等。

天枢穴

位置：脐左右旁开 2 寸。

操作：患儿取仰卧位，医者坐于其右旁或左旁，以食指或中指揉，称揉天枢。以拇指食指作拿法称拿天枢（图 159）。

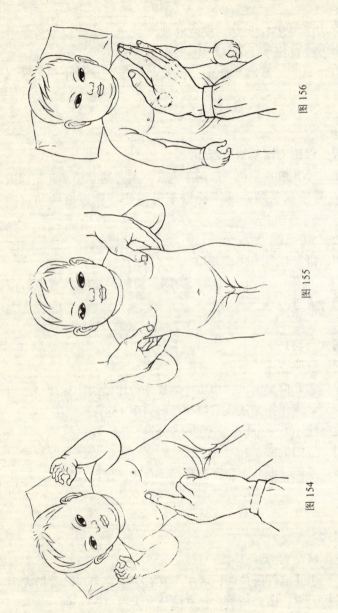

图 156

图 155

图 154

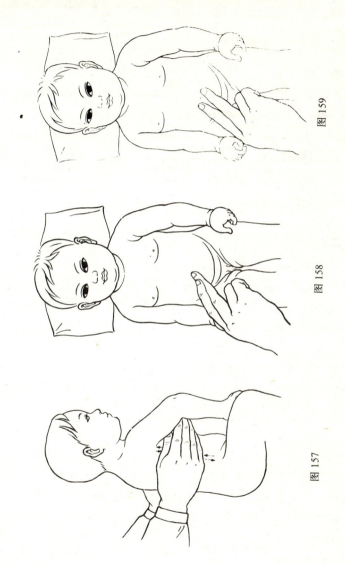

图 159

图 158

图 157

次数: 揉 50～100 次, 拿 3～5 次。

作用: 疏调大肠, 理气消滞。

主治: 泄泻, 便秘, 腹胀, 腹痛, 痢疾, 食积不化。

腹

位置: 即腹部。

操作: 患儿取仰卧位, 医者坐其右旁, 用掌或四指作顺时针或逆时针摩法, 称摩腹 (图 160)。

次数: 摩 3～5 分钟。

作用: 健脾和胃, 理气消食。

主治: 腹胀, 腹痛, 食积, 便秘, 泄泻, 食欲不振, 消化不良, 蛔虫性肠梗阻等。

腹阴阳穴

位置: 中脘穴斜向脐两旁。

操作: 患者取仰卧位, 医者站在其右旁, 用两手食、中、无名指和小指指腹或两拇指桡侧面, 自中脘穴斜向分推至脐两旁, 称分推腹阴阳 (图 161)。

次数: 分推 100～200 次。

作用: 消食化滞, 和胃降逆。

主治: 身热, 食积, 胸闷, 呕吐酸馊, 腹胀, 腹痛, 消化不良等。

肚角

位置: 脐旁 2 寸, 脐下 2 寸。

操作: 患儿取仰卧位, 医者用拇指置于腹部肚角上, 食、中指于儿腰背相对处, 然后 3 指同时用力, 向深处拿肚筋, 称拿肚角 (图 162)。

次数: 2～3 次。

作用：缓急止痛，理气消胀。
主治：寒热腹痛，腹胀，泻痢等。

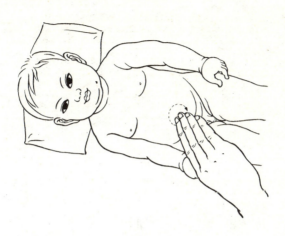

图 160

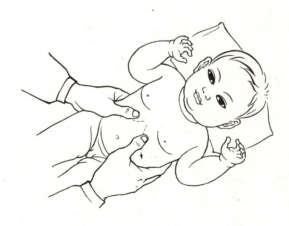

图 161

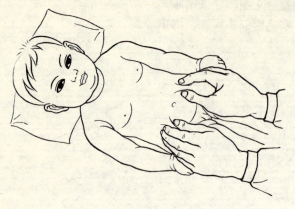

图 162

丹田穴

位置: 在小腹部, 脐下 2.5 寸处。

操作: 患儿取仰卧位, 医者坐其右旁, 以中指揉之或掌心摩之。以手揉之或摩之, 分称揉丹田或摩丹田 (图 163)。

次数: 揉 50~100 次; 摩 3~5 分钟。

作用: 培肾固本, 温补下元, 分清别浊。

主治: 遗尿, 脱肛, 尿闭, 小便短赤, 小腹胀痛, 疝气等。

10.3 背部穴位

大椎穴

位置: 在第七颈椎棘突下。

操作: 患儿取坐位, 医者站在其右旁。用右手拇指或中指对准穴位按揉之, 称揉大椎 (图 164)。

次数: 100~300 次。

作用: 清热解表。

主治: 感冒, 发热, 头痛项强, 骨蒸盗汗, 咳嗽, 气喘。

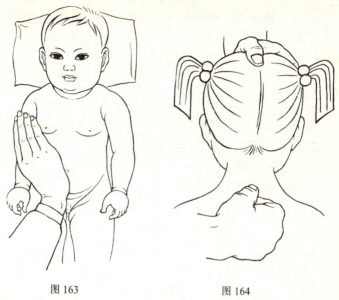

图 163   图 164

肺俞穴

位置：在第三胸椎棘突下，旁开 1.5 寸。

操作：患儿取俯卧位，医者站在其右旁。用两手拇指或食、中指对准穴位按揉之，称揉肺俞。向外揉为泻，向脊椎方向揉为补（图 165）。

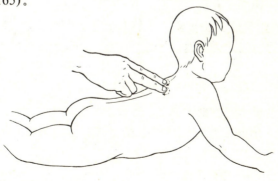

图 165

次数: 100～300 次。

作用: 调肺气, 补虚损, 止咳嗽。

主治: 咳嗽, 气喘, 胸闷, 胸痛, 发热等。

风门穴

位置: 第二胸椎棘突下, 旁开 1.5 寸。

操作: 患儿取端坐或俯卧位, 医者按风门, 用右手食、中指指端作按法或揉法, 称按或揉风门。

次数: 30～50 次。

作用: 疏风散寒, 宣肺平喘。

主治: 风寒感冒, 咳嗽气喘, 身热头痛, 项背强痛, 夜卧不安等。

腰俞穴

位置: 第三腰椎旁 3 寸半凹陷处。

操作: 患儿取俯卧位, 医者用双手拇指先按之称按腰俞, 再作揉法揉之, 称揉腰俞。

次数: 30～50 次。

作用: 通经活络, 壮腰补肾。

主治: 腰痛, 五软, 五迟, 下肢痿软不用。

(五软: 头软、手足软、项软、肌软、口软。五迟: 立迟、行迟、发迟、齿迟、语迟)。

脾俞穴

位置: 第十一胸椎棘突下, 旁开 1.5 寸。

操作: 患儿取俯卧位, 医者站在其右旁, 用两手拇指面或食、中指按揉, 称揉脾俞穴。

次数: 100～200 次。

作用: 健脾和胃, 助运化湿。

主治：呕吐，腹泻，疳积，黄疸，水肿，胃脘胀痛，消化不良，小儿慢惊风，四肢乏力等。

肾俞

位置：第二腰椎棘突下，旁开 1.5 寸。

操作：患儿取俯卧位，医者站在其右旁，用两手拇指或右手用食、中指端按揉之，称揉肾俞。

次数：50～100 次。

作用：滋阴壮阳，补益肾元。

主治：肾虚腰痛，腹泻，便秘，少腹痛，下肢痿软无力等。

七节骨

位置：命门至尾椎骨端成一直线。

操作：患儿取俯卧位，医者用右手拇指桡侧面或食、中指面自下向上作直推，称推上七节骨；反之，自上向下作直推，称推下七节骨（图 166）。

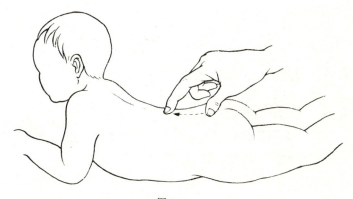

图 166

次数：100～300 次。

作用：推上七节骨能温阳止泻。推下七节骨能泻热通便。前者为补，后者为泻。

主治：推上七节骨主治虚寒腹泻，久痢，气虚下陷的脱肛，遗尿。推下七节骨主治肠热便秘、腹胀、湿热泻、伤食泻、急性痢疾。

龟尾
位置：尾椎骨端。
操作：患儿取俯卧位，医者站在其右旁。用右手拇指端或中指端作揉法，称揉龟尾（图167）。

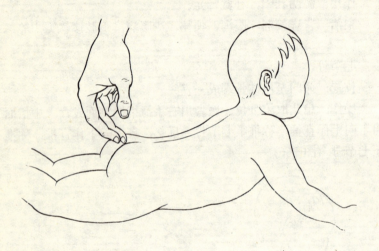

图 167

次数：100～300 次。
作用：通调督脉经气，调理大肠功能，能止泻，也能通便。
主治：泄泻，便秘，脱肛，遗尿等。

脊柱
位置：大椎至龟尾穴成一直线。
操作：小儿取俯卧位，医者站在其右旁或左旁，用食中指面自上而下作直推，称推脊（图168-1）。用两手拇、食、中指捏法，自下而上称捏脊（图 168-2)，捏脊一般每捏 3 下，再将背脊皮提 1 下，称为捏三提一法。在捏脊前先在背部轻轻按摩几遍，使肌肉放松。

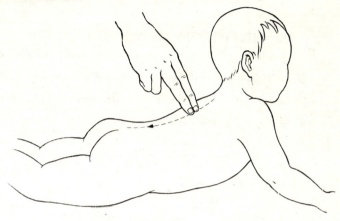

图 168-1

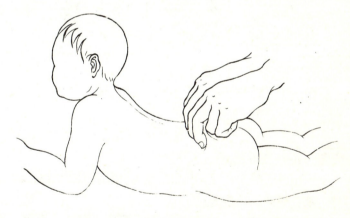

图 168-2

次数：推 100～300 次，捏 3～5 遍。

作用：推脊能清热；捏脊能调阴阳，补气血，通经络，和脏腑，培元气，强壮身体。

主治：推脊主治发热，惊风，夜啼，捏脊主治先后天不足的一些慢性疾病，如小儿疳积，腹泻腹痛，呕吐，便秘等。

10.4 上肢部穴位

脾经穴

位置：在拇指桡侧自指尖至指根处。

操作：患儿取抱坐位，医生以左手中、无名指、小指固定其左上肢，拇、食指将患儿拇指屈曲，用右手拇指自指尖推向掌根方向，称补脾经（图169）。将患儿拇指伸直，自指根推向指尖，称清脾经；来回用力推，称清补脾经。

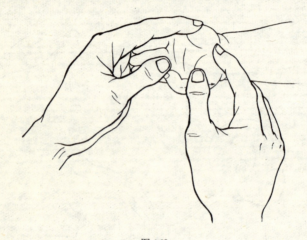

图 169

次数：100～500次。

作用：用补法健脾和胃，补益气血；用清法能清热利湿，消积导滞，消食导滞，化痰涎。

主治：体质虚弱，食欲不振，面黄消瘦，呕吐，腹泻，便秘，痢疾，黄疸，湿痰咳嗽，隐疹不透。

胃经穴

位置：在手掌大鱼际桡侧赤白肉际处。

操作：患儿取抱坐位，以左侧面对医生，医生用左手固定其上肢，暴露胃经，用右手拇指或食中指自掌根推向拇指根为补，称补胃经；向指根方向直推为清，称清胃经（图170）。

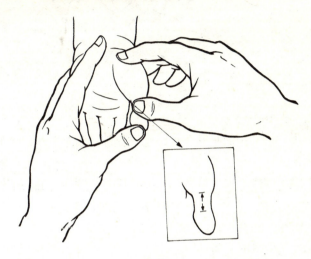

图 170

次数：100～500 次。

作用：补胃经健脾胃，助运化；清胃经清，胃泻火，降逆止呕，除烦止渴。

主治：脾胃虚弱，消化不良，纳呆腹胀，胃火炽盛的高热，烦渴，便秘，鼻衄，腹痛，呕吐，纳呆等。

肝经穴

位置：食指末端螺纹面。

操作：患儿取抱坐位，左侧面向医生，医者用左手握住患儿之手，使手指向上，手背向外，然后再以右手拇指，用推法自食指掌面末节指纹起推向指尖为清，称清肝经（图171）；反之为补，称补肝经。

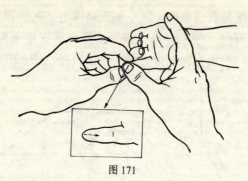

图 171

次数：100～500 次。

作用：清肝经能平肝泻火，熄风镇惊，解郁除烦；补肝经能养肝滋肾。

主治：烦躁不安，目赤，惊风，口苦，咽干，五心烦热等。

心经穴

位置：中指末节螺纹面。

操作：患儿取抱坐位，左侧面向医生，医者用左手固定患儿之手，用右手拇指面向指尖方向直推为清，称清心经（图172）；向指根方向直推为补，称补心经。

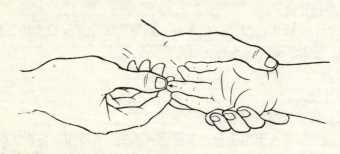

图 172

次数：100～500 次。

作用：清心经：清泻心火。补心经：补心血，安心神。

主治：心火炽盛引起的高热神昏，面赤口疮，小便短赤，五心烦热，惊惕不安；心血亏虚引起的心烦不安，睡时露睛等。

肺经穴

位置：无名指末节螺纹面。

操作：患儿取抱坐位，医者左手固定其左手，暴露无名指，用右手拇指向指尖方向直推为清，称清肺经（图173）；向指根方向直推为补，称补肺经。

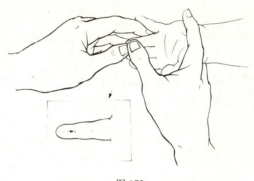

图 173

次数：100～300次。

作用：清肺经：清肺泻热，止咳化痰；补肺经：温肺止咳，补益肺气。

主治：感冒发热，咳嗽气喘，痰鸣，面白自汗，盗汗，急惊，鼻干，脱肛，遗尿，大便秘结，麻疹不透。

肾经穴

位置：小指掌面稍偏尺侧，自小指尖直至掌根。

操作：患儿取抱坐位，左侧面向医生，医者以左手握住患儿之手，使手掌向上，再以右手拇指自掌根推至小指尖为补，称补肾经；自指尖推向掌根为清，称清肾经（图174）。

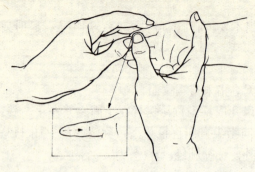

图 174

次数: 100～500 次。

作用: 补肾经: 滋肾壮阳、强健筋骨。清肾经; 清利下焦湿热。

主治: 先天不足, 久病体虚, 五更泻, 遗尿, 虚喘, 目赤, 膀胱蕴热, 小便淋漓刺痛。骨软无力宜用补法, 小肠气痛宜用清法。

四横纹穴

位置: 手掌面, 食、中、无名、小指第一指间关节横纹处。

操作: 患儿取坐位或仰卧位, 医者先以左手握住患儿之手, 使手掌向上, 手指略屈, 再以右手拇指甲, 自患儿食指依次掐至小指, 每掐 1 指, 继以揉之, 称掐四横纹; 或小儿 4 指并拢, 医者用右手拇指面, 从食指横纹处推向小指横纹处, 称推四横纹。

次数: 各掐 5 次, 推 100～300 次。

作用: 退热除烦, 散瘀结, 调气血, 消胀满。

主治: 疳积, 腹胀腹满, 气血不和, 消化不良, 惊风, 气喘, 口唇破裂。

小横纹穴

位置: 手掌面, 食、中、无名、小指的掌指关节横纹处。

操作：患儿取抱坐位，医者以左手固定其左手，使掌心向上，用右手拇指指甲，在食、中、无名、小指的掌指关节横纹处依次掐之，继以揉之，称掐小横纹；用拇指桡侧，在小横纹处推之，称推小横纹。

次数：掐各 5 次，推 100～300 次。

作用：退热、消胀、散结。

主治：唇裂、发热、烦躁、口疮、腹胀等。

大肠穴

位置：食指桡侧缘，指尖至虎口成一直线。

操作：患儿取抱坐位，医者以左手托住患儿左手，使虎口向上，以食、中 2 指夹住患儿之拇指，然后用右手拇指桡侧缘，自指尖推向指根方向为补，称补大肠（图 175），亦称侧推大肠；若向指尖方向直推为清。

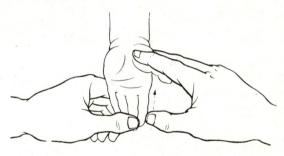

图 175

次数：100～500 次。

作用：补大肠，涩肠止泻，温中固脱；清大肠：清利肠府，除湿热，导积滞。

主治：腹泻，痢疾，便秘，腹胀腹痛，脱肛、肛门红肿。

小肠穴

位置：小指尺侧边缘，自指尖到指根成一直线。

操作：患儿取抱坐位，医者以左手握住患儿左手，使其小指尺侧向下，用右手食、中指面从指尖向指根方向直推为补，称补小肠（图176）；反之则为清，称清小肠。

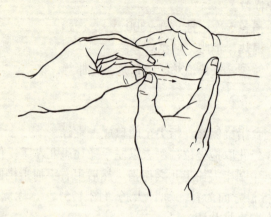

图 176

次数：100～300次。

作用：清小肠：清利下焦湿热，泌别清浊；补小肠：温煦下焦，散寒利尿。

主治：小便短赤，水泻，遗尿，尿闭，口舌生疮等。

肾顶穴

位置：小指顶端。

操作：患儿取抱坐位，医者左手固定患儿左手，使其小指尖向上，以右手用中指或拇指端按揉，称揉肾顶（图177）。

次数：100～500次。

作用：收敛元气、固表止汗。

主治：自汗，盗汗，或大汗淋漓不止，解颅等。

肾纹穴

位置：手掌面、小指第二指间关节横纹处。

操作：患儿取抱坐位，医者用中指或拇指端按揉，称揉肾纹（图178）。

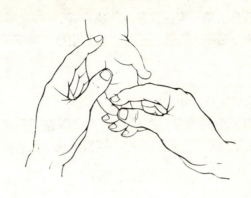

图 177

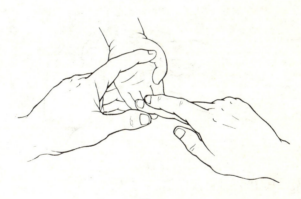

图 178

次数：100～500次。

作用：祛风明目，散瘀结。

主治：目赤肿痛，鹅口疮，热毒内陷等。

掌小横纹穴

位置：手掌面，小指根下，尺侧掌纹头。

操作：患儿取抱坐位或仰卧位，医者左手持儿左手食、中、无名、小指，然后以右手中指或拇指端按揉，称揉掌小横纹。

次数：100～500次。

作用：清热散结，宽胸宣肺，化痰止咳。

主治：痰热喘咳，发热，肺炎，口舌生疮，顿咳流涎等。

总筋穴

位置：掌后腕后纹中点处。

操作：患儿取抱坐位或仰卧位，医者以左手握患儿右手4指，以右拇指甲掐总筋，称掐总筋；以拇指或中指端按揉，称揉总筋（图179）。

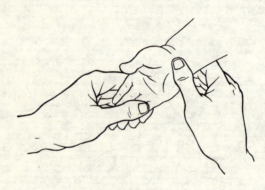

图179

次数：揉100～300次，掐3～5次。

作用：清心经热，散结止痉，通调周身气机。

主治：口舌生疮，夜啼，潮热，牙痛，惊风抽搐等症。

板门穴

位置：手掌大鱼际肌平面。

操作：患儿取抱坐位或仰卧位，医者以左手握患儿左手4指，使大鱼际向上，以右手拇指或中指端按揉，称揉板门或运板门（图180）；用推法自指根推向腕横纹，称板门推向横纹（图

181)，反之，称横纹推向板门。

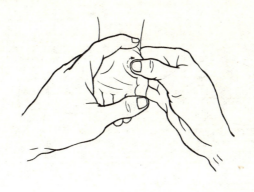

图 180

次数：100～300次。

作用：揉板门：健脾和胃，消食化滞；板门推向横纹：主止腹泻；横纹推向板门：主止呕吐。

主治：食积、腹胀、食欲不振、嗳气、腹泻、呕吐等。

大横纹穴

位置：仰掌，掌后横纹处，近拇指端称阳池，近小指端称阴池。

操作：患儿取坐位，医者以两手食、中、无名、小指固定其腕关节，以两拇指自掌后横纹中（总筋）向两旁分推，称分推大横纹，又称分阴阳（图182）；自两旁（阳池、阴池）向总筋合推，称合阴阳。

次数：30～50次。

作用：分阴阳：平衡阴阳，调和气血，行滞消食；合阴阳：行痰散结。

主治：寒热往来，烦躁不安，乳食停滞，腹胀腹泻、呕吐、痰结喘嗽、胸闷、痢疾、小儿惊吓等。

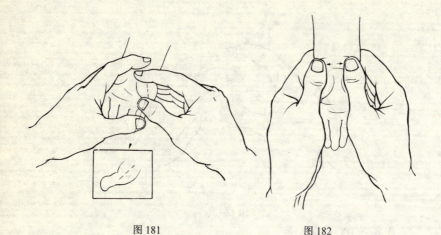

图 181 图 182

运水入土、运土入水穴

位置：大拇指根至小指根，沿手掌边缘一条弧形曲线。

操作：患儿取坐位或仰卧位，医者左手捏住患儿左手使五指并拢，用右手拇指自其拇指根沿手掌边缘，经小天心推运至小指根，称运土入水；反之，称运水入土。

次数：100～300 次。

作用：运土入水：清脾胃湿热，利尿止泻；运水入土：健脾助运，润燥通便。

主治：小便赤涩，腹胀，痢疾，吐泻，便秘，疳积，食欲不振等。

内劳宫穴

位置：掌心中，屈指时中指，无名指之间的中点。

操作：患儿取坐位或仰卧位，医者以左手握住患儿 4 指，使其掌心向上，然后右手中指端揉，称揉内劳宫；用运法自小指根起，经掌小横纹，小天心至内劳宫，称运内劳宫，又称水底捞明月。

次数：揉 100～300 次，运 10～30 次。

作用：揉内劳宫，清心热，除烦躁；运内劳宫：清虚（心、肾两经）热。

主治：发热，烦躁，口舌生疮，牙龈糜烂，内热等症。

内八卦穴

位置：手掌面，以内劳宫为圆心，从圆心至中指根横纹约 2／3 处为半径作圆周。

操作：以右手拇指桡侧面用运法，顺时针方向称运内八卦或运八卦。

次数：100～300 次。

作用：宽胸利膈，理气化痰、行滞消食。

主治：咳嗽痰喘，胸闷纳呆，腹胀吐泻等症。

小天心穴

位置：大小鱼际交接处凹陷中。

操作：患儿取抱坐位或仰卧位，医者以左手握住患儿左手，以右手中指端揉，称揉小天心（图 183）；以拇指甲掐，称掐小天心；以中指尖或屈指的指间关节捣，称捣小天心。

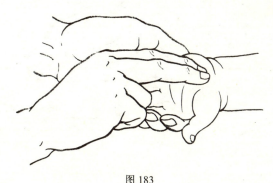

图 183

次数: 揉100～300次，掐捣各10～40次。

作用: 清热，镇惊，利尿，明目。

主治: 惊风，烦躁不安，夜啼，目赤肿痛，口舌生疮，小便短赤，疹痘欲出不透。

十宣穴

位置: 十指尖，距指甲约0.1寸处。

操作: 患儿取抱坐位或仰卧位，医者用拇食指分别固定其拇、食、中、无名、小指，然后以右手拇指甲作掐法，依次掐之，称掐十宣。

次数: 各掐5次，或醒后即止。

作用: 清热，开窍，醒神。

主治: 高热，惊风，抽搐，昏厥。

老龙穴

位置: 中指甲根近侧1分处。

操作: 患儿取仰卧位，医者以左手拇、食、中指固定其中指，使指甲暴露，医者用右手拇指甲掐之，称掐老龙（图184）。

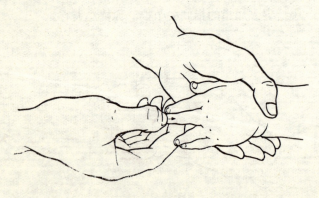

图184

次数：掐 5 次，或醒后即止。

作用：醒神开窍。

主治：急惊暴死，高热抽搐。

二扇门穴

位置：手背第三掌骨小头，两侧凹陷处。

操作：患儿取坐位，医者令患儿掌心向下，以左手食中指固定患儿腕部，无名指托患儿之手掌，然后以右手拇指甲掐之，称掐二扇门；拇指偏峰或食中指按揉之，称揉二扇门（图 185）。

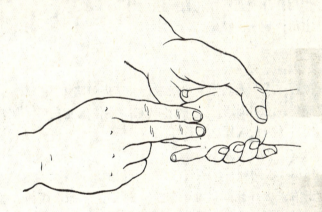

图 185

次数：掐 5 次，揉 100～500 次。

作用：发汗透表，退热平喘。

主治：风寒感冒，身热无汗，咳嗽气喘，急惊风，抽搐，眼歪斜。

左端正穴

位置：中指桡侧，指甲根旁 1 分许。

操作：患儿取坐位，医者以左手拇、食、中指，固定其中指，以右手拇指甲掐之，继以揉之，称掐揉左端正。

次数：掐 3～5 次，揉 50～100 次。

作用：止泻痢。

主治：泄泻，痢疾。

右端正穴

位置：中指尺侧，指甲根旁 1 分许。

操作：患儿取坐位，医者以左手拇、食、中指固定其中指，以右手拇指甲掐之，继以揉之，称掐揉右端正。

次数：掐 3～5 次，揉 50～100 次。

作用：降逆止呕，止血。

主治：呕吐，鼻衄。

二人上马穴

位置：手背无名指及小指掌指关节近侧陷中。

操作：患儿取坐位，医者以左手握住患儿之手，使掌心向下，用右手拇指端揉之，称揉二马。

次数：100～500 次。

作用：滋阴补肾，顺气散结，利尿通淋。

主治：虚热咳喘，小便短赤，神昏，牙痛，腹痛，睡时磨牙，遗尿，脾虚泄泻，肾虚泄泻等。

一窝风穴

位置：腕背横纹正中凹陷中。

操作：患儿取坐位，医者以左手握患儿左手，使其掌心向下，然后以右手拇指或中指指端揉之，称揉一窝风（图186）。

次数：100～300 次。

作用：温中行气，止痹痛，利关节。

主治：腹痛，肠鸣，关节痹痛，伤风感冒。

外劳宫穴

位置：掌背中，与内劳宫相对处。

操作：患儿取坐位，用指端揉之，称揉外劳宫（图187）；用拇指甲掐之，称掐外劳宫。

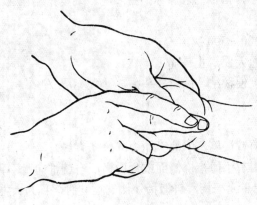

图186

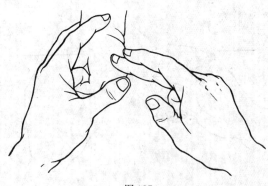

图187

次数：揉100～300次，掐5次。

作用：温阳散寒，升阳举陷，兼发汗解表。

主治：风寒感冒，腹痛腹胀，肠鸣腹泻，痢疾，脱肛，遗尿，疝气。

膊阳池穴

位置：在手背一窝风后 3 寸处。

操作：患儿取坐位，医者以左手托住患儿的腕关节，使掌面向下，用右手拇指甲掐之，称掐膊阳池；继以指端揉之，称揉膊阳池。

次数：100～300 次。

作用：通大便，止头痛。

主治：大便秘结，感冒，头痛，小便赤涩。

三关穴

位置：前臂桡侧，阳池至曲池成一条直线。

操作：用右手拇指桡侧面或食中指面自腕推向肘，称推三关（图 188）；屈患儿拇指，自拇指外侧端推向肘，称为大推三关。

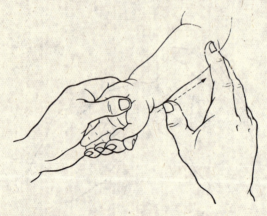

图 188

次数：100～300 次。

作用：补气行气，温阳散寒，发汗解表。

主治：气血虚弱，病后体虚，阳虚肢冷，腹痛，腹泻，斑疹，白痦，疹出不透，及风寒感冒等一切虚、寒病症。

天河水

位置：前臂正中，总筋至洪池成一条直线。

操作：患儿取坐位，医者以左手持患儿之左手，使掌心向上，将食指伸直托患儿前臂，拇指捏住掌根部；用右手食、中指指面自腕推向肘，称清天河水（图189）；用食、中2指沾水自总筋处，一起一落弹打，如弹琴状，直至洪池，同时一面用口吹气随之，称打马过天河。

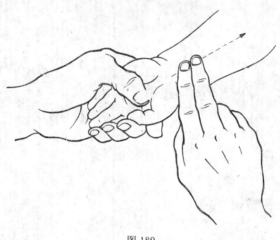

图189

次数：100～300次。

作用：清热解表，泻火除烦。

主治：外感发热，潮热，内热，烦躁不安，口渴，弄舌，重舌，唇舌生疮，口燥咽干，夜啼，惊风等一切热证。

六腑

位置：前臂尺侧，阴池至肘成一直线。

操作：以拇指面或食、中指面自肘推向腕，称推六腑（图190）。

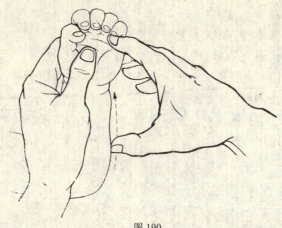

图 190

次数：100～300次。

作用：清热凉血解毒。

主治：一切实热病症，高热，烦渴，发斑，惊风，鹅口疮，木舌，重舌，咽痛，疟腮，大便秘结等症。

10.5 下肢部穴位

箕门

位置：大腿内侧，膝盖上缘至腹股沟成一直线。

操作：患儿取仰卧位，使其大腿轻微内翻外展，医者一手扶握其膝关节外侧处，以另一手食中指指面自膝盖内上缘直推至腹股沟，称推箕门。

次数：100～300次。

作用：通利小便。

主治：水泻，尿闭，小便赤涩不利。

百虫穴

位置：膝上内侧肌肉丰厚处。

操作：患儿取仰卧位，医者以左手握其踝关节，使腿轻度内翻，用右手拇指或拇食指按之拿之，称按百虫或拿百虫（图191）。

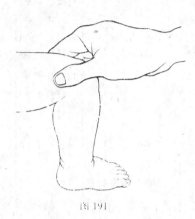

图191

次数：5次。

作用：通经络，止抽搐。

主治：下肢瘫痪，四肢抽搐。

足三里穴

位置：犊鼻穴下3寸，距胫骨前嵴外1横指处。

操作：患儿取仰卧位，医者用左手固定住其踝部，用右手拇指指端按揉之，称按揉足三里。

次数：50～100次。

作用：健脾和胃，调中理气，导滞通络。

主治：腹胀，腹痛，泄泻呕吐，下肢瘫痪。

委中穴

位置：腘窝中央，两大筋中间。

操作：患儿取仰卧位，屈膝90°，医者用左手固定其足，以右手拇指、食指、中指端提拿，钩拨腘窝中筋腱，称拿委中（图192）。

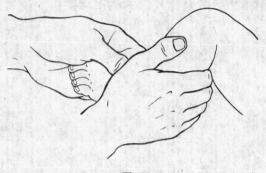

图 192

次数：5次。
作用：止抽搐，通经络，利腰背。
主治：惊风抽搐，下肢瘫痪，腰背酸痛等证。

后承山穴
位置：腓肠肌腹下凹陷中。
操作：患儿取俯卧位，医者用右手中指钩拨或以拇食指拿之，称拿后承山。
次数：5次。
作用：通经络，止抽搐。
主治：腿痛转筋，下肢痿软，惊风抽搐。

前承山穴
位置：前腿胫骨旁，与后承山相对处。
操作：患儿取仰卧位，医者用右手拇指甲或用拇指面掐或揉本穴，称掐前承山或揉前承山。
次数：掐5次，揉30次。
作用：止抽搐。

主治：惊风，下肢抽搐。

三阴交穴

位置：内踝上 3 寸。

操作：患儿取仰卧位，医者左手固定其左足或右足，以右手拇指或食指端按揉之，称按揉三阴交（图193）。

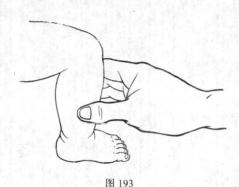

图 193

次数：100～200 次。

作用：通血脉，活经络，疏利下焦湿热，通调水道。

主治：下肢痹痛，遗尿，小便频数，涩痛不利，癃闭，惊风等症。

解溪穴

位置：踝关节前横纹中，两筋间凹陷处。

操作：医者以拇指端按揉之，称按揉解溪（图194）。

次数：50～100 次。

作用：止惊止吐泻，利关节。

主治：惊风，呕吐、腹泻，踝关节屈伸不利。

涌泉穴

位置：屈趾，足掌心前正中凹陷处。

操作：患儿取仰卧位，医者以左手托住患儿足跟，用拇指端向足趾推，称推涌泉；用指端揉之，称揉涌泉（图195）。

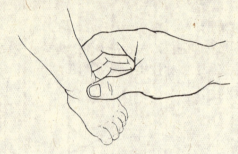

图 194

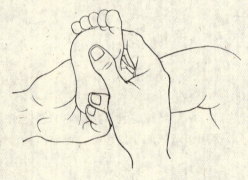

图 195

次数：推、揉各50～100次。

作用：推涌泉：引火归元，退虚热；揉涌泉：止吐泻。

主治：发热，头痛，喉痹，惊风，呕吐，腹泻，五心烦热，小便不利等症。

仆参穴

位置：足跟外踝下凹陷中。

操作：患儿取俯卧位，医者坐于床头，用拿法，称拿仆参；用掐法称掐仆参（图196）。

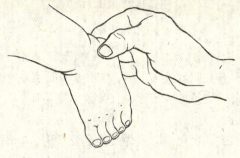

图 196

次数：5次。
作用：开窍，醒神，止抽搐。
主治：昏厥，惊风，抽搐。

11   小儿常见病症治疗

11.1   发热

体温异常升高叫做发热。除去由传染病等原因所引起的小儿发热外，其余的均可推拿治疗，且疗效迅速可靠。

病因病机

感受外邪或乳食积滞，或先天不足及后天亏乏伤及阴液，而致发热。

临床表现

外感发热：恶寒发热，鼻塞流涕，咳嗽，苔薄，指纹浮。偏于风寒者见恶寒重，发热轻，流清涕，无汗，指纹浮红；偏于风热者见发热重，恶寒轻，流浊涕，有汗，指纹浮紫。

阴虚发热：午后发热，两颧红赤，五心烦热，形体消瘦，烦躁盗汗，食少纳呆，舌红苔少，指纹紫沉。

肺胃实热：高热烦躁，掌心及胸部热甚，面红气促，脘腹胀满，大便秘结，不思饮食，渴而引饮，舌红苔黄，指纹紫滞。

治疗

1. 外感发热

(1) 治法：解表清热。

(2) 处方：推天门 300 次　推坎宫 300 次　　运太阳 300 次运耳后高骨 100 次。

(3) 加减：风寒者加按揉风池 100 次　拿肩井 2 次　　风热者加捏挤大椎 50 次　揉合谷 100 次。

(4) 疗程：每日 1 次，3 次为 1 疗程。

(5) 操作：

A. 风热用薄荷水，风寒用葱姜汁为介质。

B. 患儿由母亲扶抱位或坐位，面对医者，然后按要求施术。风热者先揉其双侧合谷穴，再用双拇指桡侧由下而上交替推天门，由印堂向两侧分推坎宫，向耳后方向运太阳穴。

C. 患儿背向医者。医者先运其双侧耳后高骨穴，风寒者再按揉风池，风热者捏挤大椎，最后拿肩井穴。

2. 阴虚发热

(1) 治法：滋阴清热。

(2) 处方：补脾经 300 次　补肺经 300 次　补肾经 300 次　揉二马 500 次　清天河水 300 次　分阴阳 50 次　运八卦 50 次　揉涌泉 300 次。

(3) 疗程：每日 1 次，3 次为 1 疗程。

(4) 操作：

A. 用温水作介质

B. 患儿由母亲扶抱位，医者持其一侧手臂，按要求施术。先于手掌部自指尖向指根方向推脾经、推肺经，由指根至指尖方向推肾经，再顺运八卦，揉二马，在腕部分推阴阳，然后由腕向肘方向推天河水。

C. 最后揉双侧涌泉穴。

3. 肺胃实热

(1) 治法：清泄里热。

(2) 处方：清肺经 300 次　　清胃经 500 次　清大肠 500 次　清天河水 200 次　推六腑 300 次　运八卦 50 次　摩中脘 3 分钟　推下七节骨 100 次。

(3) 疗程：每日 1 次，3 次为 1 疗程。

(4) 操作：

A. 用鸡蛋清作介质。

B. 患儿由母亲扶抱位，医者持其一侧手臂，按要求施术。先于指掌部由指根向指尖方向依次推肺经，推胃经，推大肠，再运八卦，然后于前臂由腕至肘方向推天河水，由肘至腕方向推六腑。

C. 患儿仰卧位，暴露腹部。医者单手蘸蛋清于腹部按顺时针方向摩中脘穴。

D. 俯卧位，暴露腰骶部。医者由第 4 腰椎推向尾椎自上而下推下七节骨。

注意事项

1. 注意区别各种不同原因所致的发热，凡感染性发热者，可选用相应的抗菌素治疗。

2. 高热特别明显时，可配合适当的物理降温疗法。

3. 对于推拿后体温又见回升者，可每日推拿 2 次。

11.2 感冒

感冒一证，一年四季均可发生，尤以秋冬明显。由于小儿生理病理特点，其发病迅速，且容易出现变证。

病因病机

小儿每值外界气候突然变化或冷热失调，均可感受风邪而发本病。

临床表现

风寒型：怕冷，微热，无汗，鼻塞流清涕，喷嚏，咳嗽，痰清稀，舌质淡红，苔薄白，指纹淡红。

风热型：发热重，微恶寒，有汗，鼻塞流浊涕，面赤咽红，咳吐黄痰，舌质红，苔薄黄，指纹红紫。

治疗

1. 风寒型

(1) 治法：祛风散寒解表。

(2) 处方：推天门 300 次　推坎宫 300 次　运太阳 40 次运耳后高骨 40 次　拿风池 10 次　揉迎香 20 次　揉一窝风 3 分钟　推三关 100 次　揉肺俞 50 次。

(3) 疗程：每日 1 次，3 次为 1 疗程。

(4) 操作：

A. 用姜水或葱水作介质。

B. 患儿由母亲扶抱位，医者持其一侧手臂，按要求施术。先在掌上揉一窝风，再自腕向肘方向推三关。

C. 患儿扶坐位，面对医者，在面部施术。先用双拇指或单手食、中指分开揉迎香，再由下而上推天门，自印堂向两侧分推坎宫，向耳后运太阳。然后令患儿背对医者，在其项颈部运双侧耳后高骨，轻拿风池穴。

D. 患儿俯卧位，暴露背部。医者指揉肺俞 50 次。

2. 风热型

(1) 治法：疏风清热解表。

(2) 处方：推天门 300 次　推坎宫 300 次　运太阳 40 次运耳后高骨 40 次　揉迎香 20 次　揉大椎 200 次　推天柱骨 200 次　清肺经 300 次　推六腑 200 次　揉小天心 200 次。

(3) 疗程：每日 1 次，6 次为 1 疗程。

(4) 操作：

A. 用薄荷水作介质。

B. 患儿由母亲扶抱位，医者持其一侧手臂，按要求施术。先由指根向指尖方向推肺经，再揉小天心，自肘部向腕方向推六腑。

C. 患儿扶坐位，面对医者，医者在其面部施术。先以双拇指或单手食、中指分开揉迎香，再由下而上推天门，由印堂向两侧分推坎宫，向耳后方向运太阳。令患儿背对医者，然后运双侧耳后高骨，自上而下推天柱骨，揉大椎。

(5) 加减：

A. 夹痰者：加揉按天突 30 次　分推膻中 100 次　揉乳根 30 次。

B. 夹滞者：加清脾经 100 次　清胃经 100 次　运板门 100次　摩腹 5 分钟。

C. 夹惊者：加清肝经 300 次　清心经 300 次　揉小天心 20 次

11.3 咳嗽

咳嗽是小儿常见肺系症候之一，多发病于春季。临床分为外感咳嗽和内伤咳嗽两大类。小儿咳嗽以前者多见，且推拿效果亦优于后者。

病因病机

1. 风寒或风热外侵犯肺，邪束肌表，导致肺失宣肃，气机上逆，则为咳嗽。

2. 肺脏虚弱或肺阴虚损，则气机不利，宣通闭塞，津液停积而为痰；脾常不足，则水谷精微不能运化，寒湿内生，反酿成痰；痰阻气逆，而致咳嗽。

临床表现

外感咳嗽：咳嗽有痰，鼻塞流涕，恶寒发热，头身疼痛，苔薄脉浮。外感风寒者见：咳痰清稀，流清涕，恶寒重，苔薄白，指纹淡红；外感风热者见：咳痰黄稠，流黄涕，发热重，苔薄黄，指纹鲜红。

内伤咳嗽：久咳不愈，身有微热，干咳痰少或咳嗽痰多，食欲不振，精神萎靡，形体消瘦。

治疗

1. 外感咳嗽

(1) 治法：祛风解表，宣肺止咳。

(2) 处方：推天门 100 次　推坎宫 100 次　运太阳 100 次　清肺经 100 次　运八卦 100 次　推膻中 100 次　揉膻中 100 次　揉乳旁　乳根各 20 次　清天突 20 次　分推肩胛骨 100 次

(3) 加减：风寒者加推三关 300 次　揉二扇门 100 次；风热者加推六腑 300 次　清天河水 300 次　推天柱骨 100 次。

(4) 疗程：每日 1 次，6 次为 1 疗程。

(5) 操作：

A. 用姜汁或薄荷水作介质。

B. 患儿由母亲扶抱位，医者持其一侧手臂，按要求施术。先在手掌部自指根向指尖方向推肺经，运八卦，风寒咳嗽者加揉二扇门。再根据咳嗽性质不同，于前臂自腕向肘方向推天河水或推三关，或自肘至腕方向推六腑。然后由下而上推天门，自印堂向两侧分推坎宫，向耳后方向运太阳。

C. 患儿仰卧位，暴露胸部。医者先以双手拇指分推膻中，然后揉膻中，揉天突，揉乳旁穴和乳根穴。

D. 俯卧位。风热咳嗽者先在项颈部由上而下推天柱骨，然后暴露脊背部，以双手拇指分推肩胛骨。

2. 内伤咳嗽

(1) 治法：健脾化痰，宣肺止咳。

(2) 处方：补肺经 300 次　　补脾经 300 次　　运八卦 300 次　　推膻中 100 次　　揉乳旁、乳根各 100 次　　揉中脘 100 次　　揉肺俞、脾俞各 100 次　　捏脊 3 遍。

(3) 疗程：每日 1 次，6 次为 1 疗程。

(4) 操作：

A. 用滑石粉作介质。

B. 患儿由母亲扶抱位，医者取持其一侧手臂，按要求施术。先在指掌部由指尖至指根方向依次推肺经、推脾经，再顺运内八卦。

C. 患儿仰卧位，暴露胸部。医者先分推再下推然后按揉膻中穴，再揉乳旁、乳根穴，再暴露腹部，揉中脘穴。

D. 患儿俯卧位，暴露脊背部。医者先揉肺俞、脾俞穴，再用掌根自上而下推揉脊柱 2 遍，然后由下而上捏脊 3 遍，最后用掌根上下轻揉。

注意事项

1. 推拿过程中注意保暖，防止受凉。

2. 内伤咳嗽，可见于多种疾病，必要时给予药物治疗。

11.4 哮喘

哮喘是指阵发性呼吸困难，以呼气延长，喉间哮鸣为特点，严重时可见张口抬肩，难以平卧。本病多发于春秋季节，推拿治疗有一定疗效。

病因病机

1. 小儿素体虚弱，肺脾肾三脏不足，水谷精津失却正常运化，而聚滞成痰，阻于气道，呼吸不利，遂成哮喘。

2. 气候骤变或寒温失调，邪袭肺脏，宣肃失常，气机壅塞，则成哮喘。

临床表现

热喘：咳嗽喘促，气急痰鸣，痰稠色黄，烦躁不安，小便黄赤，发热面赤，舌红苔黄厚，指纹深红。

寒喘：咳嗽喘促，喉间痰鸣，吐痰清稀，色白多沫，四肢不温，面色㿠白，小便清长，舌苔薄白，指纹紫红。

虚喘：喘促气短，咳声低微，言语无力，面色少华，形体消瘦，多汗怕风，食少纳呆，舌淡苔薄白，指纹色淡。

治疗

1. 寒喘

(1) 治法：温肺化痰，平喘止咳。

(2) 处方：补肺经 100 次　推膻中 100 次　揉膻中 100 次　揉天突 30 次　搓摩两胁 2 分钟　按揉肺俞 100 次　逆运八卦 100 次　推三关 100 次　揉风池 50 次　揉一窝风 50 次。

(3) 疗程：每日 1 次，6 次为 1 疗程。

(4) 操作：

A. 用滑石粉作介质。

B. 患儿由母亲扶抱位，医者取持其一侧手臂，按要求施术。先在指掌部由指尖至指根方向推肺经，再逆运八卦，揉一窝风，然后由腕至肘方向推三关。

C. 患儿仰卧位，暴露胸部。医者先分推再下推然后揉膻中穴，继之揉天突穴，再以两手掌搓摩患儿胁肋部。

D. 患儿俯卧位。医者先在项背部揉风池，然后暴露脊背部，按揉肺俞穴。

2. 热喘

(1) 治法：清热化痰，理气平喘。

(2) 处方：清肺经200次　捏挤天突100次　分推膻中30次　清大肠200次　分推肩胛骨30次　按肺俞30次　清天河水200次　推天柱骨50次　推脊20次。

(3) 疗程：每日1次，6次为1疗程。

(4) 操作：

A. 用滑石粉作介质。

B. 患儿由母亲扶抱位，医者取持其一侧手臂，按要求施术。先由指根至指尖方向推肺经，推大肠，然后由腕向肘方向推天河水。

C. 患儿仰卧位，暴露胸部。医者由两侧或上下向中心挤捏天突，然后分推膻中穴。

D. 患儿俯卧位。医者先在项背部由上而下推天柱骨，然后暴露脊背部，按揉肺俞穴，用双拇指向两侧分推肩胛骨，再由上而下推脊至尾骨处，结束手法。

3. 虚喘

(1) 治法：补肾纳气，敛肺定喘。

(2) 处方：补肺经300次　补肾经300次　推三关100次　揉丹田100次　按命门100次　揉肺俞200次　揉肾俞200次　补脾经500次　揉脾俞100次　分推膻中100次　揉天突100次。

(3) 疗程：每日1次，10次为1疗程。

(4) 操作：

A. 用滑石粉作介质。

B. 患儿由母亲扶抱位，医者取持其一侧手臂，按要求施术。先由指尖至指根方向依次推肺经、脾经，再由指根向指尖方向推肾经，然后由腕向肘推三关。

C. 患儿仰卧位，暴露胸腹部。医者先分推膻中，揉天突，然后揉丹田穴。

D. 患儿俯卧位，暴露脊背部。医者依次揉肺俞、脾俞、肾俞，最后按命门。

注意事项

本病易反复发作，推拿疗程可适当增加。

11.5 厌食

厌食是指小儿较长时间的食欲不振，纳呆，甚则拒食的一种常见病证。

病因病机

本病主要是由于平素饮食不节或喂养不当，以及长期偏食等情况，损伤了脾胃的正常运化功能。

临床表现

1. 脾失健运：面色少华，不思纳食，或食物无味，拒进饮食，形体偏瘦，而精神状态一般无特殊异常，大小便基本正常，舌苔薄白，脉尚有力。

2. 脾胃气虚：精神较差，面色萎黄，厌食拒食，若稍进食，大便中夹有不消化残渣，或大便不成形，容易出汗，苔薄净，脉无力。

治疗

1. 脾失健运型

(1) 治法：健脾助运。

(2) 处方：清补脾经各 500 次，揉板门 300 次，推四横纹 50 次，分腹阴阳 300 次，揉足三里 300 次，捏脊 5 遍。

(3) 操作：

A. 以滑石粉为介质。

B. 患儿取端坐位，医者左手固定患儿左手，先作清补脾经，揉板门，推四横纹。

C. 患儿取仰卧位，医者站在患儿的右旁，用两手拇指面自中脘穴向两边分推，再揉足三里。

D. 患儿取俯卧位，医者站在小儿的右旁，用双手拇食指从尾椎开始作捏脊至大椎，反复 3 次，至第四遍时捏至胃俞、脾俞、肝俞时，重提 1 下；再反复 1 遍，最后按揉肝俞、脾俞、胃俞。3～5 次结束。

2. 脾胃气虚型

(1) 治法：温中健脾、补益气血

(2) 处方：补脾经 500 次，推三关 300 次，揉外劳宫 100 次，运内八卦 100 次，揉中脘 300 次，捏脊 5 遍，消化不良者加补大肠 500 次，肠炎者，加清大肠 300 次。

(3) 操作：

A. 以滑石粉为介质。

B. 患儿取坐位，医者固定患儿左手，先补脾经、运内八卦；再揉外劳宫。

C. 患儿取仰卧位，医者以 1 手作揉中脘。

D. 患儿取俯卧位，医者用拇指食中 2 指同时用力捏拿皮肤，以尾椎至大椎 3 遍，第 4～5 遍时，每捏 3 次向上提 1 次，最后重按双侧脾俞、肾俞 3～5 次。

6～10 次为 1 疗程，每日 1 次，连续 6 次，休息 1 天，如不愈再作 4 次。

11.6 夜啼

夜啼是发生于 1 岁以内婴幼儿的一种常见病症，其表现为：白天安静如常，入夜即哭，甚或通宵达旦，彻夜不止，持续时间少则数日，多则数月。

病因病机

1. 脏腑受寒邪，寒凝脉络，滞泣不通，故作痛啼哭，入夜尤甚。

2. 火邪上扰，上乘于心，心火太盛，烦躁失眠。

3. 猝临惊骇，心惊气乱，神不守舍，惕惕而动。

4. 乳食过量，积滞不化，脘腹作胀而夜卧不安。

临床表现

1. 脾寒型：夜间啼哭，神怯困倦，声音低怯，面色青白，肢冷便清，腹痛时喜温按，指纹淡红。

2. 心热型：夜间啼哭，声音宏亮，烦躁不安，面赤唇红，口中气热，便秘溲赤，手足温，指纹青紫。

3. 惊吓型：面色乍青乍白，夜间啼哭，声惨而紧，神情不安，抚抱而卧，时有惊惕恐惧之状。

4. 食积型：夜间啼哭，腹部胀满，按之哭甚，厌食吐乳，大便酸臭，指纹紫滞。

治疗

1. 脾寒型

(1) 治法：温中健脾安神。

(2) 处方；：掐揉小天心 20 次，揉精宁 100 次，揉外劳宫 30 次，补脾经 300 次，推三关 300 次，摩腹 5 分钟。

(3) 疗程：每日 1 次，6 次为 1 疗程。

(4) 操作：

A. 以滑石粉作介质。

B. 患儿由母亲扶抱位，医者取持其一侧手臂，按要求施术。先自指尖向指根方向推脾经，再揉精宁，揉外劳宫，然后自腕部向肘部方向推三关。

C. 患儿仰卧位，暴露腹部。医者以单侧手掌在其腹部按顺、逆时针方向交替缓缓摩腹 5 分钟。

D. 以轻快手法掐揉小天心 20 次。

2. 心热型

(1) 治法: 清热安神。

(2) 处方: 揉精宁 100 次, 捣小天心 20 次, 清肝经 200 次, 清心经 200 次, 清天河水 300 次, 推六腑 200 次。

(3) 疗程: 每日 1 次, 6 次为 1 疗程。

(4) 操作:

A. 以滑石粉或温水作介质。

B. 患儿由母亲扶抱位, 医者取持其一侧手臂, 按要求施术。先自指根向指尖方向依次推肝经、心经, 再由腕部向肘部方向推天河水, 由肘部向腕方向推六腑, 最后揉精宁, 捣小天心。

3. 惊吓型

(1) 治法: 镇惊安神。

(2) 处方: 揉百会 10 次, 清肝经 100 次, 清心经 300 次, 清肺经 200 次, 补脾经 300 次, 揉精宁 20 次, 掐揉五指节 3 次。

(3) 疗程: 每日 1 次, 3 次为 1 疗程。

(4) 操作:

A. 以滑石粉作介质。

B. 患儿由母亲扶抱位, 医者持其一侧手掌, 按要求施术。先自指根向指尖方向依次推肝经、心经、肺经, 再由指尖向指根方向推脾经, 最后揉精宁, 掐揉五指节。

4. 食积型

(1) 治法: 消食化积和胃。

(2) 处方: 清胃经 200 次, 清大肠 200 次, 运板门 100 次, 顺运八卦 100 次, 揉中脘 3 分钟, 按揉天枢 10 次, 揉小天心 30 次。

(3) 疗程: 每日 1 次, 6 次为 1 疗程。

(4) 操作:

A. 以滑石粉作介质。

B. 患儿由母亲扶抱位，医者取持其一侧手臂，按要求施术。先自指根向指尖方向推胃经，推大肠，然后运板门，顺运八卦，揉小天心穴。

C. 患儿仰卧位，暴露腹部，医者依次揉中脘，按揉天枢。

注意事项

1. 明确诊断，排除由于其它原因，如虫积、发热等所引起的啼哭。

2. 推拿过程中注意保暖，以防受凉。

11.7 便秘

便秘是大便秘结不通，排便时间延长，或欲大便而坚涩不畅，是从幼儿到学龄儿童的一种常见病症。

病因病机

1. 气血不足：素体虚弱或久病之后气血不足，气虚则大肠传送无力，血虚则津液无以润大肠。

2. 饮食不节：过食辛热厚味，以致肠胃积热，气滞不行或热病后耗损津液，腑气不通，大便传导失职。

临床表现

1. 虚秘：便秘不畅，便干坚硬，或软、面唇㿠白，指爪无华，形瘦，气怯，小便清长，腹中冷痛，喜热、恶冷、四肢不温。

2. 实秘：大便干结，面赤身热，口臭，唇赤，小便短赤，纳食减少，嗳气泛酸，或腹部胀满，苔黄燥，指纹色紫。

治疗

1. 实秘型

(1) 治法：清热通便、顺气行滞。

(2) 处方：清大肠 300 次，推六腑 200 次，运内八卦 50 次，按揉膊阳池 50 次，摩腹 100 次（顺运），推下七节骨 200 次，搓摩胁肋 50 次。

(3) 疗程: 每日 1 次, 3 次为 1 疗程。

(4) 操作:

A. 以滑石粉为介质。

B. 患儿取坐位、医者左手固定患儿左手, 先作清大肠、推六腑, 运内八卦, 按揉膊阳池; 再以两手掌从患儿胁腋下搓摩至天枢处搓摩胁肋。

C. 患儿取仰卧位, 医者站在患儿的右旁, 用右手指面或掌心在小儿腹部作顺时针方向的抚摩, 即摩腹。

D. 患儿取俯卧位, 医者站在小儿的右旁, 用右手拇指面或食中 2 指面, 从第 4 腰椎向下推至尾椎骨端, 推下 7 节骨结束。

2. 虚秘型

(1) 治法: 滋阴润燥, 益气养血。

(2) 处方: 补脾经 300 次　清大肠 100 次　推三关 200 次揉二马 50 次　揉肾俞 50 次　按揉足三里 50 次　捏脊 5 遍。

(3) 疗程: 每日 1 次, 6 次为 1 疗程。

(4) 操作:

A. 以滑石粉为介质。

B. 患儿取坐位, 医者以左手固定患儿的左手, 作补脾经, 清大肠, 推三关, 揉二马。

C. 患儿取仰卧位, 医者按揉足三里。

D. 患儿取俯卧位, 医者用两手拇指在患儿背部从尾椎至大椎, 作捏脊法, 并在肾俞穴上按揉 3～5 次结束。

11.8　呕吐

呕吐是小儿常见的证候, 可见于多种疾病中。

病因病机

小儿先天禀赋不足, 胃气虚弱, 一旦感受外邪, 暴饮伤食, 跌仆惊恐, 脾胃蕴热、虚寒, 均可使胃失和降, 气逆于上而致呕吐。

临床表现

1. 寒吐：呕吐时发时止，遇寒加重，吐物清稀，气味不臭，倦怠无力，面白唇淡，形寒肢冷，腹痛喜暖，大便溏薄，舌淡苔薄白，指纹色红。

2. 热吐：食入即吐，吐物酸臭，或伴身热、口渴、多饮、烦躁不安、唇红、大便臭秽或秘结，小便黄、苔黄腻、指纹色紫。

3. 伤食吐：呕吐酸馊频繁、恶心、嗳气，宿食臭、吐后觉安，口气秽臭，脘腹痞闷胀满，大便酸臭或秘结，舌苔厚腻，脉滑实，指纹暗紫。

治疗

1. 寒吐型

（1）治法：温胃散寒，和胃降逆。

（2）处方：补脾经 500 次　推三关 500 次　揉外劳宫 500 次　横纹推向板门 200 次　揉中脘 300 次　拿按肩井 3～5 次　揉足三里 100 次。

（3）疗程：每日 1 次，3 次为 1 疗程。

（4）操作：

A. 以姜汁为介质。

B. 患儿取端坐位，医者以左手持儿左手，以右手推三关，补脾经，横纹推向板门，再揉外劳宫。

C. 患儿取仰卧位，医者用右手中指或掌根揉中脘，揉足三里，最后患儿取坐位，按拿肩井结束。

2. 热吐型

（1）治法：清热和胃，降逆止呕。

（2）处方：清脾经 300 次　清胃经 100 次　清肺经 300 次　水底捞明月 50 次　推六腑 300 次　揉涌泉 100 次　推天柱骨 300 次。

（3）疗程：每日 1 次，3 次为 1 疗程。

(4) 操作：

A. 以滑石粉或冷水为介质。

B. 患儿取坐位，医者固定其左手，依次清脾经，清胃经，清肺经，作水底捞明月，推六腑及推天柱骨。

C. 患儿取仰卧位，医者用左手固定患儿足后部，用右手拇指向左揉涌泉结束。

3. 伤食吐型

(1) 治法：消食导滞，和胃降逆。

(2) 处方：清板门 500 次　清大肠 500 次　推六腑 300 次 运内八卦 100 次，揉中脘 300 次，分腹阴阳 200 次　摩腹 100 次，推下七节骨 200 次　按揉足三里 20 次　捏挤天突，以局部瘀血为度。

(3) 疗程：每日 1 次，3 日为 1 疗程。

(4) 操作：

A. 以滑石粉为介质。

B. 患儿取仰卧位，医者以双手拇指从中脘向两边分推，待腹消后，以掌心摩中脘，再揉足三里。

C. 患儿取抱坐位，医者以左手清板门，清大肠，运内八卦，后再推六腑。

D. 患儿取俯卧位，医者用食中指面推下七节骨。

E. 患儿复取抱坐位，医者用双手拇、食指作挤捏法，以天突为中心，每隔 2cm 按 1 个"◇"字花，共按 5 个，儿啼哭，家长抱儿轻拍背部结束。

11.9 腹泻

婴幼儿腹泻，亦名消化不良，以大便次数增多，便下稀薄或如水样为特征。

病因病机

1. 感受外邪：感受湿邪，湿困脾阳，使脾失健运而致泻。

2. 内伤乳食：由于喂养不当，乳食无度，或恣食油腻生冷，或饮食不洁，导致脾胃损伤，而致腹泻。

3. 脾胃虚弱：小儿先天禀赋不足，或久病伤脾，脾常不足，外来因素致脾胃运化失常而致腹泻。

临床表现

1. 寒湿泻：大便清稀多沫，色淡不臭，肠鸣，腹痛，面色淡白，口不渴，小便清长，苔白腻，脉濡，指纹色红。

2. 湿热泻：发热或不发热，大便如水样，色黄褐热臭，肛门灼热发红，口渴，舌质红，苔黄腻，指纹色紫。

3. 伤食泻：腹痛胀满，泻前哭闹，泻后痛减，大便量多酸臭，口臭，纳呆或伴有呕吐酸馊，舌苔垢腻，脉滑。

4. 脾虚泻：时泻时止，或久泻不愈，便稀带有白色奶块或食物残渣，每于食后作泻，食欲不振，面色苍白，舌淡，苔薄白，脉沉无力。

治疗

1. 寒湿型

(1) 治法：湿中散寒，化湿止泻。

(2) 处方：补脾经 200 次　补大肠 150 次　推三关 300 次　揉外劳宫 200 次　摩腹 100 次　推上七节骨 200 次。

(3) 疗程：每日 1 次，3 次为 1 疗程。

(4) 操作：

A. 以姜汁或滑石粉为介质。

B. 患儿取坐位，医者固定其左手，右手先推补脾经，推三关，补大肠，再揉外劳宫。

C. 患儿取仰卧位，医者用右手指面或掌心在患儿腹部作逆、顺时针方向的摩运。

D. 患儿取俯卧位，医者用大拇指面或食中指面，在儿背部从尾骨端推上七节骨至第四腰椎结束。

2. 湿热泻型

(1) 治法：清热利湿，调中止泻。

(2) 处方：清脾经 200 次　清大肠 200 次　清小肠 100 次　推六腑 300 次　揉天枢 50 次　揉龟尾 50 次。

(3) 疗程：每日 1 次，3 次为 1 疗程。

(4) 操作：

A. 以冷水或滑石粉为介质。

B. 患儿取坐位，医者固定患儿左手，推六腑，清脾经，清大肠，清小肠。

C. 患儿取仰卧位，医者两拇指端或一手食、中二指端揉天枢。

D. 患儿取俯卧位，医者用中指端揉龟尾结束。

3. 伤食泻型

(1) 治法：消食导滞，和中助运。

(2) 处方：清脾经 300 次　清板门 200 次　运内八卦 100 次　清大肠 100 次　摩腹 200 次　揉中脘 50 次。

(3) 疗程：每日 1 次，3 次为 1 疗程。

(4) 操作：

A. 以滑石粉为介质。

B. 患儿取坐位，医者固定患儿左手，作清脾经、清板门、运内八卦，清大肠。

C. 患儿取仰卧位，医者用右手中指端或手指面及掌心，先揉中脘，再摩腹（顺逆方向的摩运）结束。

4. 脾虚型

(1) 治法：健脾益气，温阳止泻。

(2) 处方：补脾经 300 次　补大肠 200 次　推三关 300 次　摩腹 100 次　推上七节骨 200 次　捏脊 3～5 遍。

(3) 疗程：每日 1 次，6 次为 1 疗程。

(4) 操作：

A. 以滑石粉为介质。

B. 患儿取坐位，医者用左手固定患儿左手，先补脾经，推三关，补大肠。

C. 患儿取仰卧位，医者用右手指面或掌心，在患儿腹部作逆时针方向的摩运。

D. 患儿取俯卧位，医者用食、中2指面先推上七节骨，再用拇指及食、中2指捏脊，从尾椎至大椎3遍，第4～5遍每捏3次向上提1次。

11.10　脱肛

脱肛是指肛门直肠脱垂的一种症状，为儿童常见病症之一。

病因病机

小儿先天不足，病后体弱，或因泻痢日久，耗伤正气，气虚下陷；亦有因大肠积热，湿热下注，大便干结而致。

临床表现

1. 气虚：肛门直肠脱出不收，肿痛不堪，兼有面色㿠白或萎黄、形体消瘦，精神萎靡，舌淡苔薄，指纹色淡。

2. 实热：肛门直肠脱出，红肿刺痛，瘙痒，兼有口干苔黄，大便干结，小便短赤，指纹色紫。

治疗

1. 气虚型

(1) 治法：补中益气，升提固脱。

(2) 处方：补脾经300次　补肺经200次　补大肠100次、推三关300次　按揉百会200次　揉龟尾50次　推上七节骨100次，捏脊3～5遍。

(3) 疗程：每日1次，15次为1疗程。

(4) 操作：

A. 以滑石粉为介质。

B. 患儿取坐位，医者固定患儿左手，补脾经，推三关，补肺经，按揉百会。

C. 患儿取俯卧位，先操龟尾，推上七节骨，再捏脊。

2. 实热型

(1) 治法：清热利湿通便。

(2) 处方：清脾经 300 次　清大肠 200 次　清小肠 200 次　推六腑 100 次　按揉膊阳池 50 次　揉天枢 100 次　推下七节骨 50 次　揉龟尾 50 次。

(3) 疗程：每日 1 次，6 次为 1 疗程。

(4) 操作：

A. 以滑石粉为介质。

B. 患儿取坐位，医者用左手固定患儿左手，先推六腑、清脾经，清大肠、清小肠、按揉膊阳池。

C. 患儿取仰卧位，医者用食、中 2 指端揉天枢。

D. 患儿取俯卧位，揉龟尾，推下七节骨结束。

11.11　营养不良

小儿营养不良是摄食不足或摄入食物不能充分利用的结果。

病因病机

1. 摄入不足，营养失调：母乳不足、或断乳过早、或喂养不当，使营养物质的供给不能适应小儿机体的需求。

2. 饮食不节，脾胃损伤：乳食无度，或食肥甘生冷，脾胃损伤，运化失常，形成积滞，纳化无权。

临床表现

1. 小儿摄入不足，营养失调：面色㿠白无华，毛发枯黄稀疏，睡卧不宁，啼声低小，四肢不温，发育障碍，大便溏泄，舌质淡，苔薄，指纹色淡。

2. 饮食不节，脾胃损伤：形体消瘦，体重不增，腹部胀满，纳食不香，精神不振，夜眠不安，大便不调，常有恶臭，舌苔厚腻。

治疗

1. 摄入不足，营养失调型：

(1) 治法：温中健脾，补益气血。

(2) 处方：补脾经 300 次　补肺经 300 次　揉外劳 200 次　推三关 300 次　揉中脘 200 次　按揉足三里 200 次　捏脊 5 遍。

(3) 疗程：每日 1 次，12 次为 1 疗程。

(4) 操作：

A. 以滑石粉或冬青膏为介质。

B. 患儿取坐势，医者取小儿左手先补脾经，补肺经。再顺时针方向揉外劳，接着推三关。

C. 患儿仰卧暴露腹部，医者以右手 4 指顺时针方向揉中脘穴。以左手固定其下肢用右手拇指按揉足三里。

D. 取俯卧位，用捏法由长强穴至大椎穴，自下而上捏脊 5 遍，第 4～5 遍每捏 3 下再将脊骨皮重提一下。最后以双手拇指按心俞、肝俞、脾俞、胃俞各 3 次。

2. 饮食不节，脾胃损伤型：

(1) 治法：消食导滞，调理脾胃。

(2) 处方：补脾经 300 次　揉板门 300 次　运内八卦 200 次　揉中脘 200 次　分腹阴阳 200 次　推四横纹 200 次　揉天枢 200 次　按揉足三里 200 次。

(3) 疗程：每日 1 次，12 次为 1 疗程。

(4) 操作：

A. 以滑石粉为介质。

B. 患儿取坐势，医者补脾经，揉板门，顺运内八卦，推四横纹。

C. 患儿取仰卧位，医者以右手 4 指顺时针方向按揉中脘穴，再用食、中指指腹顺时针方向揉天枢穴。

D. 姿势同上，医者再以左手固定患儿下肢，按揉足三里穴。

11.12 腹痛

　　腹痛是临床上小儿常见的一个症状，可见于多种病中。腹痛在这里主要指的是由于腹部感受寒邪、乳食积滞，脾胃虚寒或虫积腹中引起的腹痛。

病因病机

　　1. 感受寒邪：由于护理不当，气候突然变化脐腹部为风冷寒气所伤，饮食当风，或过食生冷瓜果，寒凝气滞，中阳受遏，气机凝涩，失于通调，不通则痛。

　　2. 乳食积滞：由于乳食不节，暴饮暴食，或恣食生冷食物，乳食壅滞中洲，致使升降违逆，传化失职，而产生痞满胀痛。

　　3. 脾胃虚寒：由于素体阳虚，或病后体弱，中阳不足运化无权，脾阳不能运化水谷，寒湿内停，气机不畅。

　　4. 虫积：感染蛔虫，扰动肠中，或窜行胆道，或虫多扭结成团，阻止气机而致气滞作痛。

临床表现

　　1. 寒痛：腹痛暴急，上下攻冲，多呈绞痛，哭叫不安，常在受凉或饮食生冷后发生，遇冷更剧，得热较舒，面色苍白，大便清稀，舌质淡，苔白滑，指纹色红。

　　2. 食积痛：腹部胀满疼痛拒按，厌食，口气秽臭，嗳腐吞酸，矢气恶臭，大便酸臭，不消化，或腹痛欲泻，泻后痛减，夜卧不安，时时啼哭，舌苔厚腻，脉滑，指纹紫滞。

　　3. 虚寒痛：腹痛隐隐，绵绵不休，喜温喜按、面色萎黄、形体消瘦，食欲不振，易发腹泻，舌质淡，苔薄，指纹色淡，脉细软。

　　4. 虫积痛：腹痛突作，以脐周为甚，时发时止，有时可在腹部摸到蠕动的块状物，时隐时现，有便虫史，消瘦纳呆，或食异物，蛔虫窜行胆道则痛如钻顶，时发时止，伴见呕吐。

治疗

1. 寒痛

(1) 治法：温中散寒，理气止痛。

(2) 处方：补脾经 200 次　揉外劳宫 300 次　推三关 300 次
揉一窝风 300 次　摩腹 200 次　拿肚角 3～6 次。

(3) 疗程：每日 1 次，6 次为 1 疗程。

(4) 操作：

A. 以滑石粉为介质。

B. 患儿取坐势，医者取小儿左手先补脾经，再揉外劳宫，揉一窝风，然后推三关。

C. 患儿取仰卧位，医者以掌心顺时针方向摩腹，再拿肚角。

2. 食积痛

(1) 治法：消食导滞，和中止痛。

(2) 处方：补脾经 200 次　清大肠 300 次　揉板门 300 次
运内八卦 150 次　揉中脘 200 次　揉天枢 200 次　分腹阴阳 200 次。

(3) 疗程：每日 1 次，6 次为 1 疗程。

(4) 操作：

A. 以滑石粉为介质。

B. 患儿取坐势，医者取患儿的左手先补脾经，清大肠，再揉板门，最后顺运内八卦。

C. 患儿取仰卧位，暴露腹部，顺时针方向揉中脘，揉天枢穴，再分腹阴阳。

3. 虚寒痛

(1) 治法：温补脾肾，益气止痛。

(2) 处方：补脾经 300 次　补肾经 300 次　推三关 300 次
揉外劳宫 200 次　揉中脘 200 次　揉脐 200 次　按揉足三里 200 次。

（3）疗程：每日 1 次，12 次为 1 疗程。

（4）操作：

A. 以冬青膏为介质。

B. 患儿取坐势，医者取患儿左手先补脾经，再补肾经，推三关，然后顺时针方向揉外劳。

C. 患儿取仰卧位，暴露腹部，医者用中指端揉中脘，用手掌心摩脐，最后按揉足三里结束。

4. 虫痛

（1）治法：温中行气，安蛔止痛。

（2）处方：揉一窝风 300 次　揉外劳宫 300 次　推三关 300 次　摩腹 200 次　揉脐 200 次。

（3）疗程：每日 1 次，6 次为 1 疗程。

（4）操作：

A. 以石蜡油为介质。

B. 患儿取坐势，医者取小儿左手揉一窝风穴，再揉外劳穴，推三关。

C. 患儿取仰卧位，暴露腹部，医者以掌心摩腹，以掌根揉脐。

D. 患儿俯卧，医者用双手拇指按、揉肝俞、胆俞至痛止。

11.13　尿潴留

尿潴留，是指膀胱蓄有大量尿液，而小便闭塞不通的一种症状。

病因病机

1. 湿热蕴积：湿热阻滞膀胱，或肾热移于膀胱，形成湿热互结，使膀胱气化障碍，从而形成尿潴留。

2. 肾气不足：肾阳不足，命门火衰，不能化气行水，膀胱气化无权，而产生尿潴留。

临床表现

1. 湿热蕴积：小便不通或尿短而赤灼热，小腹胀满，口苦口粘，或口渴不欲饮，或大便不畅，舌质红、苔黄腻、指纹紫。

2. 肾气不足：小便不通，或点滴不爽，排出无力，腰膝乏力，怕冷，面色㿠白，神气怯弱，舌质淡，脉沉细，指纹淡。

治疗

1. 湿热蕴积

（1）治法：清利下焦湿热，开通闭塞。

（2）处方：清小肠 300 次　揉小天心 200 次　按揉丹田 300 次，推箕门 500 次　按揉三阴交 200 次。

（3）疗程：每日 1 次，1 次为 1 疗程。

（4）操作：

A. 用滑石粉作介质。

B. 患儿取端坐位，医者取其左手，先清小肠再揉小天心。

C. 患者取仰卧位，医者用中指端，掌根或四指，顺时针方向按揉丹田穴，然后将右手食、中 2 指并拢，推箕门，再按揉三阴交。

2. 肾气不足

（1）治法：温阳益气，补肾利尿。

（2）处方：补肾经 300 次　补脾经 300 次　揉二马 300 次　推三关 200 次　推箕门 500 次　摩脐 1～2 分钟。

（3）疗程：每日 1 次，3 次为 1 疗程。

（4）操作：

A. 以姜汁或滑石粉为介质。

B. 患儿取端坐位，医者以左手握住患儿的左手，先补肾经，补脾经，然后揉二马，接着再推三关。

C. 患儿取仰卧位，医者以掌心或 4 指逆时针方向摩脐，然后用食、中 2 指推箕门。

11.14　遗尿

遗尿亦称"尿床"，是指 3 周岁以上的小儿，睡眠中小便自遗。

病因病机

1. 下焦虚寒：先天肾气不足，下元虚寒，致使膀胱气化功能失调而发生遗尿。

2. 脾肺气虚：上虚不能制下，致使无权约束水道而遗尿。

临床表现

1. 下元虚寒：每在睡眠中遗尿，一夜可发生 1～2 次或更多，兼见面色㿠白，智力减退，腰膝酸软，小便清长，甚则肢冷恶寒，舌质淡，脉沉迟无力。

2. 脾肺气虚：多发于病后睡中遗尿，但尿频而量少，兼见面白神疲，四肢乏力，食欲不振，大便溏薄，舌质淡，脉缓或沉细。

治疗

1. 下元虚寒：

(1) 治法：温补肾阳，固摄下元。

(2) 处方：补肾经 300 次　推三关 200 次　揉外劳宫 100 次　按揉百会 200 次　摩丹田 200 次　按揉肾俞 100 次　按揉三阴交 100 次。

(3) 疗程：每日 1 次，12 次为 1 疗程。

(4) 操作：

A. 以滑石粉为介质。

B. 患儿取坐势，医者取小儿左手先补肾经，推三关，然后顺时针方向揉外劳宫穴，再按百会，顺时针方向揉百会。

C. 患儿取仰卧位，暴露腹部，医者以掌心摩丹田，然后揉三阴交。

D. 患儿取俯卧位，医者以拇指面按揉双侧肾俞。

2. 脾肺气虚:

(1) 治法:培元益气,固精缩尿。

(2) 处方:补脾经 300 次　补肺经 300 次　揉二马 200 次　补肾经 200 次　按揉百会 50 次　摩关元 300 次　按揉八髎穴各 5~10 次　揉龟尾 100 次。

(3) 疗程:每日 1 次,12 次为 1 疗程。

(4) 操作:

A. 以姜汁或滑石粉作介质。

B. 患儿取端坐位,医者取其左手先补脾经,补肺经,补肾经;然后揉二马,最后先按百会,再顺时针方向揉百会。

C. 患儿取仰卧位,医者以掌心顺时针方向摩关元穴。

D. 患儿取俯卧位,医者用拇指先按后揉上髎、次髎、中髎、下髎,最后揉龟尾结束。

11.15　鹅口疮

鹅口疮以口腔、舌布满白色糜点为特征。

病因病机

心脾胃 3 经郁热上行,熏蒸口舌而发为鹅口疮。

脾胃虚弱,肾阴受损,气阴两亏,水不制火,虚火上炎也可致鹅口疮。

临床表现

1. 心脾郁热:口腔粘膜充血满布乳白色片状物,面赤唇红,口臭便秘,烦躁不宁,吮乳时啼哭,流涎,尿短而黄,舌质红,苔白腻,脉滑或滑数。

2. 气阴两亏:口腔粘膜无明显充血,但有白点分布,颧红,体弱食减,精神困倦,口干不渴,便溏,小便清,舌质淡红脉细弱。

治疗

1. 心脾积热型

(1) 治法: 清热解毒, 泻火。

(2) 处方: 清脾经 500 次　清胃经 300 次　清心经 500 次　揉肾纹 300 次　清小肠 500 次　水底捞月 100 次, 揉小天心 100 次　清天河水 500 次　推六腑 300 次。

(3) 疗程: 每日 1 次, 6 次为 1 疗程。

(4) 操作:

A. 以清水为介质。

B. 患儿取抱坐位, 术者取持其左手, 先清脾经, 清胃经, 再清心经; 然后揉肾纹, 清小肠, 最后揉小天心。

C. 行水底捞月。

D. 清天河水, 推六腑。

2. 气阴两亏型

(1) 治法: 健脾益气, 滋阴降火。

(2) 处方: 补肾经 300 次　补脾经 500 次　揉二马 300 次　运内八卦 50 次　摩中脘 300 次　揉涌泉 200 次　捏脊 3～5 遍。

(3) 疗程: 每日 1 次, 12 次为 1 疗程。

(4) 操作:

A. 以滑石粉为介质。

B. 患儿取抱坐位, 术者取持其左手, 先补肾经, 补脾经, 再顺运内八卦, 接着揉二马, 揉涌泉。

C. 患儿取仰卧势, 术者用食、中、无名指指面摩中脘。

D. 患儿俯卧势, 捏脊, 最后两遍重提大椎, 按揉大椎 3 次结束。

注意事项

1. 注意保持小儿口腔清洁, 可用新黑布醮香油轻擦口腔, 防止口腔粘膜破损。

2. 切勿滥用抗生素, 特别是体质虚弱的小儿。

3. 乳母注意饮食宜清淡, 营养丰富。

11.16   近视

近视是以视近清楚而视远模糊为特征的眼病。有先天性者，系因父母有高度近视遗传而来，此类较少；有后天性者，系因青少年时期过用目力，学习读书环境光线昏暗，或因偏食体质较差等原因逐步形成。临床有假性（调节性）近视与真性（轴性）近视之分，所谓假性者，指过用目力使睫状肌疲劳，不能调节晶状体的屈光能力所致，休息后可以解除或减轻。真性者指眼轴发育过长，超过了屈光间质所能调节的范围所致，必须借助近视眼镜才能矫正。初发者，往往两者兼有。

病因病机

1. 心阳虚无力鼓动，血脉不充，气血不得上荣，目中精血不足，进而神光衰微，不能发越于远处。

2. 肝肾虚，精血不能上荣于目，目失濡养，目中神光衰微，光华不能及远。

临床表现

单纯的轻度近视，除视近清晰、视远模糊外，无其它症状，有的由于看远不清而不喜欢作室外活动而乐于室内活动。

合并有散光者，往往易引起眼疲劳，眼睛有不适感，视久可出现眼酸痛、头痛等症状，休息后可缓解。中度近视患者的玻璃体容易发生混浊，自觉眼前有星点飘动。高度近视患者更容易发生疲劳，甚至会发生单眼隐性或显性外斜，外斜最终可导致废用性近视。

治疗

轻度或中度的近视，多发生于中小学学生，由于眼肌过度紧张，肌肉收缩，水晶体变凸升高而致的近视，进行推拿治疗近期效果明显。

1. 治法：调和气血，疏通脉络。

2. 处方：揉睛明 300 次　推攒竹 300 次　天应 300 次　太

阳 300 次　四白 200 次　翳风 300 次　按风池 300 次　按揉天柱骨 300 次　推坎宫 300 次　抹眼眶上下各 100 次。

3. 操作：

患者先后取仰卧位和坐势，按要求和处方依次施术。

加减

1. 心阳虚者，以上操作必加左右揉心俞 100 次，肾俞 150 次。

2. 肝肾不足者，加揉肝俞 100 次，肾俞 200 次，足光明 100 次，揉涌泉 100 次。

注意事项

1. 每日 1 次，12 次为 1 疗程，视力有进展连续做 2～3 个疗程。其后小学生可在每暑寒假期中做 1～2 个疗程。

2. 操作者需经常修剪指甲，保持两手清洁，手法要轻柔，以患者局部有酸胀为度。

11.17　佝偻病

本病是婴幼儿时期的一种慢性营养缺乏症，多见于 3 岁以下的小儿，在 6～12 月的乳婴儿发病率较高。

病因病机

祖国医学认为本病主要由于先天禀赋不足，后天哺养失调，脾胃虚亏所致。

临床表现

早期：烦躁，夜眠不安，神情呆滞，头部及颈部多汗，胃纳不佳，肌肉松弛，发稀色黄，枕部脱发，头颅骨软，囟门久不闭合，面色萎黄，四肢懈怠，易受惊吓，便溏，舌苔薄白。

晚期：晚期骨骼有改变，方颅，囟门特大，囟门闭迟，形体瘦弱，表情呆滞，动作迟钝，出齿迟，鸡胸，胫及踝部骨骺端粗大，出现"O"或"X"形腿，脊柱的畸形等。

治疗

1. 治法：
(1) 早期：健脾补肾。
(2) 晚期：健脾补肾，矫正畸形。
2. 处方：

补脾经 300 次　补肾经 300 次　揉小天心 100 次　推三关 100 次　揉肾顶 100 次　捏脊 3～5 遍　按肾俞、脾俞、胃俞、肺俞各 3～5 次。

3. 疗程：每日 1 次，30 次为 1 疗程。
4. 操作：

(1) 患儿抱坐势，医者以左手持儿左手，依次补脾经，肾经，揉肾顶，小天心。

(2) 姿势同上，暴露患儿前臂，医者用食、中指指面推三关。

(3) 患儿取俯卧势，医者站其一旁，以双手作常规捏脊 3 遍，第 4 遍边提边捏，特别重提肾俞、脾俞、胃俞、肺俞，再用双手拇指按揉俞穴。

(4) 使有鸡胸畸形者取坐势，医者用双手相对按压在突出部位作轻柔有节律的压法 30～50 次。

11.18　脑性瘫痪

因高级神经失去或缺乏控制部分或全部脊髓神经的能力，所引起受累部位的肌肉紧张力增加，随意运动失调而致。

病因病机

本病属祖国医学五迟、五软等范围，是肝肾亏损，脾胃虚弱，筋骨痿弱，气血不得宣通，四肢筋脉、肌肉失于温养而致病。

临床表现

脑型瘫痪的病型很多，最常见的有痉挛性的两侧瘫痪或脑性偏瘫或单瘫，其次是小脑性的共济失调。

随着小儿发育，其抬头，坐立困难，四肢活动少，特别是下肢尤为明显，在被动运动时肌张力增强，肢体难于移动，卧或步行时两腿互相交叉，成剪刀步态，足趾着地肢体发生痉挛或畸型，肌肉的痉挛在企图运动时增强，在深睡时才消失。

在临床上痉挛性瘫痪有程度和范围的不同，重者受累的肢体肌肉紧张力极度增强，轻度仅有细微的运动失调，可能仅1肢受累或两上肢受累，或两下肢，或1侧上肢或四肢躯干完全受累，上肢受累时表现肩内收，肘腕屈曲，前臂旋前，拇指内收，4指屈曲握拳；下肢受累时髋屈曲，内收内旋，膝屈曲，足下垂内翻；躯干受累表现为仰或俯卧，胸腰前屈或呈侧凸畸形。部分病儿语言、视力、听力和智力障碍，体格发育不良等。

治疗

1. 治法：疏通经络，活动关节，扶脾补肾，益气养血。

2. 处方：补脾经 500 次　补肾经 500 次　揉二马 200 次运内八卦 100 次　捣小天心 50 次。

加减

1. 上肢瘫痪者加掐指甲根、指关节各 5～10 遍，揉手厥阴心包经、手少阴心经、手少阳三焦经、手阳明大肠经循行线的一部分。拿少海、内关。

2. 下肢瘫痪者，掐趾甲根、趾关节各 5～10 遍，揉足阳明胃经、足少阳胆经、足厥阴肝经及足太阴脾经循行线的一部分，拿委中、承山、昆仑、左右腰俞穴，环跳、阳陵泉等穴。

3. 操作：

(1) 滑石粉为介质。

(2) 患儿取坐势，医者以左手持其右手拇指，依次先推脾经、肾经，再运内八卦，捣小天心，复其手使手背向上，以右手拇指甲依次掐指根、指关节，以痛为度。下肢操作同。

(3) 患儿取俯卧势，术者以中指先轻揉后点手厥阴心包经、手少阴心经、手少阳三焦经，手阳明大肠经循行路线的一部分，最后拿少海、内关、下肢操作同。

（4）若患儿躯干受累时可使其俯卧，较重刺激其背部是太阳膀胱经。

（5）置患儿于坐或卧位，使其配合做各关节的屈伸，内收，内旋、外展等活动。

4. 疗程：3个月为1疗程，每日1次。

对智力正常，瘫痪轻度或中度的治疗效果较明显，一般3个月后见效；对智力不足，瘫痪较重，或严重瘫痪的效果差些，需要的时间相对长些。

11.19   肌性斜颈

肌性斜颈又称先天性斜颈、原发性斜颈，是以患儿头向患侧倾斜，颜面转向健侧为特征。临床上斜颈除了个别为脊柱畸形引起的骨性斜颈，斜视所致的视力障碍的代偿性姿势性斜颈，和颈部肌肉麻痹导致的神经性者外，一般系指一侧胸锁乳突肌痉挛造成的肌性斜颈。

病因病机

1. 因斜颈常并发其他先天性畸形，如先天性足外翻、内翻、髋关节脱位等，故有先天因素的说法。

2. 有人认为胎儿在分娩时头位不正，阻碍胸锁乳突肌中部的血液供应，最后引起肌肉痉挛而致。

3. 多数学者认为胎儿在分娩时一侧胸锁乳突肌受产道或产钳挤压，使该肌肉的血管中的血流暂时停滞，以后引起片状血管栓塞，凝血块使肌肉呈梭形肿物，逐渐形成条索状挛缩。

4. 胎儿在子宫内头位不正，长期阻碍一侧胸锁乳突肌的血运供给，引起该肌肉缺血性改变所致。

中医认为上述有道理。

临床表现

患儿出生后，或1～2周内，头向一侧偏歪，颈部一侧出现椭圆或条索状肿块，质较韧无痛，当患儿颈部转向健侧时，肿块突出明显。以后肿块逐渐挛缩紧张，质坚硬而韧，头部向患侧倾斜，日见明显，面旋向健侧，颈前痛向健侧转动受限，患儿颜面部的发育受影响，患侧腮下垂，鼻唇沟变浅，眼与同侧口角的距离患侧缩小，颅骨发育不对称，如不及时治疗，健侧颜面也会发生相应的改变，晚期病例一般伴有代偿性的胸椎侧凸畸形。

治疗

推拿治疗小儿肌性斜颈疗效确切，痛苦少，但是疗程较长，一般越早治疗效果越好。

1. 治法：活血化瘀，软坚消肿，兼以矫正畸形。

2. 处方：以患侧胸锁乳突肌肿块为主。

手法操作在风池 300 次　耳后高骨 300 次　天牖 300 次　天柱 500 次　扶突穴 500 次　肩井 100 次　风门 50 次　大杼 50 次。

3. 操作：

(1) 用滑石粉作介质。

(2) 母亲怀抱婴儿使其呈吸乳势，使其患侧颈部向上，医者先按揉风池、天柱、风门、耳后高骨、天牖、扶突穴规定次数、用拇指、食指自乳突向锁骨胸骨方向拿患侧胸锁乳突肌 3～5 遍，重点在肿块及其周围，再用拇指面揉患侧胸锁乳突肌 3～5 分钟；令母竖抱患儿，再用拇指螺纹面，揉颈椎棘突 1 分钟，然后再从风池向下沿两侧肌肉作直推各 1 分钟。

(3) 令患儿充分暴露两侧的肩胛骨，用两拇指从肩胛骨内侧缘自上向下按揉 1 分钟。

(4) 最后术者一手扶住患侧的肩部，另一手扶住患儿的头顶，使患儿头部渐渐向健侧肩部倾斜，逐渐拉长患侧胸锁乳突肌，反复进行 5～10 次。

4. 疗程：1 个月为 1 疗程，每日或隔日治疗 1 次。

注意事项：

对斜颈患儿，还要注意检查是否伴有先天性髋关节半脱位，以便及时纠正。

12 小儿推拿保健

开展小儿推拿保健能提高小儿自身的免疫功能，从而增强小儿体质，预防一些疾病的发生。小儿保健推拿操作简便，易学易懂，便于掌握。

在对小儿进行保健推拿时家长要有耐心，坚持按疗程进行，不要中途而止，一般6天为1疗程，如患儿有慢性病者可连续3～4个疗程。现介绍几种常用的保健推拿法。

12.1 安神保健法

小儿见闻易动，易受惊吓，故病多惊悸哭叫，手足动摇，神乱不安等，因此小儿的精神调摄是极为重要的；应用安神保健法，养心安神，滋阴益血。

1. 处方：揉心俞50次，抚推颈椎50～100遍，猿猴摘果30次。

2. 操作：

(1) 用滑石粉为介质。

(2) 家长左手怀抱小儿使其背向后，或使其俯卧于床，术者用右手掌心轻轻拍儿左上背部相当于厥阴俞、心俞的部位，拍时要用空掌，动作轻柔要有节奏，拍毕用拇、食指面分别按揉双侧心俞50次。

(3) 姿势同上，术者用左手中指按在风府穴上，食、无名指分别按在两侧的风池穴上，自上而下推托50～100次。

(4) 小儿取抱坐势，术者与其面对面站立，以两手食、中指夹住小儿的耳尖向上提3～10次，再用双手拇、食指捏住双耳垂3～5次（图197、198）。最后捧儿头部左右摇10～20次结束。

3. 注意事项：

睡前或下午进行治疗为好，每天操作 1 次，连续 2～3 次为 1 疗程，可连续进行 2 个疗程。

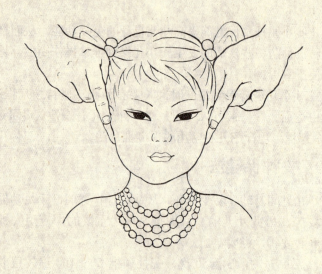

图 197

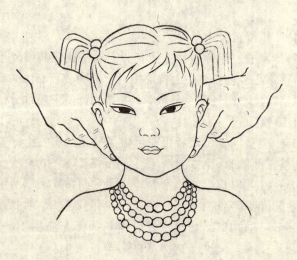

图 198

12.2 健脾和胃保健法

应用健脾和胃法能增强食欲，调理气血，提高儿童体质，可达正气内存、邪不可干的目的。

健脾和胃法可以独取1穴，也可以数穴相配。

1. 处方：

(1) 处方1：摩腹

(2) 处方2：捏脊

(3) 处方3：补脾经500次　揉足三里300次　摩腹300次　捏脊3~5遍。

2. 操作：

(1) 以滑石粉为介质。

(2) 小儿取抱坐位，术者固定其左手，补脾经。

(3) 小儿取仰卧势，术者用右手掌心摩儿腹部，从右下腹向右上腹再推向左上腹、左下腹轻轻而过再至右下腹（即升结肠→横结肠→降结肠→升结肠的方向操作）150次数后，再向相反的方向操作同样的次数，然后以左右手拇指按揉双足三里。此法可在进食后半小时进行。

(4) 小儿取俯卧势，暴露脊背，先作常规捏脊3遍，第4和第5遍捏到肾俞、胃俞、脾俞穴时各重提一下，最后用双手拇指按揉以上俞穴结束。

3. 注意事项

(1) 每天操作1次，每7天为1疗程，3天后再作下1疗程。

(2) 急性传染病期间可暂停，待病愈再行。

12.3 健脾保肺推拿法

采用健脾保肺推拿法可以增强身体的御寒能力，预防感冒的发生。

1. 处方

(1) 处方1：揉外劳宫 300 次　黄蜂入洞 50 次。

(2) 处方2：补脾经 300 次　摩囟门 100 次　推八道各 50 次　揉手足心各 50 次。

2. 操作：

用姜汁麻油为介质

(1) 外方 1 对易患感冒咳嗽者宜选用之。

小儿取抱坐位，术者用左手持儿的右手，用右手拇指揉外劳宫毕后，站在小儿前面用左手固定其后枕部，用右手食、中两指分别置儿鼻翼两旁作上下揉动称为黄蜂入洞，作规定次数后，按肩井 3～5 下结束。

(2) 处方 2 对常易伤食、感冒交替出现，或感冒发病前表现食欲旺盛的小儿尤为适宜。

A. 患儿取抱坐位，术者用左手固定患儿的左手，暴露其拇指，行补脾经。然后，用右手中指揉手心及足心。

B. 姜汁、麻油调和后涂于术者掌心，然后摩儿囟门处，手法宜轻柔，不能用力按压囟门。

C. 小儿取仰卧势，术者站在小儿一侧，用双手拇指从第一、二肋间隙的胸肋关节处向两边作分推，推毕依次再推第二、三，第三、四，第四、五肋间隙，此为推八道。最后用中指揉膻中 50～100 次。

D. 患儿取怀抱势，背向后，术者用掌心轻拍其肺俞部位。

3. 注意事项

一般宜在清晨进行，每天操作 1 次，7 次为 1 疗程。疗程间休息 3 天，可继续进行第 2 疗程。

12.4　益智保健推拿法

益智保健能促进小儿智力开发，身心健康，精神愉快。

1. 处方：

推五经 100 次　捏十王各 20 次　摇四肢关节各 20~30 次
捻 10 手指及 10 足趾各 3~5 遍　捏脊 3~5 遍。

2. 操作：

(1) 用滑石粉为介质。

(2) 小儿取坐势或仰卧势，术者以左手托儿左手使手心向上，术者右手 5 指并拢从其掌根始沿手掌顺指根向指尖推去，反复操作，称为推五经。

(3) 小儿姿势同上，术者捏其右手拇、食、中、无名小指，此为捏十王；然后摇 4 肢腕、肘、膝、踝关节，再用拇指、食指面捻儿 10 指及足趾。

(4) 患儿在家长两大腿上取俯卧势，术者以双手拇、食指面捏脊，重提肾俞、脾俞、心俞各 3~5 次，按揉前穴 3 次。然后将中指置督脉上，食、无名指分别置风门穴上，自上而下反复推 10 遍。

3. 注意事项

本法适用于 3 周岁以下的幼儿，可每日 1 次，连续 7 次为 1 疗程，疗程间休息 1 周，再做第 2 疗程。

THE ENGLISH–CHINESE ENCYCLOPEDIA OF PRACTICAL TCM
(Booklist)

英汉实用中医药大全

（书目）

VOLUME	TITLE	书名
1	ESSENTIALS OF TRADITIONAL CHIN ESE MEDICINE	中医学基础
2	THE CHINESE MATERIA MEDICA	中药学
3	PHARMACOLOGY OF TRADITION-AL CHINESE MEDICAL FORMULAE	方剂学
4	SIMPLE AND PROVEN PRESCRIPTION	单验方
5	COMMONLY USED CHINESE PATENTMEDICINES	常用中成药
6	THERAPY OF ACUPUNCTURE AND MOXIBUSTION	针灸疗法
7	*TUINA* THERAPY	推拿疗法
8	MEDICAL *QIGONG*	医学气功
9	MAINTAINING YOUR HEALTH	自我保健
10	INTERNAL MEDICINE	内科学